The Fourfold Path to Healing

The Fourfold Path to Healing

Working with the Laws of
Nutrition, Therapeutics, Movement and Meditation
in the Art of Medicine

Thomas S. Cowan, MD
with Sally Fallon and Jaimen McMillan

The Fourfold Path to Healing

Working with the Laws of
Nutrition, Therapeutics, Movement and Meditation
in the Art of Medicine

Thomas S. Cowan, MD
with Sally Fallon and Jaimen McMillan

Cover Design by Kim Waters

Illustrations by Lynda Smith Cowan, Liz Pitfield and Kim Waters

Library of Congress Cataloging-in-Publication Data

Cowan, Thomas S.
    The fourfold path to healing: working with the laws of nutrition, therapeutics,
       movement and meditation in the art of medicine
    Thomas S. Cowan, MD with Sally Fallon and Jaimen McMillan

    ISBN 0-9670897-9-4
        1. Holistic medicine   2. Nutrition
        3. Heart Disease   4. Cancer
        5. Nontoxic therapies   6. Degenerative disease
        7. Homeopathy   8. Spacial Dynamics

NewTrends Publishing, Inc.
Brandywine, Maryland 20613

www.NewTrendsPublishing.com
Order Line (877) 707-1776
customerservice@newtrendspublishing.com

Available to the trade through
National Book Network (800) 462-6420

Print Runs: 10,000, 15,000, 10,000, 10,000, 7,500

ISBN 0-9670897-9-4   978-0967089799
PRINTED IN THE UNITED STATES OF AMERICA

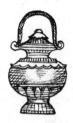

Acknowledgements

The Fourfold Path to Healing seems as though it has been in the works much of my adult life. Only with the help of numerous others would an accomplishment of this magnitude be achieved. My gratitude goes to out to many, starting with my parents, Marjorie Goodman and Warren Cowan, DDS, and my sister Marti Pels. For my whole life I have felt that they expected me to make some sort of contribution. This book is the thanks and pay back for their faith in me.

Next, to my three children Molly, Asher and Joe. It is a cliche for parents to speak about how much they have learned from their children and how humbling the whole experience of parenting has been for them. Through this yearning and struggle to do right by our children, we have the opportunity to grow into adults ourselves. That has certainly been the case for me, and for their tolerance and help I am profoundly grateful.

The next major player in my life and in the creation of this book has been Sally Fallon. Without her amazing creativity, energy and vision not only this book, but so much that I consider "good" in my life, would not have happened. Her gifts to the world of *Nourishing Traditions* and the Weston A. Price Foundation have been an inspiration and source of healing to countless thousands of people. For her efforts in spearheading this book I am truly grateful.

Jaimen McMillan has been especially generous in sharing his genius and his time to provide the section on emotional healing through Spacial Dynamics. My sincere thanks for his unique contribution.

Thanks also to Liz Pitfield for her tireless effort in creating the wonderful illustrations of Jaimen's exercises; and to Kim Waters for her unique vision that shines through the cover and text graphics.

Then come my patients, the ones in this book, the ones in the past, the current ones and the ones to come. For all of you who have taught me so much over the years I send my best wishes and my thanks for allowing me to participate in your lives.

And finally, my wife Lynda Smith, who came into my life just a short while ago. With her amazing smile and capacity for love, she has made my life the most joyous adventure any human being could ask for.

Thomas Cowan, MD, March, 2004

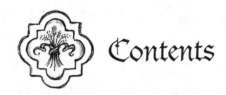

Contents

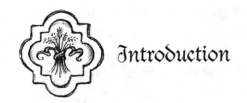

Introduction

When I began my medical practice about twenty years ago, holistic or alternative medicine was a fringe movement, regarded with suspicion by all but a handful of doctors. At that time the American Medical Association officially opposed the idea that diet had anything to do with disease and claimed that the use of herbs, vitamins and homeopathic medicines was quackery. Mind-body medicine was also on the fringe. Nevertheless, after finishing my training in family medicine, I set out in crusading style to bring the fledgling holistic approach to my patients.

In those days, I believed that the reason chronic disease was so difficult to treat was because we were prescribing the wrong medicines. It seemed to me that conditions like asthma, heart disease and arthritis resisted orthodox therapies because the drugs doctors used did little more than suppress symptoms. I imagined that if I simply gave my patients remedies that addressed the underlying causes of their diseases, they would be cured in droves.

I practiced in this fashion for about five years, using a variety of alternative therapies, such as herbs and homeopathic medicines, and although my patients were not "cured in droves," many did have wonderful results. For example, I treated more than five hundred children suffering from ear infections with natural remedies. About eighty percent of these cases cleared up without resort to antibiotics.

But twenty percent did not respond. And it is the patients who don't respond to the usual treatments that have the most to teach their doctors. I began to suspect that factors we normally don't associate with illness could be impediments to healing. Of two children treated for ear infections, for example, the one who had a calm mother cleared up beautifully, but the child with an anxious mother was still infected a week later. I used a therapy involving bee venom for osteoarthritis that worked well for some patients, while others showed no improvement whatsoever. I used natural therapies to treat two elderly women with metastasized colon cancer. One woman is alive ten years later, while the other lived only a few months.

All doctors confront the mystery of why some patients get better and others

1

don't. This mystery challenged my thinking for many years, and I began to construct a medical philosophy that encompassed more than just medicines. I began to ask detailed questions of my patients about the way they lived, the way they were treated as children, their relationships, careers, financial struggles or successes, goals, dreams, hopes and disappointments. I concluded that the use of medicines—whether conventional or natural—can be effective only in the context of the patient's story, and in conjunction with the correction of some of the "errors" in his or her life-style and way of thinking.

In accepting the premise that treatment should involve more than the use of medicines, the physician embarks on treacherous terrain. Where does he start when he wants to help his patients change their life-style and attitudes? To which sources does he turn? How can he point out the "errors" in the lives of his patients without pontificating?

During my evolution toward a more holistic practice, I relied heavily on the work of Rudolf Steiner, an Austrian mystic who founded a philosophical movement called "anthroposophy," after the Greek "human wisdom." Steiner also formulated an educational system practiced in the Waldorf schools, the second largest secular private educational system in the world. Unfortunately, his teachings in the field of medicine are less well known, partly because people remain skeptical of the way in which he obtained his knowledge, which was not the scientific method of reproducible experiments, but an intuitive process based on inspired insight. It is not my intention to explore Steiner's work in depth, but I do feel that a basic understanding of his ideas concerning the human being and the healing arts is a very necessary component of any holistic therapeutic system.

Steiner taught that the human being has four "bodies" or spheres of activity, and that human beings enjoy good health when these four spheres are in harmony or balance. These four interlocking bodies are (1) the Physical Body, (2) the Life-Force Body, (3) the Emotional Body and (4) the Mental Body. They correspond to the four "kingdoms" and the four "elements" of the medievalists as follows:

1. Physical Body	Mineral Kingdom	Earth Element
2. Life-Force Body	Plant Kingdom	Water Element
3. Emotional Body	Animal Kingdom	Air Element
4. Mental Body	Human Kingdom	Warmth Element

According to Steiner, each of our four bodies reflects one aspect of our total being, and each is governed by specific rules. The Physical Body is the substance or matter of which our bodies are composed. It corresponds to the mineral realm and the

...an to a house, then the Physical Body corresponds to ...ch the house is built. If the bricks are faulty and the ... unsound. We need a sound Physical Body if we are ...y sense. It will come as no surprise that the health ...ed to the food we eat. Thus, a wholesome diet is ...ve must build complete and long-term healing. ... other therapies will provide little benefit.

...ly, we rise above the level of mere substance to ... The etheric realm pertains to the way physi- ...ur metaphor of the body as a house, imagine ...king it her own. This is a picture of the Life- .... The Life-Force Body corresponds to the ...body that we hope to affect when we give ...dicines like herbal extracts and homeo- ...are carried in the fluids of the body—the ...he way cells communicate, help achieve ... of the various organs to each other.

...pt of the four bodies intuitively, there actually ...ur the existence of non-physical-life-force bodies in
all l... ...plant, animal and human. Harold Saxton Burr, a professor of
anat... ...ﾟ Yale University, spent many years researching what he called "fields of
life" or "L-fields," describing them as the blueprints of all life. He proposed that all
living things were molded and controlled by "electrodynamic fields" that we can map
and measure. Invisible and intangible, they are analogous to magnetic fields that
cause iron filings scattered on a card held over a magnet to arrange themselves in the
magnet's force field pattern at both poles. Burr described these fields or bodies in the
scientific terms of electromagnetism but it is easy to imagine them as fluid or watery,
giving off an electromagnetic signal just as underground water gives off an electromagnetic signal that can be perceived by a dowser.

The third body, according to Steiner, is the realm of emotions or feelings and the
dwelling place of the soul. In our house analogy we can compare the Emotional Body
to the way the enlivening person has decorated the house—the inviting porch, welcoming garden, interior decorations and all the touches that make a home personal.
Houses can be sunny or gloomy, cluttered or tidy, corresponding to the many moods
and life-styles that characterize the human race. There is no doubt that our moods
and life-style affect our health, just as the decorations of a house determine whether
or not it is a pleasant place to live.

It is the Emotional Body that is first affected by the kind and quality of our relationships. Many of my female patients with gynecological or intestinal problems could not heal until they made major changes in the relationships they had with parents or partners. In fact, I had three cases of women with highly abnormal pap smears that recurred in spite of surgical treatment. The problems cleared up only after they had a major reconciliation with their spouse or got a divorce. In my male patients, I have seen career worries cause health problems that immediately resolved when the patient achieved success in his field.

The Emotional Body corresponds to the air element and the animal kingdom. Unlike plants, whose movement is limited to the circulation of internal fluids, animals move through the outer world on their own volition. Thus, movement and exercise belong to this realm. Consider, for example, the simple act of standing up straight and tall and how this affects our mood and outlook. The way we move, including how we exercise and the sports in which we engage, affects our sense of well-being, our emotions and hence our health.

The fourth and final realm that I address in the prevention and treatment of illness is the realm of the ego or spirit, which we will call the Mental Body. This realm is the habitation of that unique part of each of us, the part that gives individuality and continuity to our life. In our house analogy, the Mental Body corresponds to the visitors coming and going into the house, their conversations, ideas and thoughts. These visitors stand for the Mental Body that can travel freely inside and outside the house, exchanging, communicating and recognizing the guests as others. While the emotions stem from the soul, our perception of these emotions and how they are used is the proper concern of the Mental Body.

Many diseases reveal themselves as a distortion of our warmth or Mental Body. Sick children, for example, usually have increased warmth or fever as their individual Mental Body participates in their struggle against disease. Later in life we often get colder—our hands and feet feel cold—leading to hypothyroidism or even cancer, a disease intimately associated with a loss of warmth and its ability to confer immunity. Women, however, experience hot flashes, which may be interpreted as a manifestation of the Mental Body working gently to separate her from the domestic life to which she has submerged her individuality, and push her into the world of work and community service. Often the warmth body becomes abnormally distributed so we have pockets of warmth. This is the metaphorical description of a rheumatic patient suffering from "hot" joints; or the patient suffering from eczema who experiences a fiery feeling in the skin.

The idea that we must seek healing on a number of levels is one that today is widely accepted; in fact, it forms the underlying philosophy of all holistic medicine. The problem lies in discovering the appropriate course of action to take in each of the spheres or levels that comprise the human being. Even when we accept the fact that man must be healed on many levels, things can go very wrong. Recently I spoke with a professional in the publishing business who became interested in his health after he suffered a massive heart attack. He accepted the concept of holistic healing but the life-style changes he had made, although endorsed in many popular books, were getting him no closer to his goal of vibrant health; in fact, they made him grumpy and tired. He had given up junk food for a lowfat vegetarian diet; he took handfuls of vitamin pills; he walked on a treadmill every morning and evening; and he practiced relaxation therapy to help him deal with stress. Everything he did would get a nod of approval from the gurus of the burgeoning holistic movement; unfortunately, each of his choices was counterproductive.

The appropriate and effective approach to healing the different levels that comprise the human being is the subject of this book: Right diet for healing the Physical Body; beneficial medicines or therapies for the Life-Force Body; healing movement and exercise for the Emotional Body; and effective thinking activity for the Mental Body, activity that moves the human spirit forward in its evolution toward meaning, service and health.

So how do we determine the right diet for human beings? There are literally hundreds of books about diet and nutrition on the market, most of which suggest a diet low in fats and high in plant foods and complex carbohydrates. Some writers recommend large amounts of lean meat while others suggest a completely vegetarian diet. One school of thought promotes all raw foods; others recommend various systems of food combining. The authors of these books present many theories to explain why these diets *should* work; but *in practice*, the typical modern diet systems presented in our popular books have never been used by traditional groups of healthy human beings.

The one book on nutrition that actually presents a description of people who are healthy, and that gives an account of the diets that healthy people eat, is *Nutrition and Physical Degeneration* by Weston A. Price. During the 1930s and 1940s, Price traveled to isolated corners of the globe and studied the diets of tribes and villages that had no contact with western foods. His book has inspired many workers in the field of medicine and nutrition, including myself. It was on reading Weston Price's book that I decided to become a doctor, and it is the book to which I always return when questions of nutrition arise.

Price's book is important for two reasons. One is that it shows, through the medium of photography, how healthy people *look*. They have broad faces, flawless straight teeth and muscular, well-formed physiques. Second, it describes the characteristics of their diets, which can be summed up in two words: nutrient-dense. The diets of isolated healthy peoples were extremely rich in minerals and vitamins, including certain vitamins found only in animal fats. In fact, it was the foods rich in animal fats that these people valued most highly for good health, stamina, freedom from disease and ease of reproduction. None of the groups he studied consumed a lowfat vegetarian diet, none ate all of their foods raw, and none practiced any system of food combining.

The book that translates Price's findings into practical recipes for modern Americans is *Nourishing Traditions* by Sally Fallon. Along with Price's masterpiece, her book serves as a companion to this volume, and the dietary principles she elucidates can serve as a general guide to all who seek better health.

As for supplements, I use a variety of concentrated food-based sources of nutrients instead of synthetic vitamins. Many of the products I recommend were developed by Dr. Royal Lee, a colleague of Dr. Price. These principles are discussed in detail in Chapter 1 and form the basis of the dietary recommendations found in the various disease chapters of this book.

When the physical body is supported by a good diet, the medicines we take can help fine-tune the organizing principles of our bodies. They can facilitate the circulation of fluids, help the cells communicate better, bring the various organs into equilibrium and restore hormonal balance, all of which come under the purview of the Life-Force Body. Most orthodox drugs merely suppress symptoms and in the process inhibit rather than facilitate balance and movement within the body. The result is side effects, often worse than the original disease.

In Chapter 2, we will explore a number of therapeutic principles, including the use of herbs, homeopathic medicines and various other therapies that affect the Life-Force Body. These principles are the gift of a number of great minds in the field of medicine, including Rudolf Steiner, Samuel Hahnemann and Edgar Cayce.

Movement and exercise belong to the realm of the Emotional Body and are discussed in Chapter 3. We express our emotions in the way that we move, and the kind of movement and exercise we engage in can make a real difference in our ability to heal. I don't believe that using a treadmill for 30 minutes each day confers the same benefits as creative, coordinated exercise like T'ai Chi, fencing, dance or tennis. Whenever possible, movement and exercise should be performed in the open air, as this realm corresponds to the air element.

We will also discuss specific movements that can help with specific emotional conditions that our body translates into disease. Many of the movements that I prescribe are inspired by the work of Jaimen McMillan, founder of the Spacial Dynamics movement and author of Chapter 3.

Although the Emotional Body is the seat of the emotions and the realm of the soul, the proper domain for soul work is the Mental Body for, as I have said, our perception of our emotions and the use to which they are put is the proper stuff of our cognitive faculties.

Many books on holistic medicine urge readers to "get in touch with their feelings," implying that the road to health requires that we become less inhibited, more spontaneous, more demonstrative of our emotions. Programs to deal with unpleasant feelings like anger, depression or stress often recommend "releasing" negative emotions through playacting or meditation. The fallback position when these programs don't work is drugs, and the widespread use of antidepressants and similar medicines tells me that such programs aren't particularly effective, especially in the long run.

The Mental Body is essentially the realm of meaning and as I gain experience as a doctor, I realize how important it is for my patients to access this meaning in their quest for health. The proper activity of the Mental Body is not feeling but focused meditation or *thinking*, an activity for which the human being is uniquely qualified. The Mental Body does not "get in touch with our feelings" but observes those feelings in a detached and objective way. And it is through thinking about our lives—our situation, our experiences, our relationships, our mission and, of course, our emotions—that we discover the purpose of our lives and very often, at the same time, come to a better understanding of why we are sick.

There is no greater joy in life than to have purpose, to know what your life means. Some find this meaning through their families and other relationships. Others meet their destiny through their work or through activities like music and sports. Those who have discovered the purpose of their lives—through observation, through study, through thinking—can expect to achieve vibrant health and longevity, not only because they make sensible use of food, medicines and exercise, but also because they cultivate a healthy Mental Body, one that integrates and remains in balance with the three lower bodies.

A basic meditation or thinking exercise that stimulates the Mental Body and helps it grow is given in Chapter 4.

The goal of medicine should be healing on all levels and all of us are moving toward that goal. The wise physician no longer dispenses drugs to treat a catalog of symptoms. She realizes that the medicines she prescribes and the therapies she recommends must be aimed at specific imbalances. She knows that diet, life-style, exercise and the life of the mind must all be addressed for true healing to occur.

But it is not enough to merely embrace these holistic principles. The patient needs accurate information and effective advice. The purpose of this book is to provide, for each of the four realms of the human being, rules and guidelines that work; and to stimulate the Mental Body, dwelling place of the human spirit, to become its own wise physician through the exercise of that activity that makes the human being uniquely human—focused meditation, which is deliberate and objective thought.

Part 1:
The Fourfold Approach

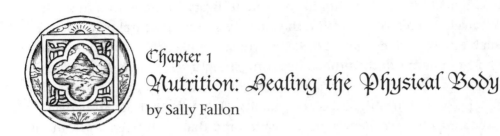

Chapter 1
Nutrition: Healing the Physical Body
by Sally Fallon

*O*rthodox medicine, in fact, virtually all of modern science, recognizes the physical world as the only reality and the physical body as the only part of the human being that is real and that can be treated. Drugs, surgery, exercise and even psychiatry all aim at "fixing what's broke" in the physical body. Ironically, the role of food—the body's only physical source of energy and building materials—is usually ignored or relegated to an afterthought. Yet the most fundamental requirement for a healthy physical body is food to supply what the body needs and, it goes without saying, food that does no harm.

What kinds of foods does the body require, and what kinds of foods should we avoid? The opinions given in today's popular books range from strict vegan to an all-raw meat diet, from anything-goes to rigid rules of food combining. How can we find our way to the correct information through this forest of conflicting claims?

Scientists and writers who formulate modern diet systems begin with theories and then apply them to people in the hope that these theoretical diet plans will lead to good health. A better approach is to start with people who are healthy, and who have been healthy for many generations, and then find out what kinds of food they have eaten. This entails determining the parameters of good health, and then finding groups of people that conform to those parameters and whose dietary patterns have been stable for many years, something that would be almost impossible to accomplish today. Fortunately, just such a study was carried out in the early part of this century, when there still were groups of isolated peoples in various parts of the globe.

WESTON A. PRICE

Weston A. Price was a prominent dentist and researcher during the 1930s and 1940s who became interested in determining the factors fundamental to healthy dental development. His specific way of addressing this question was profound, mainly because of its remarkable simplicity. He simply asked the following question: Are there any people or groups of people alive who have perfect teeth, that is, who do not suffer from cavities, gum disease or orthodontic troubles—all the dental diseases that he saw in the patients who came to him for treatment. Every summer for a number of years, Price traveled to remote places on the globe in search of dental perfection. He found 14 such groups—tribes, clans or villages whose members all exhibited remarkable freedom from decay, and who had beautiful straight teeth including room for their wisdom teeth—a condition virtually unknown in America today. He then studied their general state of health and dietary habits. He found that dental perfection invariably accompanied excellent general health, and that such freedom from disease and physical imperfection could be explained by the food they ate. Those groups who abandoned their traditional diets in favor of what Price called the "displacing foods of modern commerce," namely imported foodstuffs made from white sugar and white flour, or condensed and canned foods, quickly developed rampant tooth decay. Children born to those who changed their diets had more narrow palates, crooked or crowded teeth, and a reduced immunity to disease.

The message of Dr. Price is this: the quality of our food determines in large part the quality of our lives. And the quality of what we eat is determined by every step that goes into production and processing—the feeding of the animals, care of the soil, preservation, storage and even cooking methods.

A diet rich in readily available nutrients allows the bones to mineralize properly, particularly during gestation and early development, and gives the teeth immunity to decay throughout the stresses of life. Not surprisingly, he found that the native diets that conferred such good health on healthy, so-called primitive groups were rich in minerals, particularly calcium and phosphorus, necessary for healthy bones and teeth. What *is* surprising about the work of Weston Price is his discovery that these healthy diets always contained a good source of what he called "fat-soluble activators," nutrients like vitamin A and vitamin D, and another vitamin he discovered called Activator X or the Price Factor. These nutrients are found only in certain animal fats. Foods that provided these nutrients were considered sacred by the healthy groups he studied. These foods included liver and other organ meats from grazing animals; fish eggs; fish liver oils; fish and shellfish; and butter from cows eating rapidly growing green grass from well-mineralized pastures. Price concluded that without a rich supply of these fat-soluble nutrients, the body cannot properly use the minerals in food. These fat-soluble nutrients also nourish the glands and organs to give healthy indigenous peoples plenty of immunity during times of stress.

NUTRIENT-DENSE FOODS

What Dr. Price's work teaches us is that the absolute fundamental requirement of healthy diets cannot be found in pasta, nor vegetable juices, nor oat bran, nor olive oil, but only in certain types of animal fats. These fats come from animals who consume green, growing organisms (such as grass and plankton), or who consume other animals that have consumed green, growing organisms (such as insects). What is tragic is the difficulty in finding such foods today. Most of our dairy cows spend their entire lives in confinement and never see green grass; chickens are kept in pens and fed mostly grains; pigs are raised in factories and never see sunlight; even fish are now raised in fish farms and given inappropriate feed, like soy pellets.

Even worse, most people avoid these foods today because medical spokesmen claim they cause cancer, heart disease or weight gain, even though a number of highly qualified scientists have admirably refuted these charges. Suffice it to say that the patient who is afraid of consuming foods containing animal fats and cholesterol will make no headway in his efforts to improve his diet as these foods are absolutely vital for good health.

The list of foods that supply substantial amounts of fat-soluble vitamins (vitamin A, vitamin D and the Price Factor) is relatively short:

> Butter, cream and whole milk products (milk, cheese, yoghurt, etc.) from cows on green pasture
> Organ meats (liver, kidneys, heart, brain, etc.) from cows on green pasture
> Lard from pigs raised outside (who then make vitamin D and store it in their fat)
> Eggs from chickens and other fowl raised outside or fed insects
> Shellfish (oysters, clams, mussels, crab, shrimp, lobster)
> Fish eggs
> Wild oily fish, such as salmon, sardines and anchovies
> Fish liver oils, particularly cod liver oil
> Insects (for those who have the courage to eat them!)

Your first step in the quest for good health is finding some or all of these foods. Shellfish are readily available in many locations, and good-quality cod liver oil can be obtained by mail order. Most European cheeses, and a growing number of artisanal American cheeses, come from herds allowed to graze. Local chapters of the Weston A. Price Foundation can help you find milk products and other animal foods locally from cows, chickens and pigs that are raised outdoors.

Quality counts in all the other foods that comprise the diet as well, including meats, seafood, poultry, grains, legumes, nuts, vegetables, fruits, oils, sweeteners and seasonings. Plant foods should be organic or, even better, biodynamic, grown in mineral-rich soil.

DO NO HARM

The degradation of the American food supply—from factory farming to industrial processing—is so pervasive that it requires some effort to find good quality foods; and the same effort must be applied to avoiding foods that are overtly harmful. The list of harmful foods begins with refined sugar and white flour, which provide plenty of calories but which have been shorn of the nutrients that naturally occur in sweet foods and in grains. To digest and assimilate sugar and white flour, the body must draw on its own reserves of vitamins and minerals, leading to depletion and deficiencies. In addition, sugar and white flour cause glucose to enter the bloodstream very quickly. When the body tries to compensate for this rapid rise in blood sugar, diabetes, hypoglycemia and adrenal insufficiency can result. These conditions open a veritable Pandora's box of unpleasant conditions—from allergies to depression.

This does not mean we should not eat sweet foods—the tongue has tastebuds for sweetness and they must be satisfied, at least occasionally, with desserts made from whole foods and nutrient-dense sweeteners, such as raw honey, maple syrup, maple sugar and dehydrated sugar cane juice. And whole grains can be prepared in such a way that they are just as pleasant to eat as products made from white flour.

Note that our list of acceptable sweeteners does not include fruit juice. While some people can eat whole fruit frequently without ill effects, fruit juice is concentrated, refined sweetness, just like white sugar. Even worse, fruit juice is composed primarily of fructose, which studies show to be more damaging to the body's biochemistry than white sugar.

More than 2,000 additives have been approved for use in American foods. The effects of these additives are synergistic and cumulative. That means that if we consume one or two additives in small amounts, we are unlikely to have any ill effects; but when we consume many types of additives frequently, their adverse effects are multiplied.

The most dangerous additives in the food supply are toxic to the nervous system, namely MSG and aspartame. MSG gives food a meaty taste without the use of meat; and aspartame gives food a sweet taste without the use of any food-based sweeteners. In effect, these substances trick the tastebuds, and these tricksters can play havoc with the central nervous system. Almost 100 symptoms have been attributed to consumption of MSG and aspartame, including seizures, nervousness, blood pressure fluctuations, headaches, multiple sclerosis and Alzheimer's disease. Aspartame is used in diet drinks and sugarless gum; MSG is found in literally thousands of products, often labeled innocuously as "spices" or "natural spices." Anything labeled "hydrolyzed" contains MSG. Hydrolyzed vegetable protein and hydrolyzed soy protein form the basis of many sauce and soup mixes, including the soup base products used in restaurants to make "homemade" soup.

Modern soy products must be included in our list of foods to avoid, as well as any type of protein powder. These are not whole foods, but are proteins that have been separated from the components in our food needed for their assimilation. In addition, modern high-temperature processing over-denatures many of the proteins and causes the formation of carcinogens. And unfermented soyfoods contain high levels of substances that block mineral absorption and interfere with protein digestion. The phytoestrogens in soy are potent endocrine disrupters that can depress thyroid function and cause other problems with the endocrine system, particularly in growing children.

Caffeine and other stimulants found in coffee, tea, chocolate and soft drinks have effects that are similar to sugar. They give the body a temporary lift by stimulating the production of adrenaline and raising blood sugar levels. When used frequently they can cause adrenal exhaustion leading to chronic fatigue and many other problems.

Finally, one more category of harmful foods belongs in our list—refined and hydrogenated vegetable oils, including oils from cottonseed, safflower, soy, corn and canola. These oils are completely new to the human diet and have been implicated in a host of illnesses, from cancer to heart disease. In their liquid form they are invariably rancid from high-temperature processing, which means that they provoke damaging oxidation reactions in the body; when made solid by the process of hydrogenation, these oils pose other dangers, particularly on the cellular level where they interfere with thousands of complex chemical processes.

FATS AND OILS

Our bodies do, however, need certain high-quality fats and oils, partly because these fats and oils carry important vitamins, and partly because they supply different types of fatty acids that the body uses both for energy production and for building cell membranes.

The three main types of fats, or fatty acids, are saturated, monounsaturated and polyunsaturated. Saturated fats tend to be solid at room temperature and occur mostly in animal fats including butter, and in tropical oils, like coconut oil. Saturated fats perform many important functions in the body, from strengthening the immune system to providing energy for the heart. Butter and coconut oil provide a special category of saturated fats, called short- and medium-chain fatty acids, which have antimicrobial properties; that is, they fight against pathogenic organisms in the gut, thereby protecting us from disease. There is no need to avoid saturated fats for fear of heart disease. The great increase in heart disease (as well as cancer and other degen-

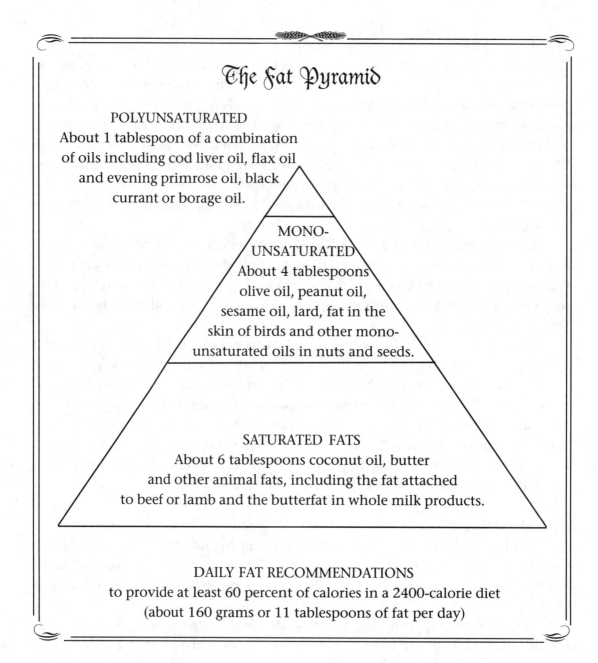

The Fat Pyramid

POLYUNSATURATED
About 1 tablespoon of a combination
of oils including cod liver oil, flax oil
and evening primrose oil, black
currant or borage oil.

MONO-
UNSATURATED
About 4 tablespoons
olive oil, peanut oil,
sesame oil, lard, fat in the
skin of birds and other monounsaturated oils in nuts and seeds.

SATURATED FATS
About 6 tablespoons coconut oil, butter
and other animal fats, including the fat attached
to beef or lamb and the butterfat in whole milk products.

DAILY FAT RECOMMENDATIONS
to provide at least 60 percent of calories in a 2400-calorie diet
(about 160 grams or 11 tablespoons of fat per day)

erative diseases) has paralleled the increasing use of processed vegetable oils, not animal fats.

Monounsaturated fats tend to be liquid at room temperature but go solid when refrigerated. They are found mostly in olive oil, peanut oil, sesame oil, avocados and nuts like almonds, cashews and pecans. Monounsaturated fatty acids pose no problems when consumed in moderation, but can cause numerous problems in a diet that does not also contain saturated fat.

The body does need good quality polyunsaturated fatty acids, but only in small amounts. They are found in many foods and also in cod liver oil, flax seed oil and in evening primrose oil, black currant oil or borage oil. Cod liver oil not only provides vitamins A and D but also important fatty acids called docosahexaenoic acid (DHA) and eicosapentaenoic acid (EPA), both of which play critical roles in cellular metabolism and in the functioning of the brain and nervous system. Similarly, flax oil provides an important polyunsaturated fatty acid called alpha-linolenic acid (ALA) and the final three (evening primrose, black currant and borage oils) provide gamma-linoleic acid (GLA), which, like DHA and EPA, plays an important role in cellular metabolism. These special fatty acids simply do not occur in modern processed foods and many health conditions improve when we add them to our diets in supplement form.

We are all familiar with the USDA food pyramid, which suggests whole and refined grains as the basis of our diet, with smaller amounts of fruits and vegetables, and very small amounts of animal foods and fats. This is not a concept we endorse— it results in a diet too high in carbohydrates and deficient in saturated fatty acids and the nutrients found exclusively in animal foods. Instead, we propose a different pyramid, one that will provide guidelines for fat consumption. The basis of our pyramid is saturated fats from animal foods and tropical oils. The middle band represents moderate amounts of monounsaturated fatty acids while the peak represents small amounts of polyunsaturated oils.

These recommendations are the exact opposite of establishment guidelines, which recommend only small amounts of saturated fats and large amounts of unsaturated fats and vegetable oils. The USDA guidelines reflect the priorities of the food industry, which reaps greater profits using liquid and partially hydrogenated vegetable oils rather than the more expensive animal fats and tropical oils. But many studies have shown that high levels of polyunsaturated oils can be harmful; we also know that the body cannot use and store the polyunsaturated fatty acids effectively without ample quantities of saturated fat. Many disease conditions will right themselves simply by redressing the kind and balance of fats in the diet.

DIGESTION

The nutritive elements in our food do us no good if the body cannot assimilate them. Rudolf Steiner consistently emphasized the importance of good digestion. The process of breaking our foods down to their smallest components—mineral ions, vitamins, simple sugars, individual fatty acids and individual amino acids—is more than just a biochemical phenomenon, he said. Optimal health is achieved only when "every trace of outer life" is removed from our food. The digestion of meat, said Steiner, "drives out everything which the foods represent in the animal body. In addition, everything that belongs to the plant food, by virtue of having been part of a living plant, must be driven out." If we are not successful in stripping our foods of their foreign nature, the effects of the animal and plant natures continue to operate in man to a certain extent. The result is disease.

Once our food is fully digested, and the resulting components enter the blood and lymph, it then takes on the characteristics of the human being, including those of the Emotional and Mental Bodies, and provides us with true nourishment.

A fundamental tenant of the Fourfold philosophy is that food preparation and processing should make our foods easier to digest. Unfortunately, most food processing techniques, such as canning, preserving in sugar and chemicals, pasteurizing and irradiation, make food much more difficult to digest. When we consistently eat foods that are difficult to digest, we compromise our vitality because the body is forced to expend a great deal of energy in merely breaking the food down into individual components. And anyone who has taken care to prepare his food in such a way as to make it easier to digest reports greatly increased energy, because the body does not have to work so hard at digestion.

The most important digestive aid in our food is salt. Salt activates an enzyme that begins the digestion of carbohydrates in the saliva, and many other digestive enzymes in the gut; and salt provides chloride the body needs for hydrochloric acid, for the digestion of meats. Unfortunately, commercial salt is highly refined, stripped of vital trace minerals and adulterated with additives. We recommend unrefined Celtic sea salt, which comes from unpolluted waters off the coast of Brittany. It is moist and light grey in color. Other unrefined salts are beige or pink—but not white. Whiteness in salt, like whiteness in sugar, means that it is refined, and the minerals removed.

The gelatin in homemade bone broths is another aid to digestion. Homemade broths or stocks also provide an abundance of minerals in a form that is very easy to assimilate. Homemade bone broth makes an excellent tonic; it can also be used to prepare delicious and satisfying soups, stews and sauces.

Grains, nuts and legumes contain anti-nutrients that render these foods very difficult to digest, but the process of digestion can begin before we consume them with preparation techniques that involve soaking, sprouting and sour leavening. Nuts contain enzyme inhibitors that can interfere with digestion. They can be neutralized by soaking raw nuts in salt water for 6-8 hours and then dehydrating the nuts in a warm oven or dehydrator. (We call nuts prepared in this way "crispy nuts.") A few basic recipes for grains and nuts are given in Appendix A. Many others are provided in *Nourishing Traditions*.

Before the days of refrigeration and canning machines, man preserved much of his food through the process of lacto-fermentation. A lacto-fermented food we are familiar with is old-fashioned sauerkraut, made not with vinegar but simply with salt and pounded cabbage. Pounding releases lactic acid, which is nature's best preservative. Almost any food can be preserved by lacto-fermentation to make a condiment, chutney or beverage. Even meats can be preserved in this way. In fact, dry cured sausages are actually fermented foods as are fermented milk products like cheese, yoghurt, buttermilk and kefir. In milk-drinking cultures, the adults usually consume a fermented version of cow, sheep or goat milk because the fermented version is easier to digest.

The wonderful thing about lacto-fermented foods, beside the fact that they taste good, is that they aid digestion by supplying lactic acid and friendly organisms to the digestive tract. They are the perfect digestive aid, delivered in a delicious package, particularly synergistic with rich, fatty foods.

Lacto-fermented beverages include fermented fruit juices and various types of kvass, a sour drink from Russia. Bread kvass is an effervescent soft drink sold by street vendors and beet kvass is a medicinal drink that provides numerous benefits. These beverages are easy to make in modern diets and should be part of everybody's diet.

Other digestive aids include dilute apple cider vinegar and Swedish bitters, which are especially valuable as part of high-fat diets.

RAW OR COOKED?

The concept of digestibility can serve as a guide when we consider whether our foods should be eaten raw or cooked. Grains and legumes are indigestible in their raw state and should be well cooked, or fermented for a long time. Nuts must be roasted or prepared by soaking and dehydration, as described above, or they cause irritation and indigestion. Many vegetables are difficult to digest in their raw state, often because they contain toxins that block thyroid function, interfere with mineral absorption or irritate the digestive tract. Green leafy vegetables and cruciferous vegetables like broccoli and cabbage belong in this category. Cooking neutralizes these antinutrients and makes these vegetable easy to eat. (Fermentation also neutralizes these substances, as in cabbage made into saurkraut.) Raw salads can be very beneficial but if your digestive apparatus is compromised, even these should be avoided.

On the other hand, it's best to consume milk products in their raw state. Pasteurization destroys enzymes that promote ease of assimilation and digestion; and pasteurization also makes many nutrients less available, particularly vitamins B_{12} and B_6.

As for meat and fish, traditional cultures consumed these animal foods both raw and cooked. Many nutrients are more available in raw fish and meat, but cooking actually breaks down the proteins in such a way that makes the amino acids easier to absorb. Thus, a well balanced diet includes meat and fish that are both raw and cooked.

Several dietary gurus have promoted various systems of food combining to facilitate digestion. One school of thought claims that meat and carbohydrate foods should not be combined in the same meal because the body cannot easily digest both at the same time. Yet Dr. Price did not discover any food combining rules among the populations he studied. In fact, the indigenous peoples of the Amazon basin always ate their meat with bananas!

The human digestive tract is admirably equipped to digest proteins, carbohydrates and fats all at the same time. In fact, it is impossible to separate these components in our diet. All plant foods contain proteins and fats, and even meat contains carbohydrates in the form of glycogen.

Most food combining systems are very restrictive, forcing people to be unnecessarily fussy about their foods. With proper choices and preparation, proteins, carbohydrates and fats can be eaten together in the same meal, in delicious combinations of traditional fare.

VITAMINS PILLS OR SUPERFOODS?

Food is our best medicine but very often we need strong medicine. The typical alternative or complementary treatment loads the patient down with synthetic vitamins in the form of pills and powders. Synthetic vitamins are fractionated forms of the vitamin complexes that occur naturally in foods. Because they are concentrated and simplified, the body cannot use them as well the more complex, naturally occurring versions. Larger amounts of synthetic vitamins are needed to obtain the desired effects, and in large amounts they can cause many biochemical imbalances and drug-like side effects.

Several recent studies have shown that taking synthetic vitamins can actually be harmful, thus challenging a practice suggested in virtually all the books written about health and nutrition over the past 40 years. The first study, published in the *New England Journal of Medicine*, April 1994, showed that supplementation by synthetic beta-carotene in smokers increased the rate at which these individuals contracted lung cancer—exactly the opposite results the researchers expected. The second study, described in the *Los Angeles Times*, March 3, 2000, showed that high-dose vitamin C supplementation can accelerate the progression of atherosclerosis by increasing the rate of intimal thickening. Intimal thickening refers to a progressive increase in the thickness of the inner lining of artery walls, which is now considered one of the causes of heart attacks and strokes. "High-dose vitamin C supplementation" was defined as the ingestion of 500 mg of ascorbic acid daily for many years, a practice in which literally millions of Americans engage. The final and perhaps most daunting report was the Los Angeles Atherosclerosis Study, published in *Science* 2001, which concluded that 500 mg vitamin C ingested daily is genotoxic, which means that synthetic vitamin C can interfere with DNA and potentiate the growth of malignant tumors. While these results—all of which were reported in the mainstream media—were shocking to most people in the alternative health field, they represent a stunning confirmation of what the true nutritional pioneers such as Weston Price and Royal Lee had said all along.

Dr. Royal Lee was the father of natural vitamin treatment. He argued for years that ascorbic acid, commonly referred to as vitamin C, does not provide us with what our bodies need. In fact, even the discoverer of vitamin C, Dr. Albert Szent-Giorgi, never claimed that ascorbic acid was the antiscorbutic or scurvy-curing agent found in lemons and other natural foods. He maintained, as did Royal Lee, that the "whole complex of substances found in vitamin-rich foods is the active ingredient that can cure scurvy" and that this complex of substances is not at all the same as the isolated chemical ascorbic acid. Vitamin C is actually a complex of nutrients that includes bioflavonoids, rutin, tyrosine, copper and other substances known and unknown. Ascorbic acid functions as the preservative for this complex, serving to keep it together in the plant tissue, preserving its integrity, freshness and color. Ascorbic acid is not a food for us; that which it preserves is our food. It is the whole vitamin C complex that prevents scurvy, supports white blood cell function and stimulates collagen production, thereby preventing tissues from bleeding. Furthermore, since we need the whole complex in order for it to have a nutritional effect, when we take a lot of vitamin C, we actually become more deficient in the other parts of vitamin C complex. This is because as we ingest excessive amounts of only one part, we liberate stores of the other components, rapidly depleting their supplies. Thus, high-dose supplementation, or any supplementation of ascorbic acid, actually makes us deficient in this vital nutrient—not a good nutritional strategy.

This well-documented phenomenon for ascorbic acid holds true for all the other vitamins. High vitamin A levels in the tissues are associated with reduced cancer rates, but ingesting high doses of the synthetic beta-carotene, the precursor of vitamin A, actually increases the rate of lung cancer because when we flood the body with beta-carotene, the production of true vitamin A is blocked. Synthetic vitamin D (vitamin D_2) has the opposite effect of vitamin D_3 naturally occurring in food—it causes softening of the hard tissues, such as the bones, and hardening of the soft tissues, such as the arteries.

The perverse effects of synthetic vitamins were exactly predicted by Royal Lee, who founded a company to supply whole food extracts instead of chemical, fractionated vitamin supplements. His first product, called Catalyn, was derived from the following whole foods: defatted wheat germ; carrots; nutritional yeast; bovine adrenal, liver, spleen and kidney; ovine spleen; dried pea (vine) juice; dried alfalfa juice; mushroom; oat flour; soy bean lecithin; and rice bran extract. Catalyn and similar products are still available today through doctors under the Standard Process label. The company organically farms more than one thousand acres of mineral-rich fertile soil, created when the retreating glaciers moved mountains of earth across the Kettle Moraine area in Wisconsin. They are excellent products for helping patients balance body chemistry and restore nutritional deficiencies.

Dr. Weston Price also understood that we need to obtain our nutrients from foods rather than from vitamin pills. He always encouraged his patients to pay close attention to the quality of the food they ate and to take whole food extracts such as cod liver oil, rich in vitamins A and D, and high vitamin butter oil, a product obtained from high-vitamin butter using a process of low-temperature centrifuging, which he developed. Other "superfoods" include wheat germ oil for vitamin E; nutritional yeast and bee pollen for most of the B vitamins; desiccated liver for vitamin B_{12}; and certain powdered fruits such as rose hips, acerola berries and amalaki (a fruit from India) for vitamin C complex.

It is a humbling fact that in spite of the many discoveries of modern science, we still have very little idea which factors in food need to be present in order to facilitate the promotion of optimal health. All we can really do is eat the best quality food, and let our intestines, liver, pancreas, blood and cells sort out the biochemistry.

A word on cod liver oil: this is the most basic supplement in the Fourfold Healing approach. It supplies not only a concentrated source of vitamins A and D (which the body requires in much greater amounts than we can obtain in a western-style diet) but also special fatty acids called EPA and DHA, needed for a host of processes on the cellular level. EPA and DHA are particularly important for the function of the brain and nervous system. The amount of vitamins A and D in various brands of cod liver oil can vary considerably. In general, cod liver oil supplies 5000 IU vitamin A per teaspoon, but some high-vitamin varieties provide 10,000 IU per teaspoon. The basic recommended dose for adults and children over the age of 12 is one that supplies about 10,000 IU per day, and about 5000 IU for infants and children under 12. For many conditions of disease and stress, this dose can and should be higher.

The best and most inexpensive way to take cod liver oil is in liquid form. It can be added to a small amount of fresh juice or water, mixed thoroughly and swallowed quickly to avoid the unpleasant oiliness and taste. Capsules are also available and an eye dropper works well for giving cod liver oil to infants and small children. Virtually all cod liver oil imported into the US comes from Norway where it is thoroughly tested for any traces of pesticides, mercury and other contaminants. Cod liver oil in the US must pass very strict standards and is a safe and pure product. One important caveat, however, is to include plenty of good quality saturated fats, especially butter, in your diet if you are taking cod liver oil. Saturated fats work synergistically with highly unsaturated EPA and DHA. Weston Price found that he only got good results with cod liver oil when he gave butter concurrently.

THE CALCIUM FACTOR

Weston Price discovered that primitive diets contained the various minerals at levels many times greater than the amounts found in western diets—particularly calcium. Calcium, of course, is the principal component of bones and teeth; it also plays a part in nerve transmission and muscle contraction. When calcium stores are low, we tend to be irritable and suffer from cramps.

Calcium also helps the body maintain the proper balance between acid and alkaline. Proponents of vegetarianism claim that consumption of animal foods will make the body too acid. However, Price did not find any evidence of over-acidity in primitive peoples consuming animal products almost exclusively and that was because they had a plentiful supply of calcium in their diets.

Many foods contain some calcium but there are actually only two food types that supply an abundance of calcium in a form the body can easily absorb—raw dairy products (milk, yoghurt, cheese, and so forth) and bone broths. Cultures that do not consume dairy products include bone broth in the diet, often with every meal. Even better is the inclusion of both, a characteristic of most traditional European diets. Remember that your body cannot absorb calcium without adequate amounts of vitamins A and D from animal fats. If minerals, especially calcium, are the bricks out of which the body is built, vitamins A and D are the mortar.

An easy test for calcium status is to measure the pH of the saliva—slight alkalinity is a sign that the body is absorbing and utilizing calcium and other minerals. The test should be taken morning and evening for at least a week and the results recorded. Occasionally certain foods will give anomalous results, but in general, a pH reading of 6.8-7.0 indicates good nutrient status and good overall health. Those with a salivary pH of 6.6 and below generally have health problems and cancer patients usually have acidic saliva readings in the range of 5.8. (For more detailed instructions, see Appendix B.)

EATING TO LIVE AND LIVING TO EAT

Rudolf Steiner warned against any dietary formulations, such as food combining, blood type diets or rigid guidelines, that separated individuals from their fellow men during meal times. For man, eating is a social activity, much different for humans than for animals. While animal nutrition is completely instinctual, man has developed a culture of eating that raises him above the animal stage. Animals feed, but humans eat. For man, the activity of eating involves far more than just putting food into one's mouth. It invokes the pleasure of many senses—smell, touch, taste, sight and even hearing—and affects the life of the soul and the mind, as well as the Physical and Life-Force Bodies.

The activities of cooking and eating combine ritual, talent and social skills. And just as regaining and maintaining health require achieving balance between opposites, so the provision of food for the physical body also requires a healthy balance between two extremes—one that pays no attention to food at all and one that makes a fetish out of eating.

Primitive man spends much of his effort engaging in hunting, foraging and food preparation; modern man eats on the run and devotes almost no time or thought to his food. The very first lesson to be learned about feeding the physical body is that food preparation cannot be left to others, especially not to large corporations whose motive is profit, not quality. The challenge to modern men and women involves melding a certain amount of time for food preparation and meals into a busy life-style along with a recognition that the way we cook and eat has a profound effect on the quality of our life, our state of health and the nourishment of the mind and soul.

SUGGESTED READING

Nutrition and Physical Degeneration by Weston A. Price, DDS
Nourishing Traditions by Sally Fallon
The Dynamics of Nutrition by Gerhard Schmidt
Know Your Fats by Mary G. Enig, PhD
The Cholesterol Myths by Uffe Ravnskov, MD, PhD
Nutrition Almanac by Lavon J. Dunne
The Untold Story of Milk by Ron Schmid, ND
The Yoga of Eating by Charles Eisenstein

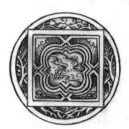

Chapter 2
Therapeutics: Healing the Life-force Body

The Fourfold Path to healing relies on the work of several geniuses in the field of medicine. We have already learned about the contributions of Weston A. Price, Rudolf Steiner and Royal Lee, whose insights into the optimum diet, the process of digestion and the use of food concentrates form the backbone of this book.

When choosing remedies for specific disease conditions, we turn once again to the work of Rudolf Steiner, along with that of two others—Edgar Cayce and Samuel Hahnemann.

RUDOLF STEINER

We have already looked at Steiner's principle of the four bodies of man, the principle that forms the basis of the Fourfold healing approach. Steiner also discussed a second principle, adopted from the great German philosopher and physician Paracelsus, that of the three poles or systems of the human organism. These systems

---

Rhythmical System

Attribute: Harmony and Balance/Feeling
Endpoint: Health
Function: Homeostasis
Substance: Blood

Nerve-Sense System

Attribute: Thinking
Endpoint: Sclerosis
Function: Catabolism (breaking down)
Substance: Clear Fluids

Metabolic System

Attribute: Willing
Endpoint: Inflammation
Function: Anabolism (building up)
Substance: Cloudy Fluids

---

describe *activity* or *movement* within the four bodies—Physical, Life-Force, Emotional and Mental. These poles of activity—the Nerve-Sense System, the Rhythmical System and the Metabolic System—as shown in the diagram on page 25.

In this model, health comes about through balanced rhythmical activity or movement, right down to the level of the organs and cells. It is a rhythm that follows the path of a lemniscate or figure eight, flowing between catabolism and anabolism, thinking and willing (or activity). The result is homeostasis, defined as a state of physiological equilibrium produced by a balance of functions and chemical composition within the organism. Many, if not most, diseases can be seen as an imbalance in this healthy rhythm, with too much emphasis on either the Nerve-Sense pole or the Metabolic pole. This model also serves as a useful construct for determining the proper therapies or medicines for a specific illness.

Two organs obviously based on rhythm are the heart, which beats, and the lungs, which breathe, but all the organs follow a daily or monthly rhythm, alternating activity and rest. We can contribute to the body's complex and subtle rhythms by following certain rhythms in our daily lives, such as regular periods of nightly sleep and daily activity, regular meals, regular rhythmical excretion and bowel movements, regular rhythmical activity of our limbs and even regular observance of festivals throughout the year. When our activities become anti-rhythmical—whether they be eating, sleeping, elimination or exercise—we risk disrupting the rhythms of our organs and cells. Steiner taught that the loss of healthy rhythm leads to either too much sclerosis or hardening, originating in the Nerve-Sense System, or too much inflammation and swelling coming from the Metabolic System.

The Nerve-Sense System is associated the activity of thinking, with the head and with clear fluids. This comparison may seem odd, but consider that the thinking process is one of coolness and clarity. That is why the fluids of the head, such as those in the eye and in the spine are crystal clear in their normal state, like the mineral quartz or silica. When these fluids are healthy and clear, the thinking process can proceed without hinderance. On the other hand, the fluids of the Metabolic pole are cloudy and thick. The cloudy fluids of the lymph are normal for the abdominal area, which is the center of the Metabolic System.

Excessive or deficient activities of the Nerve-Sense or the Metabolic systems can also manifest as improper activity in the "wrong place." When a superabundance of cloudy fluids fills the head as in hay fever, for example, we suffer from stuffiness in the nose and throat and reddening of the eyes. Under these conditions, we find it difficult to think clearly. The head area should have a certain stillness and clarity so that thinking can proceed without hinderance. However, clarity and stillness are not appropriate for the abdomen. If the qualities of the Nerve-Sense System have too much influence in this area, we suffer from a hardening or contraction process, leading to cramps, spasms or even gall stones.

Many of Steiner's therapeutic recommendations derive from this model of three poles or principles governing the human organism, and I have found it a very useful construct in determining which preparations and treatments to prescribe for specific disease conditions. For example, kidney stones, according to Steiner, are caused by an overexuberant mineralization process in the kidneys. Gall stones, gout and hardening of the arteries are likewise the result of mineralization that is too "exuberant." On the other hand, if we have too little mineralization, we get rickets or osteoporosis. A thorough understanding of this concept of mineralization is crucial to the successful use of medicinal remedies.

EDGAR CAYCE

The second pioneer of twentieth century holistic medicine is Edgar Cayce. A simple, uneducated man with no medical background of any sort, Cayce seems a most improbable choice for the title of medical genius. But I have found invaluable guidance in the insights that "came through" him. Early in his life, Cayce discovered that he had the ability to go into a trancelike state and, in a slightly difference voice, speak of things about which he had no conscious experience. Working completely without showmanship, commercialism or hucksterism, he exercised his talents as a "sleeping prophet" for the rest of his life. All of the readings were transcribed by his faithful secretary Gladys Davis and are now available to researchers on CD-ROM from the Association for Research and Enlightenment (ARE) in Virginia Beach.

The body of material left by Cayce is vast. It contains much that is specific to various individuals and their diseases, and much of a more general philosophical nature. I would like to describe a few basic points that seem to emerge from the thousands of readings.

First of all, Cayce often traced the etiology of disease in later life to upsets or traumas that occurred much earlier and even, sometimes, to events that seemed irrelevant. Thus the process of healing often involved revisiting certain events to which the individual had attached little or no importance, or may even have forgotten. Such work by the patient is tantamount to our efforts to heal our Emotional and Mental Bodies.

When it came to prescribing specific remedies, Cayce taught that good health depended on a harmonious relationship between the sympathetic and parasympathetic nervous systems, which together make up the autonomic nervous system. Unlike the central nervous system, which controls thinking and conscious muscle activity, the autonomic system controls functions like heart rate, breathing, digestion, sexual urges and so on. Clearly these functions are not normally under our conscious control. The sympathetic nervous system promotes "fight or flight" responses while the parasympathetic nervous system plays the role of nourishing and healing. The Type A, hard-driving or skittish person typifies a condition of over-activity or stress in the sympathetic nervous system. Such individuals often suffer from nervous disorders, insomnia, frequent infections and heart disease. The more laid-back individual with parasympathetic dominance is prone to low blood pressure, depression and particularly allergies and asthma, conditions in which there is an excess of mucous in the head and lungs.

Cayce's readings suggest that the autonomic nervous system also registers and processes emotions and traumas, and is somehow connected with one's "drive" or ability to accomplish things in life. Often in a reading he would trace a problem with an organ—say a digestive organ—to an emotional or physical trauma that occurred many years earlier. He claimed that such events could "switch on" the sympathetic nervous system, thereby promoting the "fight or flight" response—even when such reactions were inappropriate—and overwhelm the more passive, nurturing functions of the parasympathetic system.

According to Cayce's model, an imbalance resulting in dominance of the sympathetic system can become more and more fixed. In essence, the "fight or flight" syndrome becomes the habit of the person's unconscious makeup. Years of living with such an imbalance, in which excessive sympathetic activity dominates the more healing activities of the parasympathetic system, can actually starve the organs, resulting in such diseases as hypertension, adrenal insufficiency, colitis and chronic fatigue. On the other hand, years of living with parasympathetic dominance typically manifests as hypoglycemia and hypothyroidism, as well as blockages and constrictions in certain organs which are, in essence, smothered by over-attention.

Cayce's philosophy bears many resemblances to Paracelsus' notion of the three poles of activity in the human body. The sympathetic nervous system corresponds to the Nerve-Sense pole and the fight-or-flight response that it engenders is essentially catabolic, in that it uses up energy. The parasympathetic nervous system corresponds to the Metabolic pole. This is the nurturing tendency that helps organs build up and heal. Thus, we can add these two opposing principles to our chart as shown opposite.

Both Steiner and Cayce attributed many illnesses to early events that trigger excessive activity either in the Nerve-Sense/Sympathetic nervous system or the Metabolic/Parasympathetic nervous system. They suggest that an emotional life that is unbalanced—either deficient or overstimulated—can lead to lack of balance in the physical body and even the destruction of the very organs that nourish us. Both Steiner and Cayce viewed the physical body as part of a complex in which the quality

Rhythmical System

Attribute: Harmony and Balance/Feeling
Endpoint: Health
Function: Homeostasis
Substance: Blood

Nerve-Sense System
Sympathetic Nervous System

Activity: Fight or Flight
Attribute: Thinking
Endpoint: Sclerosis
Function: Catabolism (breaking down)
Substance: Clear Fluids

Metabolic System
Parasympathetic Nervous System

Activity: Nurturing
Attribute: Willing
Endpoint: Inflammation
Function: Anabolism (building up)
Substance: Cloudy Fluids

of the emotions played a vital, if unrecognized, role. These ideas are now accepted as a tenet of the holistic health movement. Truly, both Steiner and Cayce were pioneers in the healing arts and in what is now referred to as mind-body medicine.

If we accept that many illnesses are due to either excessive sympathetic or parasympathetic activity, resulting in either the starvation or smothering of certain organs, then one of Cayce's primary intervention strategies begins to make sense. In essence, he suggested that imbalances due to destructive emotions need to be "washed away" so that the nutritive organs can regenerate. Thus, along with dietary changes, exercise and massage, he often suggested castor oil packs over certain organs.

Although completely ignored by the orthodox medical establishment, castor oil and castor oil packs constitute an ancient remedy that has been in use for at least three thousand years. The profound positive benefit of castor oil is probably the reason practitioners during the Middle Ages called it the Oil of Christ. The packs incorporate two important therapeutic principles. The first is warmth, especially warmth over the metabolic organs, which may have been denied warmth due to excessive activity of the sympathetic nervous system or, put another way, a misplacement of the nerve-sense activity. It is the oil in plants that stores the most calories or heat and that can burn with gentle, warming flames. The second principle is detoxification. Castor oil seems to be able to increase the flow of bile, particularly in the liver. This gentle stimulation and draining in turn helps the liver perform its detoxification tasks, and stimulate more excretion through the bowels. When you apply the castor oil pack over a diseased organ, the organ gets warmer almost immediately. More blood flow comes to the area, thereby flushing out toxins. The lymph—the garbage-collection system in our bodies—begins to circulate more quickly. Spasms and pain are relieved and, in time, the organ gets healthier. For example, properly applied, castor oil packs can relieve menstrual cramps. If used on a regular basis, the packs will also allow the uterus itself to become healthier.

The unique configuration of the fatty acids in castor oil gives it excellent emollient and lubrication properties. In addition, these fatty acids have a number of reaction sites that allow them to bond with a great variety of other substances. Paradoxically, castor oil is also extremely stable. I like to think of castor oil as representing the stable, balancing and integrating influence of the ego or warmth body, imparting nourishing heat to organs that have been starved due to over-activity of the sympathetic nervous system, and gentle detoxification to organs that have been smothered by over-activity of the parasympathetic nervous system.

Castor oil packs are a vital element in the therapies I use for a number of disease conditions. They require a certain amount of patience because results are not always immediate, but then the imbalances that cause disease do so only over time. They are a gentle, non-invasive method for beginning the process that restores balance and harmony to the body.

SAMUEL HAHNEMANN AND HOMEOPATHY

Samuel Hahnemann was a German physician, chemist and Renaissance man who lived in the latter part of the 18th century and early 19th century. He was a brilliant, intuitive scholar and an expert in many fields of knowledge. His career spanned an era that can be considered the Dark Ages for medicine. Traditional wisdom and healing philosophies, including the doctrine of the four humors, were giving way to the development of scientific inquiry. New ways of thinking about the human body were replacing older, intuitive paradigms. Unfortunately, in the early stages of this development, the treatment was often worse than the disease, such as amputations without anesthetics, brutal use of forceps for difficult births and administration of extremely toxic drugs like mercury. Improved surgical methods, sanitary procedures, insulin and better drugs were still at least one hundred years away. In fact, medicine was in such a quandary that one of the most popular "schools" of medicine at this time was the Nihilistic School, which claimed that physicians could do little to alter the course of any disease. Therefore, the predominant task of the physician was to make an accurate diagnosis for the patient and then give a prognosis—no treatment, just a prognosis.

Remnants of this thinking continue to this day, as doctors still assume that their major task is to diagnose and give a prognosis. Of course, we demand and expect a treatment that will alter the prognosis. Yet, the foreboding dictums of the Nihilistic School still linger—many patients are told that there is no cure for their particular disease. The notion that nature and destiny will prevail continues to be more widely accepted than the belief that we have the innate ability to heal ourselves.

Because treatments were limited during Hahnemann's day, many physicians actually became astute diagnosticians, able to accurately describe illnesses and their natural course or progression. This set the stage for Hahnemann's discovery of homeopathy, a discovery that is profound in its implications for the understanding of illness and health—and even of life itself. Today we have only scratched the surface of homeopathy's potential to advance the practice of medicine and relieve the suffering of disease.

The central tenet of homeopathy is the principle of "like cures like," which Hahnemann discovered while treating a patient for malaria. Drawing on his vast knowledge of botany and botanical pharmacology, Hahnemann took note of the fact that quinine, an extract from the bark of a Peruvian tree, exactly reproduces the symptoms of malaria in a healthy person. Paradoxically, quinine was also reputed to be an effective treatment for malaria. His own experiments confirmed that the extract was indeed a cure for this debilitating disease.

He then began to investigate whether the like-cures-like principle could be applied to other diseases. Hahnemann would note the symptoms that occurred when people were poisoned by various toxic substances. Belladonna poisoning, for example, caused dilated pupils, rapid pulse and fever. He methodically tested hundreds of substances by giving them to healthy subjects and noting in great detail their reaction. This methodology, known as "homeopathic proving," was one of the first scientific attempts to discover in an objective way the effects of various herbs, minerals and animal extracts on human beings.

Hahnemann then used these various substances to treat diseases according to their symptom patterns. He used belladonna, for example, to successfully treat a child whose symptoms of scarlet fever were exactly those of belladonna poisoning—dilated pupils, high fever and a characteristic skin rash. Similarly, he used mercury, which when ingested causes bloody diarrhea, to cure the various intestinal diseases so common in his era.

Homeopathy remedies are specific to the person, not the disease. Two patients with scarlet fever may, in fact, have different symptoms and therefore require different remedies, a principle totally at odds with the kind of disease-oriented medicine practiced today.

The second major principle that Hahnemann discovered is the principle of "potentiation." As you can imagine, the substances that Hahnemann worked with were some of the strongest poisons known to man. Obviously, if he were to use them to cure his patients, he would have to use them in such a manner that he did not poison them instead. He solved this dilemma intuitively in his discovery of "potentiation," a process in which the poisonous substance is mixed with water, shaken for a certain length of time, and progressively diluted until what remains is only a few parts per million. Usually, Hahnemann diluted one part of the original medicine with nine parts of water. After rhythmically shaking the solution for three to five minutes—a process called "succussion"—he would repeat the dilution process with one part of the solution and another nine parts water. The process of dilution and succussion was continued until only a minute amount of the original substance remained in the solution. Hahnemann discovered that highly diluted medicines acted more powerfully than full-strength or even moderately diluted medicines. In addition, the poisons lost their toxicity and so caused no side effects.

Hahnemann found that the principle of potentiation also worked for minerals. Sulphur, for example, can be a good treatment for dry, flaky skin. But highly potentiated sulphur is a remedy for the opposite condition—swollen or suppurating skin.

It is easy to subject the principles of homeopathy to scientific scrutiny—in fact, in numerous studies the homeopathic medicines have proved to be very effective in treating disease. The difficulty is in understanding how the medicines work. "More dilute, more potent" just does not make sense to the modern mind. Many have suggested explanations, and there are numerous texts on homeopathy for the reader who wishes to explore the subject more deeply.

The explanation I offer is this: We know through the work of Einstein and other physicists that the substances we find on earth, be they of mineral, plant, animal or human origin, consist not only of physical matter but also of a kind of compressed energy. Each substance, each mineral, each plant and even each person, possesses a very particular kind of energy with unique characteristics and a unique biography. This biography and these characteristics form what can be called the "essence" of the particular substance. If we extract these essences, we can use them for healing. These essences are discovered through the homeopathic proving of symptoms; and they are liberated through the method of homeopathic potentiation.

In using the homeopathic metal preparations, we are guided once again by Rudolf Steiner, who revived the medieval view of correspondences. Traditional cultures assigned a quality or "essence" to each of the heavenly bodies, based on the length of their cycles and other properties. Then, invoking the philosophy of "as above, so below," they linked the qualities of each planet with the metals found in the earth, and with the organs of the human body, as summarized below:

Sun	Gold	Heart
Moon	Silver	Reproductive Organs and Brain (reflection)
Mercury	Mercury	Lungs, Large Intestine
Venus	Copper	Kidneys
Mars	Iron	Gall Bladder
Jupiter	Tin	Liver
Saturn	Lead	Spleen

We use the same process of correspondences in choosing the many other essences that Hahnemann discovered to be useful for various diseases.

The use of homeopathic "essences" to cure diseases is, in fact, a way of restoring balance to the body, either through a kind of reprogramming using highly dilute poisons, or the redressing of certain biochemical tendencies using mineral solutions. As such, homeopathy dovetails very well with the principles that Steiner and Cayce described. And because the treatments have no side effects, we can, each one of us, make use of them in our quest for healing.

Homeopathic preparations are now readily available in pharmacies and health food stores throughout the United States. The wise physician will make homeopathic medicines an integral part of his practice.

HERBAL EXTRACTS

The use of herbs as medicines is a practice as old as the human race itself. Medicinal herbs are mentioned in all traditions, in all cultures, in all locations, and herbal medicine is still the most widely used healing modality, even in modern times. When using herbal medicines, the practitioner can draw on many rich sources of information, including the traditions of Chinese medicine, Ayurvedic medicine, Native American medicine and so forth. There is also a voluminous body of scientific literature on the use of herbs. Many of the studies were carried out at the most prestigious universities of our day. The book I have found most useful in combining tradition with science is *Principles and Practice of Phytotherapy* by Kerry Bone and Simon Mills.

In these pages I hope to add to the rich history of herbal medicine by incorporating Rudolf Steiner's method of inquiry into the nature of herbs. This means that in addition to presenting the traditional uses of specific herbs and the scientific studies that justify such uses, we will also try to understand the "essence" of each plant used as a medicine. Using observation, inspection, study of life habits, smell, taste and so forth, we will try to understand what each medicinal plant is trying to teach the human being and what it corresponds to in humans. Many examples will be given throughout the chapters in Section II. We will discuss the essence or distinguishing characteristics of a variety of compounds to show why mistletoe, for example, is a good treatment for cancer, or echinacea is a good treatment for infectious disease.

Plants contain a complex mixture of known and unknown substances, as well as the forces or "essences" that operate in homeopathic medicines. Just as isolated or synthetic components of food can never nourish us, so too isolated or synthetic components of herbs can never provide the benefit that we can obtain from the herb itself. Digitalis leaf is not the same as the so-called active ingredient digoxin. For if we make the mistake of using only the chemical digoxin as our medicine, we omit the other components of the digitalis leaf, some of which produce nausea and vomiting if we take too much. Use of the isolated chemical digoxin in conventional medicine, rather than digitalis leaf as an herb, has resulted in the death of thousands of patients from digitalis overdose, because the built-in protective components have been removed.

Of course, the so-called active ingredients in plants must be present or they will be ineffective as medicines. The active ingredients of echinacea are called alkylamides, substances that improve immunity and numb your tongue upon ingestion. Without alkylamides the medicine probably won't work. But echinacea is even more effective and safe if the alkylamides remain in the context of the whole plant extract, including all of its known and unknown substances, and all its aspects both substantial and subtle.

This understanding then leads us to consider how our herbs are grown and prepared. The herbs we use as medicine must be allowed to grow in their natural way, in their natural habitat. They must be extracted so that both the active ingredients as well as the entire plant extract remain in the medicine. And, finally they should be used in amounts that have been shown by tradition and modern research to have therapeutic benefit. This amount is often far higher than the doses commonly suggested in herbal textbooks

The company that meets all these requirements is Mediherb from Australia. Founded by the master herbalist, Kerry Bone, they produce concentrated whole herbal extracts with rich smells and tastes, analogous to the whole food extracts of Standard Process and providing similar therapeutic effects.

PROTOMORPHOGENS

The scientific and medical world has been swept up by the promises of the genetic revolution whose benefits, according to almost daily reports, are imminent. One of the high points of this revolution was the human genome project, which was supposed to determine the precise role of every human gene, especially as they relate to disease. Funded with huge amounts of taxpayer money, the project actually came out with some perplexing findings. We all learn in high school biology that there is a central dogma in genetics, an inviolable rule upon which all the rest of genetics is based. This central dogma states that each living being has a set of DNA, or genetic material that, except for mutations, is fixed and immutable. This DNA translates itself into an organism through the creation of RNA, which is then translated into proteins that carry out all the functions needed in growing and maintaining a living entity. This central dogma teaches us that us that this process is unidirectional, that the direction is always DNA to RNA to protein, never the other way around. By mapping the human DNA we learned which specific gene, or sequence of DNA, coded for each protein. Scientists believed that it was only a matter of time before we would learn to manipulate the DNA to produce proteins more to our liking. The human genome map was to be our guide.

The reality, however, turned out much differently. Scientists had already discovered at least 200,000 human proteins. To their surprise, the human genome project revealed only about 30,000 genes (a few more than fruit flies). Thus, DNA does not determine proteins in a one-to-one correspondence. The central dogma of genetics has proved to be false.

The relationship between DNA and protein can best be explained by analogy. In the game of Scrabble, each player makes words from a set of letters, each of which is assigned a numeric value. The words the players form are like the proteins, the letters are like the DNA. While the letters are necessary to make the words, no one would say that the letters determine the words produced. That is accomplished by the savvy or insight of the player. Nor do the letters determine the outcome of the game. My wife, who spent 17 years as an editor and who is an expert with words, always beats me in Scrabble (I am not an expert in words) no matter which letters she draws. Similarly, the qualities and quantities of proteins produced by the cells are not determined by the DNA. Rather the cell and the organism as a whole, in some as yet undetermined way, uses the DNA to fashion the proteins it needs.

As part of Royal Lee's research, he studied the nucleoproteins that reside in the nucleus of our cells and that influence the functioning of both the individual cells and the gland or organs from which those nucleoproteins originated. He termed these cellular determinants "protomorphogens." He claimed that each organ or gland has a unique protomorphogen and that these protomorphogens were similar across the various species. Thus, the nucleoproteins from a cow's adrenal gland are similar to the nucleoproteins from a human adrenal gland. He then postulated that sick or stressed organs spill their nucleoprotein content into the bloodstream. This spillage causes the immune system to react by producing antibodies to these nucleoproteins in order to remove them from the blood. Sometimes, this antibody response becomes overly enthusiastic and the immune system attacks the intact cells in a misguided effort to remove the protomorphogens inside the cells. Lee believed such antibody attack was an integral step in any disease process, a kind of autodigestion, which actually prevented the organ from healing after the initial inciting event. It is worth noting that this theory of protomorphology was formulated before the "discovery" of what we now call autoimmune disease. In fact, they describe the same phenomenon. However, Lee claimed that this autoimmune, or self-digestion process occurs as an integral part of many disease processes, not just the classic autoimmune illnesses.

Lee proposed to heal the diseased organ by providing the nucleoproteins of the same organ from a different species. He theorized that the immune system, centered as it is around the intestines, would preferentially attack the orally ingested nucleoproteins and leave those from the sick organ alone. This would break the cycle and allow the body to heal. He called this process "oral tolerance therapy," and he developed the technology to isolate the nucleoproteins from the various glands of cows and pigs.

Protomorphogen therapy, then, has two essential underpinnings. First, you are supplying those "determinants" that control the functioning of the targeted gland. This would be analogous to having a poor Scrabble player like myself study the dictionary. And secondly, you break the cycle of autoimmune disease, thereby giving the organ a chance to heal.

In the following chapters you will find that I often combine three specific therapies to help glands and organs heal—the appropriate protomorphogen extract, a homeopathic dilution of the metal that corresponds to the organ or gland in question and, finally, the herb or plant extract that has been used historically to restore function to a particular organ.

WHAT IS DISEASE?

One of the most important lessons I have learned during my years in the practice of medicine—and one of the most important ideas that I strive to convey—is that most, if not virtually all, of the "dis-eases" that I see in my patients are best understood as the body's attempt at self-correction, or self-healing. For example, if you get a splinter in your finger but don't take it out, eventually it will form pus and the body will expel the splinter. Some would call the pus an "infection," but a better description is "self-correction," the body's attempt to rid itself of a foreign body. Treating the "infection" with antibiotics or even with herbs is not only foolish but counterproductive. The only reasonable therapy is to help the splinter come out. Similarly, gall stones, which are little cholesterol deposits, occur only in individuals who do not consume the right kinds of fats—they eat either processed vegetable oils and *trans* fatty acids, or they follow a lowfat diet and consume very little fat at all. Since these diets do not supply the body with the nutrients it needs, it is forced to make and store them. It does so in the form of cholesterol stones. This is not a disease, it is an adaptive strategy. I know this is so because whenever I have been able to convince a patient with gall stones to eat a normal diet containing adequate amounts of traditional fats, the stones dissolve. I have the ultrasounds to prove it. Provision of adequate fats in the diet obviates the need for the body to form stones, thereby solving the problem.

Literally all "dis-eases" can be seen in this light and it is only when practitioners understand the true nature of human illness that they can make the right treatment decisions. When we work against this wisdom, when we do not recognize or honor it, whether in the realm of conventional or alternative medicine, the result is failure and misery for the patient. The human body is an incredible wisdom-filled vehicle for the unfolding of the human spirit. The practitioner who does not recognize this fact risks making things worse rather than better for his patients.

In his ground-breaking work *Non-Violent Communication*, Marshall Rosenberg describes a method of nonviolent communication that relies on careful, compassionate listening. Likewise, the vast majority of the treatments and therapies I recommend can be classified as nonviolent or nontoxic therapies. However Rosenberg also elaborated on what he calls the "protective use of force." Even if you espouse the principles of nonviolent communication, if someone has a gun and is about to shoot your friend, you simply disarm the person with whatever means necessary, no questions asked. You do so for two reasons. The first, and most obvious reason, is to protect your friend from harm. The second, less obvious reason, is to protect the attacker from harming another human being, for whatever reason. In this situation, using force to disarm a person is not violence, it is protection! Similarly, in the practice of medicine if the bacteria that manifest in the body to "biodegrade" poisons get out of hand and threaten the life of the patient, I prescribe a course of antibiotics to kill them, no questions asked. This is the protective use of force. I understand that while saving a life, I am also causing harm, although not doing violence. The healing work needs to come later.

The arsenal of orthodox medical therapies is best seen in this light, to be used only for protection—antibiotics when the proliferation of bacteria becomes life-threatening, removal of a gall bladder if a stone is stuck and endangering the life of the patient, removal of a tumor if it is depressing or disrupting some vital function. These are protective measures only; they have nothing to do with healing. Healing must come later, with dietary changes and supportive nontoxic therapies described in this book, but only after the patient is out of danger.

CHOOSING THE RIGHT MEDICINE

Most of us would agree that the best training for children consists in gentle education. When children engage in behavior that is selfish or destructive—as all children do occasionally—our first choice in corrective measures would consist of a calm and rational explanation about why the child's behavior is innappropariate. At the same time, of course, the parents and all who care for the child should set an example of balanced and considerate behavior and create an environment filled with nurture and love.

If the child's actions put him or others in immediate danger—if the child runs into the street, for example—we act quickly and decisively to pull him back. This is not punishment, but the protective use of force.

Let's apply this metaphor to the treatment of an illness such as asthma, which, as we shall see in Chapter 6 of Part II, is fundamentally a disease of adrenal insufficiency. Our first step in the treatment of this disease is to create a picture of health that can serve as a goal, equivalent to explaining appropriate behavior to a child. Various therapies would include carefully chosen food supplements, protomorphogens, herbs, homeopathic remedies, massage and so forth to help fortify and "reeducate" the adrenal glands and put the body more into balance. A nutrient-dense diet, appropriate movement or exercise and a certain discipline applied to one's thinking provide the environment in which such medicines can work, equivalent to good example and a supportive environment that adults should provide.

If the condition does not respond to these measures, then the next step is to begin cortisone therapy—the equivalent of the protective use of force because cortisone therapy, although often helpful in suppressing symptoms, always comes with side effects. A more extreme example would be the removal of an organ that is so diseased it is actually killing the patient.

The problem with modern orthodox medicine is that treatment all too often begins with strong medicine. In many instances orthodox medicines like cortisone are absolutely necessary and lifesaving. The important thing to keep in mind, however, is that drugs like cortisone are not educational in the least; in fact, they *never* lead to healing. They may allow a patient to survive, but they will never help him overcome his asthma. In fact, just the opposite occurs. When the patient tries to reduce or eliminate these types of medicines, he finds that the underlying illness is no better and the affected organ (in this case the adrenal gland) is weaker than when he started the therapy. The side effects for prolonged use of steroid drugs include osteoporosis, cataracts and diabétes, but the worst side effect is the damage done to the body's ability to heal itself.

My main disappointment with conventional medicine is not that we don't have the answers to all of today's illnesses, for this is a daunting task, but that we have stopped looking for solutions that truly heal instead of just managing symptoms, and that we have confounded emergency action with long-term healing. Most physicians still cling to the central tenet of the Nihilistic School of medicine, and do not believe that it is possible to educate the patient in such a way that he can actually overcome his illness. Instead, doctors begin with measures that suppress symptoms and even deny the possibility that patients engage themselves in the process of education and restoration. In medicine today, one never speaks of techniques for improving liver function, or enabling the thyroid gland to regulate its own hormone production. If a patient has gall stones, we remove the gall bladder and tell him that his disease is cured; if he has a tumor in the colon, we remove a portion of the colon and tell him that his cancer is cured. But surgery and other extreme measures are no more a cure than imprisonment is a cure for murderous behavior.

We have lost faith in this amazing organism, the human being, to overcome its own illnesses, and we have forgotten that true healing involves education and change. In the process, the joy has gone out of the practice of medicine, and patients have been relegated to the status of mere victims, rather than pilgrims on the path to health.

SUGGESTED READING

Principles and Practice of Phytotherapy by Kerry Bone and Simon Mills

Non-Violent Communication by Marshall Rosenberg

There is a River by Thomas Sugrue

The Science of Homeopathy by George Vithoulkas

Portraits of Homeopathic Medicines by Catherine Coulter

Fundamentals of Therapy by Rudolf Steiner and Ita Wegman

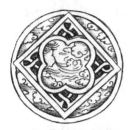

Chapter 3
Movement: Healing the Emotional Body

by Jaimen McMillan

Some of the most popular books available to consumers today deal with the subject of emotions and health. Most present the theories of one or more psychologists and offer a variety of systems for self-analysis and psychotherapy to help us recognize and deal with the emotional scars that cause suffering and disease.

In spite of the materialistic orientation of modern medicine, most people recognize that the immaterial emotions do indeed have an effect on the physical body. One popular book goes so far as to explain specific diseases as the result of specific emotional problems—lung disease is caused by sorrow, for example, while thyroid problems result from misuse of the spoken word. To heal these diseases, the author suggests positive affirmations and new ways of thinking.

While these systems have many good points and have helped many people, Steiner's description of the fourfold human body suggests a different approach to emotional healing. As we have discussed, the Physical Body corresponds to the mineral kingdom; the Life-Force or Etheric Body corresponds to the watery realm of the plant kingdom; the Emotional or Soul Body corresponds to the animal kingdom, which breathes air and moves in space; and the Mental Body, unique to man, is the seat of the spirit. It corresponds to the higher vibration of fire and the electric activity of integrative thinking.

An integrative approach suggests that when we set out to heal our *emotions*, the most appropriate starting point is the realm of *motion*—movement and exercise. This is because the way we move is dictated by how we feel. Our "body language" tells people whether we are happy or depressed, centered or hysterical, constricted or free. If we can alter our body language, if we can consciously change the way we move through space, we can actually change the way we feel, and even the way we think. When people change their relationship to movement, to their bodies and to the surrounding space, this has a surprising influence on their emotional and physical health.

As an example, consider the movements of an autistic child. All autistic children move in the same way, even though they have probably never seen other autistic children. The backwards and forwards motion of the torso and the jerking, uncoordinated movements of the limbs indicate chaos and disruption of both the metabolism and the nervous system. Great progress can be made with autistic children through movement therapy.

Each illness has its own gesture. If we can create new gestures, we can break the vicious cycle of illness and healing can take place.

The Emotional Body actually moves in three interpenetrating spaces: the space within your body, the form of your body-space, and the space, roughly an arm's length around your body. Even the subtlest shift in the relationship of these spaces to each other will elicit a feeling. According to this theory, the shift in these spacial relationships comes first, and the experience of having a feeling follows. It is impossible to have a feeling without first "being moved." It is the movement in the spaces which causes the feeling in the first place. The feeling we experience is indeed then an "emotion," that is "from motion" or "out of motion."

In this chapter, we will study emotions as dynamic movements at the stage just before they become functioning feelings. We will be employing techniques to encourage the interplay of the human being's four bodies. Using the discipline of Spacial Dynamics, we will experience how a new relationship to motion and emotion may create a living continuum between Physical Body, Life-Force Body, Emotional Body, and Mental Body that are sometimes worlds apart.

Spacial Dynamics is the the study and discipline of enhancing the growing human being's relationship to his or her body and surrounding space through appropriate movement and gestures. These spacially oriented movements are used worldwide in therapy, stress management, movement ergonomics, educational and artistic support, world-peace efforts and personal transformation.

The adjective for space has two accepted spellings, "spatial" and "spacial." We use the lesser-known spelling, spacial with a 'c' throughout, to call attention to this new area of research. This unique approach to exercise can help form the Physical Body, re-form the Life-Force Body, transform the Emotional Body and inform the Mental Body.

A DYNAMIC, NOT A STATE

What is health? Health is often called a state of being, implying that is is something static and unchanging. However, health is a process involving balance and change. Health is not a *state* of being, it is a dynamic—you are always on an *interstate*!

Our modern western civilization tends to delude us with the promise of "possessing" perfect health. We therefore often go to great lengths to squelch the first symptoms of any illness. We may go even further by exalting everything youthful and despising all things associated with old age. We view illness as something we fear; aging as something to delay at all costs and death as the ultimate failure. But anyone who promises that you will never get sick, will always stay young or will never die is either lying or trying to cheat you. In every cell and at every moment, life and death processes are active simultaneously. The cycle of life is in constant movement, and the soul rides the tides of life's ebbs and flows. Sickness, gentle aging and death are not only unavoidable, but are real gifts for soul development.

The modern effort to "stay" healthy may not only be impossible, it may even be a stealthy cause of unnecessary infirmity itself. Dynamic change is the pattern of life. Nothing is stationary—everything is in constant flux. Living organisms spring to life, flourish, fall and die—spring, summer, fall and winter. "Stay" too long in a given state and you will no longer be part of the whole. Symptoms will appear in an attempt to draw you back into the rhythm of life. We need to be aware of what various symptoms are telling us and learn to guide these symptoms gently towards balance with adjustments in our diet, our therapies and above all our movements. Rhythmical life is one of the best educators. Without proper training, the forces that create the symptoms do either too little or too much. In both cases, life itself is threatened. If symptoms are repeatedly suppressed and aren't allowed to manifest (for example in fever), the body can later succumb to unwanted cancerous growth. If symptoms get out of control (for example in auto-immune diseases where one's defense system attacks one's own body), cells and organs can become victims of the body's unchecked attempt to achieve wholeness.

The word "health" comes from the word "whole." In this holistic view, we can experience illness as an opportunity to generate spaces for transformation, create supportive rhythms and move towards balance. Symptoms of illness, then, are not enemies but friendly movements that guide us again towards wholeness. Constantly ignoring or, worse, suppressing the symptoms is like being lost and closing your eyes to warning signals and signposts. Creating spaces for "wholing" to take place is an important step in allowing the processes of building up and tearing down to do their work. All these processes are spacial processes that require forms and rhythms for healing to occur. Healing involves re-balancing that which takes place in the spaces between formation and annihilation.

One of the greatest threats to health in our society is the emphasis on self-sufficiency. We are taught that we are strong when we need nothing and no one. But no person is an island. No organism lives in a vacuum. In fact, a healthy organism is one that has a vibrant interaction with its environment. This successful interplay is called synergy; it is no less than the dance of life. The glorification of isolated independence is a major reason for the epidemic of alienation and loneliness that prevails in our society. These soul states are simultaneously expressed in a compartmentalization of the physical body and a lack of connection with others. This sense of lack becomes locked into various body parts and expresses itself through certain gestures, ultimately leading to a sense of separation of the four bodies—Physical, Life-Force, Emotional and Mental.

Opening these dammed-up body parts and organizing the dynamics that weave the areas together brings an immediate sense of release—a feeling akin to "coming home." At the same time, this spacial allocation of different movements for hand, limbs and trunk allows for increased awareness and interest in your surroundings. These gestures allow you to remain an individual, while recognizing healing interdependence in connecting yourself to the world around you.

Our emotional lives can be very puzzling until we learn that the soul is a riddle that has more than one answer. The soul has the ability to have contradictory feelings at the same time. For many people, these contradictory or changing feelings are uncomfortable or confusing. That is because we may unnecessarily hold on to a limited identity or ideal. We can change this vision of ourselves and instead define ourselves as beings in flux, born of opposites, born to move from stage to stage of development. This change involves some risk. It entails letting go of what we know and have. Learning to move on from limiting emotional states helps free the Emotional Body, the spacial envelope of the soul. The poet William Blake expresses this concept beautifully:

> He who binds to himself a joy
> Does the winged life destroy;
> But he who kisses the joy as it flies
> Lives in Eternity's sunrise.

INTEREST

The soul's major movement is interest. "Interest" comes from the Latin *interesse*, "to be in between." The healthy Emotional Body builds a bridge between the inner and the outer world. In healthy interest, you remain neither within your body nor lost in the object of your curiosity. You are spacially—and literally—located in-between. Interest builds this third space, which allows for an objective subjectivity. It also frees the body and bodily functions from the direct influence of the activity. Through the space within which it moves, the Emotional Body needs to give and receive, have its needs addressed and address the needs of others, be recognized, and meet other souls.

Young children today are increasingly showing symptoms of lack of interest, lethargy and paralysis of the will.

"I don't feel like it!"

"That's no fun!"

"I'm bored."

They exhibit an extreme and alarming difficulty in doing anything they don't feel like doing at that very moment. This state begins with lack of interest, slides to boredom, and ends in sluggishness and despair.

A baby is rightfully concerned with its immediate needs. It lives in a sucking space, drawing in the nourishment, warmth and attention it needs to survive. As a child grows, its Emotional Body requires nurture as well, including the nurturing experience of Mother Nature. Her loveliness and consequence are equally good teachers. The soul sustenance that Mother Nature provides gives the child a rosy glow.

There are countless ways to cultivate the growing Emotional Body in children. Singing songs, storytelling, drawing, painting, music, handclapping games, children's eurythmy, dancing and Spacial Dynamics activities are all ways to encourage and enrich the growth of the child's Emotional Body. This expansion of the child's space is a prerequisite for the healthy development of interest, interaction and the ability to initiate and direct its own activities.

The two-dimensional world of TV and computer screens has flattened the feeling world of our youth. The early and excessive exposure to virtual reality does not offer a viable space for social exchange and healthy communication. The Emotional Body has become deflated and distanced, making it difficult for young people to experience the full range of their feelings. Many of "their" feelings have been forced upon them from the outside. Most dangerously, they have acquired the majority of these feelings unconsciously. The ever-present media have programmed them as to what to consider desirable, chic, and "in." The Emotional Body has experienced a fall from grace, leaving it haphazardly hungry, and embarrassingly indiscriminate.

MOVING WITH GRACE

Most of us are constantly mis-using our bodies. If the body space is too constricted and cramped, the result is exhaustion, pain and, ultimately, dis-ease. We feel our own effort and the result is strain. On the other hand, when we learn to move beautifully, the result is strength, and we are rewarded with endurance, effectiveness, and ease.

"Initiating the spacial dynamic" is a term that we will use for the changes in our relationship to space that precede any activity we do. In this chapter we will learn not only to perceive these subtle stirrings in the space around us but also to select and direct the dynamic that we find most appropriate for a given activity. It is possible to become an architect of your own actions, to design the space that you require for any given activity.

Many books on psychology and health urge readers to imagine or visualize the results they desire. The world of imagination and thought are too often relegated to the head, but it is possible to imagine with your heart, your mind and even your limbs. This is an important step in including the whole human being in a given activity. When it comes to changing our movement, then, visualization is not enough. We need to do more than visualize—which concentrates on a picture and relies heavily on the sense of sight. Imagination should employ as many senses as we can muster. True imagination goes beyond the activity of sight, the sense that dominates in the forming of an image. We are most successful when we learn to "imagine" with every sense.

"Being in the zone," "getting into it," and "going with the flow" are phrases that best capture the feelings we have in those moments that defy description, moments when we are truly in "another space." Each moment, each movement, requires a unique dynamic. Learning to initiate the spacial dynamic that best fits a situation allows for a feeling of ease and frees the doer to experience greater range and depth of feeling. We can initiate the movement of our space *before* the physical body moves and prepare the stage for the drama of the coming act.

The practice of directing our actions in this manner will develop a new sense for movement. This new sense will require us to use an integrated set of capacities so that the expression of our imagination, thinking, feeling and willing will become more effective as well as more alive and aesthetic.

A healthy emotional life reflects itself in graceful, easy movement. In fact, the way we move not only reflects the way we feel, it can *determine* the way we feel. Each disease and psychological complaint that afflicts the human body and soul manifests as characteristic movements. Similar ailments have similar movement patterns. When these limiting movement patterns take on a life of their own, the disease becomes locked in and chronic, and the effects of a healthy diet and appropriate therapies will be compromised. Indeed, an illness is chronic when a vicious cycle involving runaway habits define the person. When we learn to wear our bodies and movements with ease and choose our own spacial patterns, we will stop wearing down our bodies and our psyche with unnecessary strain and dis-ease.

In this chapter I will outline a few movement principles that can be applied in any activity. These principles were derived from years of studying anyone doing anything well. Applying the correct dynamic in space lent a mastery to their deeds. For example, the carpenter works with the grain for more effect with less effort; the kayaker uses the currents of a stream to navigate with increased ease. Application of these principles creates energy, fosters interest, eases pain and provides a greater sense of well-being.

The following qualities will be present in any movement that we recognize as masterful:

1. The movements will be economical—they are efficient because there is no superfluous or wasted motion.
2. The movements will be invigorating, giving an increased sense of well-being, both for the mover and the observer.
3. The movements will be beautiful.
4. The movements will create an enhanced state of awareness.
5. The principles once mastered in one activity will then be available for application to any and all activities of life.

GRAVITY, LEVITY AND RHYTHM

The Emotional Body needs to experience both gravity and levity in order to enjoy the full dimension of feelings. Gravity is the recognized point–centered force that exerts a pull towards the middle of the earth. Levity is the lesser known counter-force to gravity. It is gravity "turned inside out." Levity's form is an inverted sphere; its force is the opposite of gravity's insistent tug towards the point. Levity's complementary force, an invitational draw from a surrounding sphere, can be sensed in the rising sap in a sequoia or in the crocuses pushing up from beneath the snow towards the early spring sun.

Gravity is accepted as a force by science because it is a measurable "given." Levity on the other hand is, by nature, infinite and thus cannot be measured by instruments that are limited. Levity is not a "given." It is an invitation. Levity follows certain laws, just as gravity does, but we must approach it differently to study its characteristics. Euclidean geometry operates within the set laws of gravity, measurable according to a point-centered model of the earth. The 200-year-old science of Projective Geometry, developed by the French mathemetician Desargues, is also an exact science which, in addition to the basics of Euclidean geometry, adds infinity as a premise. Projective Geometry explains many phenomena that cannot be explained within the parameters of Euclidean geometry. It allows the student to experience the laws of levity and of infinity through disciplined thinking. Similarly, the artist can have a direct soul experience of the laws of levity when she responds to the beckoning of the endless possibilities that occur in the artistic process.

The discipline of Spacial Dynamics engages the forces of both of gravity and levity as well as a third element, rhythm. Gravity and levity are playmates. The result of their interplay is rhythm. The Emotional Body discovers new dimensions when the Physical Body breaks out of rigid movement patterns and learns new dynamics in the pulsing spaces thus created.

The infinite is the world of never-ending possibilities, the unborn. The finite world is the world that has become; it is already dying. Swinging on the pendulum between gravity and levity, the soul can participate in the processes of dying and living, of departing and being born. This may seem an obvious concept, even child's play—think of young children building a tower of blocks and knocking it down again! For us as adults, it is possible to enter into the world of being a child again, following the invitation to venture out with an open mind into ever-widening spaces.

PRIMARY AND SECONDARY MOVEMENT

Let's begin by recognizing the vital difference between primary and secondary movement, a key concept of Spacial Dynamics. For example, a jet plane flying across the sky can do so only because of the backward thrust of its engines. We will call this causal force, which goes largely unnoticed, the *primary* movement. The *secondary* movement, in this case the jet changing location across the sky, is not the active agent, but the passive side effect of the engine's backward primary movement force. We will call the result of the primary movement the secondary movement. The secondary movement is what we see, but it is actually the by-product of primary movement, the unrecognized impulse behind a given activity.

Those who have a particularly challenging time learning to move, dance or even exercising correctly—tend to be those who concentrate on the secondary movement. They have their eyes fixed on a goal and go directly at it looking for results. These attempts are doomed to failure, however, because they are demanding secondary movements, which are outcomes, and neglecting primary movements. Trying to execute the last steps before the first ones are taken is a sure way to trip up. A movement goal we set our sights on (a secondary movement) can only come about by doing something quite different. Exercise done "head on" and carried out solely for the effects will soon become robotic and monotonous. Such disengaged activity requires more and more drive towards the illusive goal. This misplaced force makes the Emotional Body "clumsy," and can even lead to paralysis of the will when the drive wears out.

The natural athlete and dancer move with supernatural grace, fulfilling the principles of displacement as if by instinct. Movement is what we see, but displacement is the unobserved or invisible activity that creates movement. The activity of displacement works in the opposite direction to movement. Thus, to jump in the air, we must first bend down and then push our feet into the ground. We are actually displacing the earth, and the result is a motion upwards. If we try to jump without initiating this force in the opposite direction, we can actually hurt ourselves. When we lift something, or even when we stand up, we are in effect pushing down. Push-ups are more effective and less tiring if we consider that we are not pushing ourselves up, but pushing into the ground, a movement initiated solely by relaxing the elbows. When we run we actually push down and backwards, as though we were trying to spin the earth like a giant ball beneath us. Good runners look as though they are standing still, with the earth rotating under them in a backwards direction.

The drawback of PE or Physical Education is that it merely teaches us the physical motions of sports or exercise. On the other hand, Movement Education or ME teaches displacement. If we fix our attention on displacement, the resulting movement happens in a natural and graceful way, but if we try to concentrate on the end effect itself, we merely "go through the motions" and the results are awkward and counterproductive.

If we push computer keys with a motion that confines force to the fingers, and from an angle that prevents an efficient countermotion (in this case, keeping the fingers straight and raising them at an angle from the hand) the result is fatigue and carpal tunnel syndrome; whereas if we position ourselves so that the hands can make a gentle curve above the keyboard to allow the fingers to draw up minimally above each key, if we can concentrate on the finger's point of contact on the key, then the keys will go down with greater ease. Even better, if we imagine the spacial dynamic of the keys pulling themselves down away from the fingers, typing is achieved with a joyful sense of ease and freedom.

The story is told of a young man and an old man chopping wood. The young man thinks the work involves a show of muscle power. He sweats and strains and soon sits down exhausted. But the old man continues to chop wood with an effortless rhythm that seems to have a life all its own. "You are working," he says to the lad, "but my axe is doing the work." Similarly, the carpenter who whistles while he labors imagines that the wood pulls the nail in for him; the cook admires the cucumber as it parts into slices at the instruction of her knife point; the violinist allows her friend the bow to glide across the strings as if pulled by an invisible thread.

When properly performed, any activity can be done with greater ease. When someone says, "I hate Activity X," he or she is probably not doing it correctly. When we learn to perform Activity X with the right spacial dynamics, it can become a pleasurable, even a joyful experience.

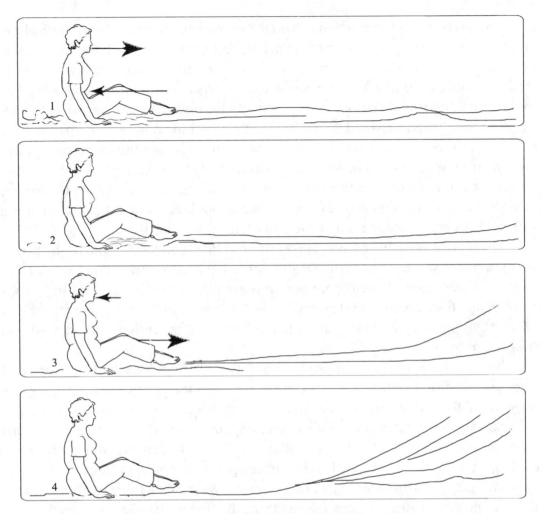

BREATHING EXERCISE

Imagine you are sitting on a beach and an ocean wave breaks and swirls in around you.

1. At this moment, allow the abdomen to draw in as the air exits.
2. As the water comes to a stop and prepares to change direction, gently pause in a moment of stillness and silence.
3. Then as the water moves out to sea and gathers into a new wave, inhale silently, allowing the air to fill the abdomen.
4. As the wave swells and prepares to come towards the shore again, enjoy another moment of stillness and silence.

This exercise has a calming effect on the Emotional Body and establishes a relationship between the inside and outside spaces. This is a fundamental exercise for any condition or disease, as breathing is the basic rhythm of life.

The difference between action that remains imprisoned within the physical body and movement that stretches across space is the difference between strain and strength. This is true of any motion—typing on the computer, drawing a bow across violin strings, cutting a cucumber, hammering nails or felling a tree with an axe. Body-bound effort is torture for the Physical and the Emotional Bodies but strength, born of the rhythm between gravity and levity, begets exhilarating mastery.

BREATHING

Even the smallest of movements creates a countermovement. The process of breathing, for example, will be most natural when the opposite movements are brought into play. Conversely, the more consciousness one brings to one's body in the process of breathing, the less natural and the more cramped it will become.

Imagine you are sitting on the beach at the water's edge, looking out to the sea, with the waves rolling in. Exhale as a wave surrounds your legs and hips with swirling white foam flowing behind you. Pause ever so slightly as the water lingers, before it begins its return journey. Now create the dynamic of the forceful pull of the water back to the sea. Let your abdomen be drawn out with the departing wave, your lungs will fill with air as your belly silently widens with the swelling of the ocean. Pause as the next wave hovers, then exhale like a sigh as the new wave breaks at your feet yet again. You have joined in the cyclic drama of the rhythms of life.

Thus, there are four steps or phases to breathing. There are two still moments, the pauses between inhalation and exhalation, and there are two active moments, the in-breath and the out-breath. As breathing has four stages, so does the wave: the incoming breaking of the wave, the transitional period as the wave dissipates, the drawing back of the wave and the building of the wave again. We often think of a wave as having only two phases, but the in-between spaces in breathing and the ocean waves, although less noticeable, are what provide the rhythm. It is in these transitional, quiet spaces that the Emotional Body is enlivened. A day that has us panting to make it from one moment to the next stifles both the Physical Body and the Emotional Body.

Normally we conceive of the in-breath as being the active component and the exhaling the passive, but in this dynamic, the out-breath is active while the in-breath is the action that follows your relaxation. Your breathing then creates a countermotion to the waves of the sea—when the water goes out you inhale, and when the sea waves come in, you exhale.

Now do the exercise again, paying attention to the motions of your body. Did you feel your chest or shoulders rise up with the in-breath? If the answer is yes, your motions are actually counterproductive to breathing with maximum efficiency and

DOWNRIGHT-UPRIGHT

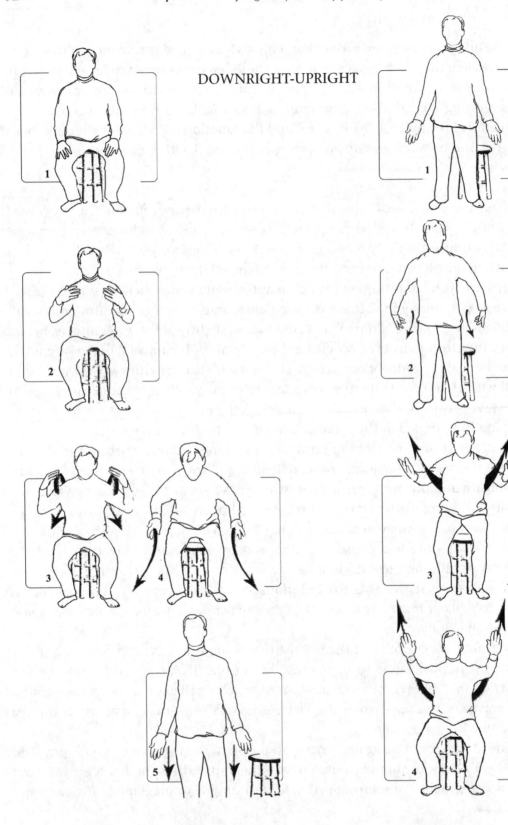

ease. The shoulders and upper chest should remain where they are and the lower ribs, abdomen, and lower back should expand three-dimensionally. As you breathe in, the abdomen should expand because it is creating space for the air—just as the wave expands to become the sea again. Then when you exhale, the abdomen should contract and empty just as the ocean pours its water on the shore. Through this rhythmical breathing we can experience a release of unnecessary tensions and surges of renewed energy.

DOWNRIGHT-UPRIGHT

The simple acts of sitting down and standing up become graceful and serene if we contemplate the opposite action, the displacement. Try balancing the act of sitting with an upward motion of the hands, and the act of standing with downward motion of the hands, an exercise we call Downright-Upright. In sitting, the force of gravity on the lower body is balanced by an expression of levity in the upper body; and in standing the expression of levity in the lower body is balanced by the force of gravity in the upper body. Your "down-right" position can be achieved through an

---

DOWNRIGHT-UPRIGHT

To go from "downright" to "upright":
1. Sit on the front edge of your chair, your feet flat on the floor, shoulder width apart.
2. Bring your hands up to the shoulder area circling slowly behind and around your shoulders into a. . .
3-4. . . . large movement of the hands downward, performed simultaneously with the act of pushing down with the soles of your feet.
5. End with your hands down and your body upright. The body becomes "upright" as a countermotion to "standing down."

To go from "upright" to "downright":
1. Stand comfortably with your hands at your sides.
2. Your hands begin a small gesture behind your body.
3. Then swing your hands and arms forward and up in a large gesture while the hips pull the trunk down.
4. The hands are up—you have glided from the upright position to a sitting position. The upward movement of the hands and arms acts as a countermotion to the torso moving down. Your hands have reached their highest position at the moment that your weight is firmly on the stool.

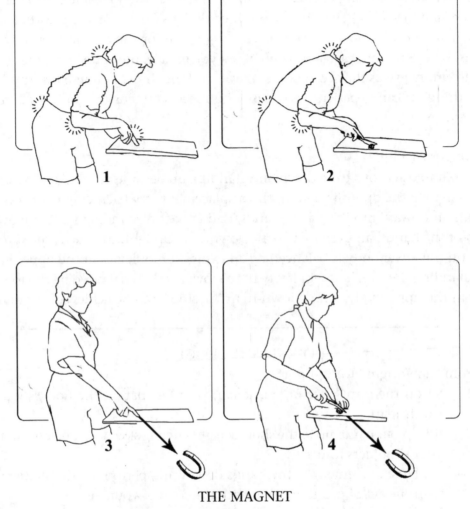

THE MAGNET

In practicing the Magnet, the Emotional Body experiences a response to a peripheral stimulus, independent of one's emotional state. It is particularly beneficial for neurological diseases because the body experiences the origin of a movement not in the nerve but from an outside stimulus. The movement is a release rather than an effort.

1. Press your finger into the board with a constricted, pushing motion.
2. Place vegetables on a board and cut or chop them with a tense, pushing motion.
3. Then, visualize a magnet pulling your finger, noting the relaxation of tension in the shoulders, arms, back and neck.
4. Now, imagine a magnet underneath the board pulling the knife across the space between you and the vegetables, allowing the cutting to proceed with ease.

upward lift and your "up-right" posture can be achieved by the active movement of a downward pull. In sitting, pull from your lower back, your sacrum, and in standing pull from your heels. You can do the essence of this exercise anywhere, many times per day. It helps your Emotional Body experience the feeling of "getting back on your feet again," thus helping counteract feelings of depression.

Now try cutting some vegetables on a board. Notice how tiring this can be if the act of cutting is done as a tense, pushing motion. But when we vizualize a magnet pulling the knife through the vegetables, we accomplish the task with ease.

Consider the Grounding Exercise on page 56 as another example of how primary and secondary movements work. It shows how easy it is to pull someone forward and off-balance if they are busy with the secondary movement, that is staying up, as in Figure 2. Her body space has the dynamic of "straining up." However, it is very difficult to pull her off balance when her body space expresses the gesture of the primary movement, "going down," as in Figures 3 and 4. By redirecting the body space gesture downward into the ground, her body takes on the position of maximum mechanical advantage.

A perfect example of the concept of displacement in the mechanical world is the pulley, which allows us to lift an object in an upward direction with a downward pull on a rope. In the Pulley Exercise, pages 58 and 59, we first allow the head to relax and sink down through the pull of gravity; it is raised again by a downward tug on the spine, just as pulling down on a rope through a pulley lifts an object up.

In the Physical Body, this exercise creates increased blood flow to the head, brain and sinus cavities and stimulates increased fluid in the intervertebral discs. The result is improved flexibility of the spine and an improved blood supply to the entire body. In the Emotional Body, the rounded gesture at the moment of greatest release gives an experience of being protected and safe. The moment of reaching the upright position lets you fully experience the feeling of having your heels on the ground and being ready to face the world.

Proper posture also strikes a balance between gravity and levity. Actually, "posture" is a misleading word because it implies something that is posed or still; "carriage" is a better description because it involves movement and balance—like the elegant horse-drawn carriages of old. There were no straight lines in those carriages—they were made up of beautiful curves which carried them smoothly over uneven roads.

Healthy carriage involves two interweaving gestures, as shown on page 60, one that begins in the front shoulder area, comes up over the shoulders and then down, the Carriage Down motion, which brings the torso into an upright position; and the other that begins from underneath the bottom and comes forward, the Carriage Up

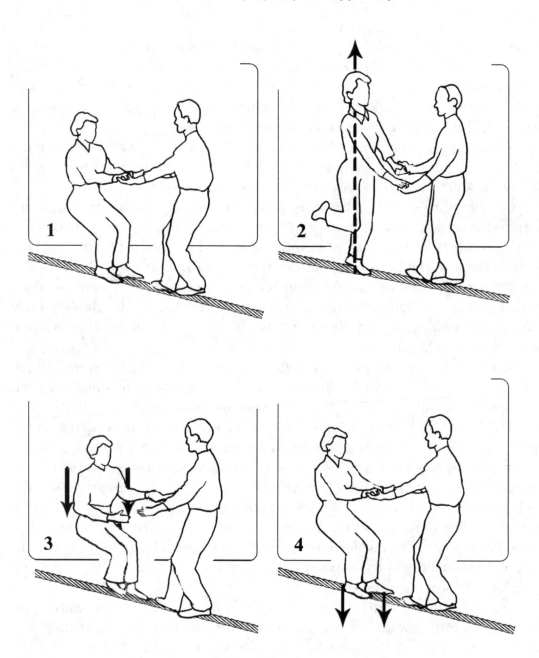

GROUNDING EXERCISE

motion, which brings the lower body into a forward position. Together these two movements create a gesture that allows the individual to face the world with flexibility and confidence.

THE CONCEPT OF SPACE

It may seem a strange concept that we can move gracefully and naturally through the vibrant medium of space by concentrating on the opposite movement, and that this action of countermotion can have a beneficial effect on our emotional life. Actually, people who do things very well can differentiate the spaces in which they live. They recognize—either consciously or unconsciously—that as they live in the space of the human body, they can also be present in other spaces.

Athletes often speak of "the zone," indicating a transcendental time and space in which he or she performs at peak levels. When an athlete is "in the zone," magic seems to happen. In basketball, for example, we speak of Magic Johnson and Air Jordan. These athletes have achieved true mastery through a kind of intense concentration that produces relaxed, flowing movement. Another basketball star, Larry Bird,

---

GROUNDING EXERCISE

The Grounding Exercise provides the Emotional Body with a sense of settling down, adding stability and strength in the growing connection with the earth. It is good for problems of estrogen dominance, hypertension, and cancer, as well as against timidity and losing your temper.

1. Place your feet one behind the other, as on a tight rope, and join hands with a partner. Create the spacial dynamic of mercury rising in a thermometer within your body as your partner and you slowly pull harder and harder.

2. As much as you try to stay on the tightrope, you will find your partner will easily pull you off balance when your mercury is rising. This movement is analogous to "being up-tight," "blowing your top," or "flying off the handle."

3. Then, begin again as in Figure 1. Release one hand and slowly move this hand in a downwards motion to indicate the spacial dynamic of the mercury sinking in the thermometer down through your feet and into the earth.

4. Join hands again. The partner will feel your strength increase as your mercury sinks. You will feel a quiet, "rooted" stability.

This is not "magic." Your body has taken the position of maximum mechanical advantage (best relationship to gravity, best angle of your joints, most advantageous muscle tension, etc.) all by adjusting the downward relationship of your space to gravity.

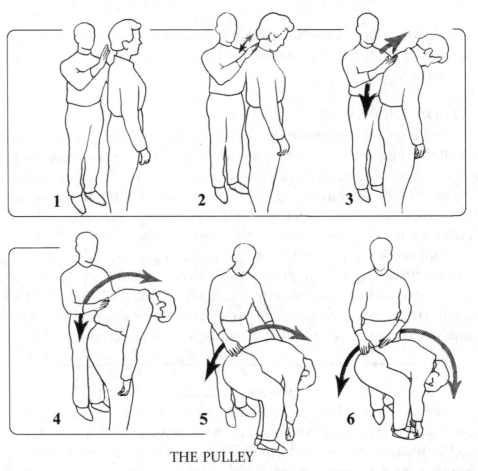

THE PULLEY

The Pulley juxtaposes the two basic building blocks of life, the curve and the straight line, as the body interacts rhythmically with the pull of gravity and the invitation of levity in balanced posture. You can do this exercise on your own, but it can be helpful to have a friend give you assistance in the beginning. The light touch of a friend moving his hand successively down the spine gives orientation from which you can relax as your head goes down. The friend now reverses this process and moves his hand from the sacrum slowly up. This time he pulls down on each successive vertebra like a pulley; and each vertebra comes into the column one by one.

In the Emotional Body, the rounded gesture at the moment of greatest release gives an experience of being protected and safe. In the moment of reaching the upright position you experience the feeling of having your feet on the ground, ready to face the world. In the Physical Body, the Pulley increases circulation to the head, brain and sinus cavities, and stimulates an increase of fluid in the discs between the vertebrae. The result is improved flexibility of the spine and improved blood supply to the entire body. The Pulley can help prevent neurological diseases, and is good for hypertension, adrenal disorders (especially asthma) and chronic fatigue.

1. For Stage I, begin in a standing position.
2. Create space between the first and second vertebrae.
3. Allow the head to become heavy and tilt downwards, much like the initial phase of dozing off during a lecture.

4-6. Repeat the release between the second and third and each following pair of vertebrae all the way down to the sacrum while relaxing the knees. The head changes from its vertical position to a hanging position through relaxing the small muscles between the respective segments of your spine.

7. For Stage II, begin by exerting downward pressure along the sacrum (analogous to tugging on the pulley rope).

8-10. The spine will begin to slowly unfurl, vertebra by vertebra, and approach a balanced upright carriage (8, 9, 10).

11. Keep the head relaxed and heavy until the very end. Resist the temptation to lift your head upwards in the accustomed manner.

12. Let the head slowly take its position as a secondary movement, the result of the downward pulley effect of the shortening of the back muscles.

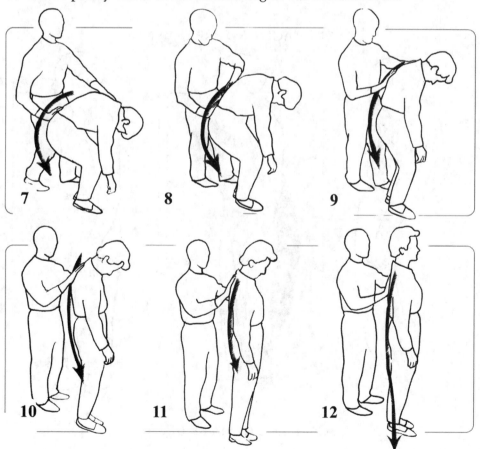

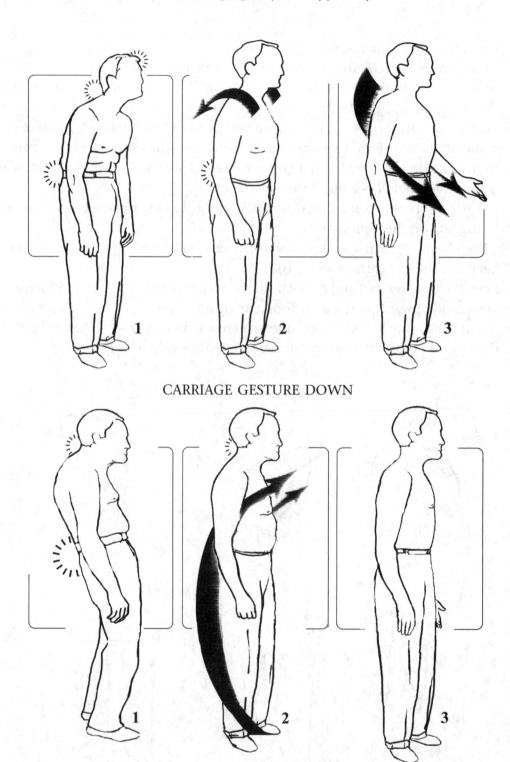

CARRIAGE GESTURE DOWN

CARRIAGE GESTURE UP

was famous for his "look." When he had that look, his opponents knew that he would score at least thirty points in the game. Larry's projection of himself over space was such a reality that it was impossible to stop the ball.

It may be useful to think of this paradox in an allegorical way. America is a nation obsessed with finding personal happiness. But the person who sets out to find happiness rarely succeeds. He or she may achieve occasional and temporary satisfaction through financial success or a busy social life, but rarely true happiness. Happiness comes to those people who concentrate on the opposite—who do things for others, who set out to produce beautiful paintings or delicious meals, or who engage in projects that bring beneficial change to the world. Such people not only contribute to a better world as a result but also achieve unexpected happiness. These are the people who move through life with ease, in spite of obstacles and misfortune.

We are aware of our thoughts and feelings through living in the Physical Body. Most of our destiny dwells on the outside, however. The people we meet, the situations we encounter, the challenges and opportunities that stir us to action—all these are "out there" awaiting our response. We meet our destiny in the outer world. But if we identify solely with the physical body, if we, like the body builders, become "muscle bound," we actually become a captive of our bodies and unable to perceive the destiny that is trying to come toward us.

Likewise, if we view the body as a machine with only a finite amount of energy at its disposal, we may find ourselves paralyzed, unable to respond with the energy that our destiny demands. The law of conservation of energy holds true only on the level of the physical universe. Through the emotions and through creative thinking we constantly create energy, and we can use this limitless energy for the accomplishment of our goals. True movement is akin to swimming—it buoys us up and carries us forward. When we respond to something out there—music for dancing, a task that needs doing, a worthy goal, the creations of our imagination—this response creates movement outside of the body, movement that provides energy rather than movement that saps our strength.

Healthy movement does not originate in the body. The muscles that enliven the face with a smile, or the corrugator muscle that knits the brow into a frown, move in response to stimuli from the outside world. These movements *use* the Physical Body but do not have their origin in the physical. Joyful, graceful, healthy movement follows when we learn to enliven the space around us in such a way that our muscles are invited to follow movements that correspond to smiles rather than frowns. We tend to think of our muscles as organs that initiate movement inside the body when in fact we can develop them to perceive and follow movement outside the body.

People who have a talent for meeting their destiny perceive it coming towards them and react with enthusiasm and energy. They *meet* their destiny with a spacial jump, just as the ball that leaves Larry Bird's hand *meets* the hoop towards which it was aimed. These are the individuals whose lives are studded with fortuitous encounters, "coincidences" and opportunities. This talent can be developed by practicing ME, which has to do with "me," rather than PE, and learning to move in a way that connects us with events in the world around us.

Those who limit themselves by identifying with the body, and with tiring or confining movement, will be blind to their destiny. They may also feel bored, isolated and alienated. They may turn to drugs, sex and life in the fast lane in an attempt to escape the confinement of the Physical Body, but once they get "out there," they cannot perceive the true nature of what is happening around them and their destiny is likely to pass them by.

As mentioned earlier, many books on psychology and health urge readers to visualize the results they desire. This is an important step that includes the whole human being in a given activity. When it comes to changing our movement, however, visualization is not enough. We need to do more than visualize—which is based on the sense of sight and is intellect-centered. We must both visualize and create the space around ourselves that we need in order to accomplish a particular gesture or goal. In a sense, we must create the dynamic of the jump spacially before we do the physical jump that others can see. This is the secret of our finest athletes, as well as of those that regularly accomplish their goals. We say that these people "lead a charmed life." The magic is their own creation, as they use space as the tool to sculpt the gestures that are born in the imagination.

Space is an often overlooked factor in this mysterious relationship between psyche and body, and the balance between illness and health. Both science and psychology typically ignore spacial aspects in their approaches. It is a classic case of not seeing the forest for the trees. The forest is the space that embraces and includes the individual trees. It is the space that weaves the individual trees together. Photographers, poets and those who appreciate a walk in the woods all experience the space within the forest as a source of nourishment.

Human beings can learn to live in different spaces. Most of us live in spaces that we haven't chosen and we have no idea of the shapes, forms and gestalt that we carry about with us. Yet, we can learn to change our space, and by changing our space we can alter the way that we feel, and even how others feel about us.

Introducing the spacial element provides a plausible continuum between what is often perceived as a duality between emotions and body. Space can show you how you affect this body-mind connection and how to slowly shape it into a healthy and mutually supportive system. Adding space to the body-mind equation bridges apparent differences and helps form a living continuum. We can slowly learn to shape space into a healthy support system through imagination and movement. Movement connects human beings with the space around them.

Spacial Dynamics is built upon the following premises:

1. You have a body. This body is a space. You can inhabit this body-space.
2. You have spaces around the body. You can inhabit these spaces.
3. In healthy movement, the body and the surrounding space build a continuum.
4. In order for the body to move, the space around it has to move first. It is possible to learn to move the space around the body and then to follow that space.
5. Each activity requires a unique body/space relationship and movement dynamic between the two.
6. The blockage or neglect of a space results in a corresponding lack of ease.
7. Lack of use, misuse or disuse of any space can negatively affect health and lead to dis-ease.
8. Proper use of the body-space continuum brings wholesome ease.

Every disease or condition contains a spacial component. A myriad of influences can hinder a harmonious relationship between the body spaces and the surrounding spaces. But with regular use of the proper dynamic, ease can become the new pattern. Whenever you feel caught by a particular emotion, don't try to fight it. Feel its gesture. Slowly move this gesture away from your body until you can experience it at arm's length. Then, create a second gesture of your own choice, placing it in the space across from the first gesture to the second. Go back to the first soul gesture, then to the second gesture you created. Move back and forth freely between these two gestures in space. The first emotion will no doubt attempt to pull you back into your body and hold you captive. If you attempt to fight or argue with an emotion that has you in its stranglehold, you will choke. Don't struggle; instead create space. You can't always change an emotion, but you can learn to change gestures, in space, before they enter your body. The new gesture that you create will also elicit an emotion. These two emotions can exist, side by side. In fact, the interaction of these two gestures is a good remedy against mediocrity. Move your attention to your ability to change gestures and you've taken a deep breath of fresh air. Every time you create a space, you have created a world. You no longer have to be bound to one limited gesture, one restricted reality. By generating alternative gestures you are fashioning healing spaces.

For example, when something seriously angers you, the space within the Physical Body gushes upwards and expands. The neck swells, the face reddens. If this movement were to continue upwards into and through your head, the result would be "losing it" or "blowing your top," like a volcano. With some practice however, it is possible to redirect this surge downwards before you experience anger. Begin with an accompanying hand gesture that descends slowly, clearing your head and your surrounding space on the way to your feet. Later you will be able to redirect your spacial dynamic without the use of your hand. Learning to objectively observe such movements and consciously alter them in this way will give you freedom from unwanted gestures that can traumatize and tyrannize your Emotional Body.

We can also create gestures or spaces that counteract the invasion of space that we experience when someone utters a hurtful or insulting remark. The result often creates a real pain in the solar plexus, as if we have been punched in the stomach. Our space has been invaded, even dented like the side of a car is dented in an accident. The antidote is the expansion of this space by imagining a plunger creating a vacuum and pulling it back to normal from the outside, much as one pulls a dent out of a fender. We cannot start from the inside, from the hurt; rather we start on the outside and pull the hurt away.

Any emotion has gone too far when it holds sway over the others for an extended period of time. When you get caught in such a state, feel its gesture. Then create another gesture of your choosing. To the extent that you have previously practiced determining your own space, you will begin to recognize the spacial changes that precede the inappropriate soul experience. You can then designate and create the spacial relationship that you find appropriate. The moment that you begin creating the freer spacial relationship, you will find that the accompanying discomfort, fear or pain begins to decrease. This approach to emotions allows you to *have* the feelings and not *become* them—to change the feelings, not change into them.

Spacial Dynamics refers to five main spaces:

1. Body Space: the space the body lives in.
2. Personal Space: the space the Physical Body and the Emotional Body live in.
3. Interpersonal Space: the shared space of personal interaction.
4. Social Space: the space where shared human activity takes place.
5. Suprapersonal Space: no longer a place but a condition of consciousness where the individual is aware of being present in the Physical Body and in infinite space simultaneously.

THE BODY SPACE

The **Body Space** is the first space that a young child has and learns to live in;

and this is not a given. It has to be learned. Babies learn to control their eyes, their heads, their hands, and slowly work downward towards their feet, gradually filling in their body space.

Many events elicit memories. We say that certain buildings, favorite spots and old haunts are "loaded with memories." We reminisce with songs, poems and people. But some specialists maintain that memory is located in specific parts of the body. Stimulating an area of the brain while performing an operation, for example, may bring forth recollections of long-forgotten events. The discipline of Spacial Dynamics suggests that memories are also imprinted on the space in and around the physical body.

For example, I have had numerous patients who were suffering from the lingering symptoms stemming from concussions. It struck me that the space around their head seemed somewhat "dented" on the side of the head where they received their injury, and it appeared to protrude like a bump on the other side. By imagining that the dented side is being warmed by the sun, the patients were able to draw out the dented space while the bump on the other side simultaneously receded. Their headaches lessened or disappeared entirely as they were able to feel the space around their heads in a three-dimensional balance again. The experience of "being underwater," or "having cotton in front of their eyes" or "feeling clouded" all vanished as they were able to keep a quiet space around their heads, a distance similar to that of a NASA space helmet. Interestingly, in the process of filling out the spaces again, those who had suffered from concussions often briefly relived the trauma associated with the injury.

We can become aware of our Body Space with the Body Space Imagination, shown on page 66, which allows you to completely fill the space of your physical body. You can do this vizualization at any time, in any situation. With some practice, you will be able to re-create these spaces at will, in the midst of your everyday life.

PERSONAL SPACE

Personal Space surrounds the physical body. The proper use of personal space allows individuals to remain separate and yet to venture forth towards a common meeting ground. When we meet people, we greet them at the border of our personal space. We allow those we like and with whom we are intimate to enter into that personal space, but when strangers or antagonists get too close, the central nervous system reacts with nervousness and irritability, even with faltering speech or stuttering. We say that someone "gets under our skin" or is "in your face" when he invades our personal space around the head.

Every part of the world has an unwritten code respecting distance and gesture

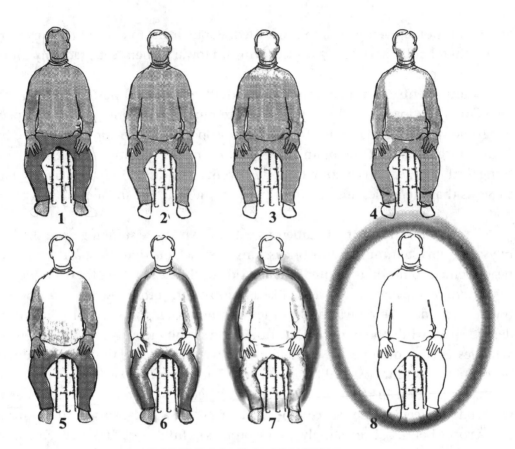

BODY SPACE IMAGINATION

1. Sit in a comfortable position in a location that will give you a minimal number of distractions (phone off, radio off, television off, computer off) and close your eyes.
2. Now begin with the space within your head. Clear it. Experience it as a three-dimensional chamber like a crystal-clear lake within a cave.
3. Flow down the inside of the neck like a tributary undisturbed by any tensions or blockages. This streaming goes right under the collarbone and shoulder blades.
4. Fill the chest cavity with space that allows for rhythmical breathing that laps against the ribs.
5. The lower torso and reproductive organs allow the gentle tidal tugging of the moon downward from the other side of the earth.
6. Create a hollow space in the bones of your arms and legs.
7. Let the space beneath your limbs draw all the tension and knots from your shoulders, upper arms, hands, and fingers.
8. Now live in these different spaces you have created within your body, singly, then one after another; then all at the same time as one vessel. With practice, you will be able to recreate and visit these spaces at will, even in the midst of everyday life.

for greetings. Germans shake hands with a straight arm and at considerable distance. Americans stand closer to each other than Germans when they shake hands, and do so with a curved arm. Americans from California will often place their left hand over the handshake or on the shoulder. Spaniards hug each other when they meet. The French kiss each other on each cheek, but with bodies separated.

Some people experience true fear and anxiety when other individuals approach their personal space too closely. Some terrible occurrence in the past may have brought the Personal Space to a state of constriction and because they have continued to express the gesture of constriction, they continue to experience fear and panic. If they can change their gesture—their gait, their carriage and bearing—they can escape the vicious cycle of fear and panic. A good place to start is the Personal Space Gesture, shown on page 68.

The German word for fear is *Angst*. *Angst* has the same root as *eng* which means "narrow" or "tight." This is an accurate description of the sufferer's personal space at the times when he experiences discomfort, nervousness, trepidation and even panic occurs. We might even say, "There is nothing to fear but 'near' itself."

Fear represents a constriction of your personal space. I have worked with countless patients who have been able to turn the movement of fear around. In the moment they were able to change the direction of their imploding space, fear disappeared. This is not a miracle cure—there is a real tug of war for the direction of this space. The process of *wholing* begins when a patient learns that he can direct what is happening to him. Of course, there are things we cannot change, but don't let what you can't change stop you from changing what you can. Altering even one gesture can transform you from a passive pawn to an active architect of your future.

INTERPERSONAL SPACE

The **Interpersonal Space** connects us to other individuals. We all know the phrase, "It takes one to know one." Gregory Bateson, the eloquent scientist and biological philosopher, one of the early developers of the science of cybernetics, put it differently: "It takes two to know one." This phrase brilliantly illumines the important role of the "other" in the process of self-knowledge—for both parties. Proper use of the Interpersonal Space allows for both individuals to remain separate, exactly where they are, and yet simultaneously to venture forth towards a common meeting ground. Here we have the paradox of both individuals living in their houses, yet going out of their houses and meeting each other, without having ever having left their individual houses. This is the spacial dynamic of human freedom and the spacial paradigm for healthy social interaction.

The Wrestling Stance, pages 70-71, helps us define that personal space neces-

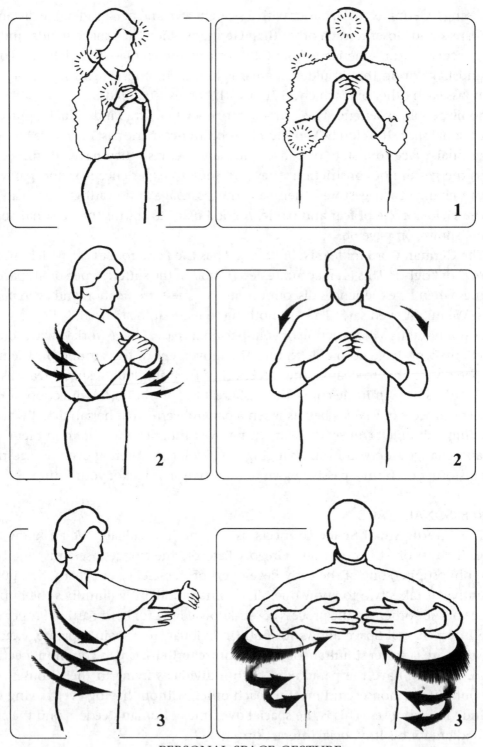

PERSONAL SPACE GESTURE

sary for "two to know one." Two people lock hands and one pushes forward to invade the other's personal space. If the one defending her personal space meets the "invasion" directly, with forward pressure, the "aggressor" easily comes into her personal space. The result is tension and strain. If, instead, she meets the pressure by visualizing her personal space in front of her, she "defends" her personal space and is able to meet the other on equal terms.

An exercise we call Penguin Wrestling, pages 72-73, also helps us honor our own personal space. Two participants face each other and interact by clapping each other's palms. When one participant has a personal space that is constricted, the other "invades" it easily, to the point of creating instability and fright, knocking her backwards like a penguin. However if the participant first defines her space and then deflects the oncoming force by opening her hands in a welcoming gesture, she actually deflects the "invasion" and can meet the other without fear, maintaining her own space with balance and ease.

I had the honor of meeting a wonderful woman in Europe who had served selflessly as a doctor for thirty years. She had recently received a diagnosis of aggressive pancreatic cancer and had requested some help in coming to grips with this merciless illness. I noticed that the space in her upper abdominal area was "caved in," like a time-worn rut. After showing her how to fill out her personal space in this area with the Personal Space Gesture, her posture changed dramatically. She experienced a slight lessening of the pain, her breath was deeper and her color and clarity noticeably improved.

PERSONAL SPACE GESTURE

The Personal Space Gesture is a prerequisite for helping the Emotional Body define and enlarge the area we call our own. This new personal space allows you to meet what is coming to you from the outside world with confidence and grace. It is an excellent exercise for cancer, depression, problems of progesterone dominance, diabetes, weight loss and neurological problems.

1. Start with a tense and constricted gesture, hands to the chest, head tucked down and shoulders tense—the gesture of a fearful person with a very small personal space.
2. Then slowly relax the shoulders, arms and head, bringing the arms and hands down to describe a space swelling beneath them.
3. Use your arms and hands to define a new personal space about two feet in front of you, as though your arms are surrounding a large column. Imagine your ribs expanding to encircle this new space, as shown in Figure 3, a gesture of embracing.

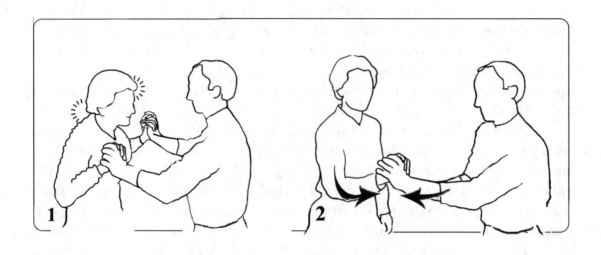

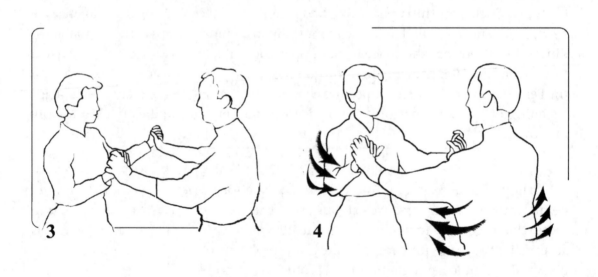

WRESTLING STANCE

WRESTLING STANCE

The Wrestling Stance helps us to define that personal space necessary for "two to know one." It strengthens the Emotional Body by preventing the invasion of the personal space, and helps you to meet what comes to you at the borders of your personal space. It is helpful for cancer (the Life-Force Body is given space to hover, not crowd), diabetes (the balance of the outer and the inner), weight loss (the body image is experienced as including the personal space and the full feeling is no longer dependent on large amounts of food), depression (the world is held at bay and gives you a fighting chance) and heart disease (especially for men as it helps counteract the feeling of "squeezing the heart," or for women of taking everything "to heart").

1. Two people lock hands. Here the man pushes forward to challenge his partner's ability to maintain personal space under pressure. If the one defending her personal space meets the "invasion" directly, with forward pressure, the "aggressor" easily comes into her personal space. The result is tension and strain.
2. Now round your arms to create a ring or circle between you and your partner.
3. Repeat the exercise, this time defining your personal space with your rounded arms.
4. You can now meet the other on equal terms, preventing invasion of your space.

Now repeat the exercise with the partners changing roles.

Then do the exercise again, this time as each partner simultaneously attempts to help the partner learn to maintain the personal space under pressure.

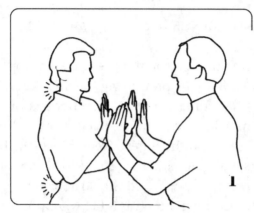

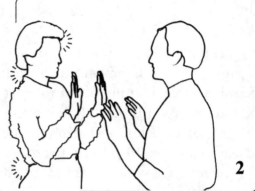

PENGUIN WRESTLING

Penguin Wrestling helps the Emotional Body maintain its space under attack, with balance and ease. It is so named because of the humorous, balance-challenging Penguin-like position of the "wrestlers," feet together at an arm's length from each other. In this exercise one learns to deflect negative gestures, verbal attacks and unfortunate situations, without taking them personally.

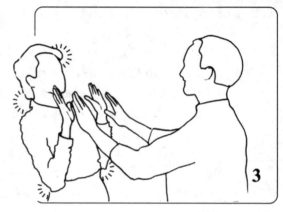

The participant can either clap his partner's hands or remove his own hands quickly at any time. Besides helping those who are withdrawn to stand on their own two feet, it is an effective exercise for taming the "bull in a china shop." It creates the ability to "stand your own ground." Penguin Wrestling is excellent for cancer, heart disease, weight loss, depression and anxiety.

1. In Phase I, the woman demonstrates a practiced contracted personal space.
2. Even the thought of the challenge from the other brings on instability and fright.
3. They interact by clapping each other's palms with moderate force. The woman loses her balance and her "Penguin" feet retreat.
4. The challenge from the partner is experienced as a personal affront.

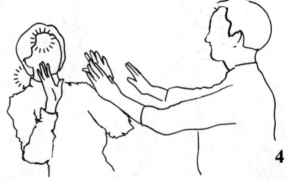

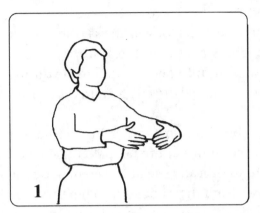

In Phase II, we do the exercise with an expanded personal space.

1. The participant first defines her space.
2. The participants interact again by clapping the palms.
3. This time she deflects the oncoming force like the prow of a ship that parts the water.
4. She no longer feels "invaded" or "injured." She meets the force objectively at the border of her personal space. She realizes that she can determine to what extent she takes things personally.

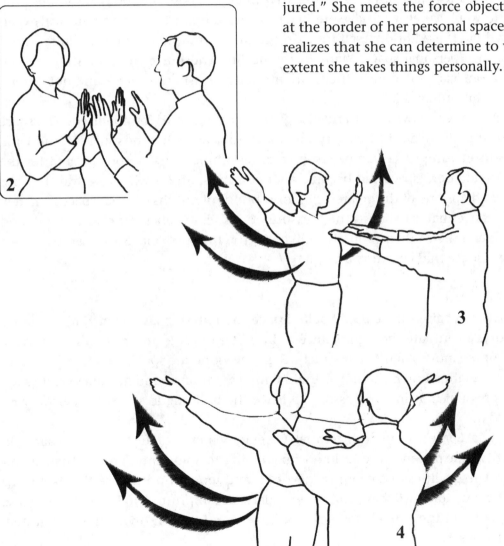

Looking into the distance she remarked that if she ever recovered from this illness she didn't think she could carry on as a doctor any longer. She said she didn't feel that she could continue to take other people's pain and illness from them to herself. I gently pointed out the gesture the well-meaning doctor had made during her proclamation. She was not aware that she had pointed directly toward the cancer-affected area of her abdomen.

A stunned silence fell over the room as the good doctor, her husband and I realized what had been happening. In her total commitment to her patients she had unconsciously taken on their infirmities. More specifically she had been making the spacial gesture of drawing her patients' illnesses from their bodies into her own. We will never know just how the cancer that finally claimed her body began, but her patients would surely also have profited from her loving attention and medical expertise without this additional self-inflicting gesture had she maintained a "buffer zone" of her own personal space. Many in the healing and nurturing professions would profit from learning to meet their patients' illnesses where they are and not unconsciously take them on.

How often do we feel stranded high and dry, our souls immobilized? The space that surrounds us may be that very supportive substance that the soul is yearning for. This surrounding space can be a source of refreshment, even nourishment for the soul. In addition, space can become a vibrant medium on which we travel to our goals. Perhaps one of the greatest misconceptions of our time is that space is merely the distance that separates—the measure of our separateness from the world, and from each other. When properly enlivened, the Interpersonal Space can become a living essence that connects us.

SOCIAL SPACE

Human beings have used **Social Space** to mark the passage of time, enhance memory, accentuate the significance of important events and raise consciousness. Some of the most magnificent structures in the world are spaces dedicated to devotion, meditation and initiation. Certain temples, churches and mosques create such an impression that it is impossible to leave the building as the same person who entered it.

Social Space is infused with ritual. Ceremony increases the possibility that individuals will experience the feeling of belonging to something greater than themselves. The qualities of solemnity, devotion and repetition increase the likelihood that the individual will have this ceremonial space imprinted on his personal space. The quality of the ritual resonates and lingers on in the individual as a cultured, sacred space.

Rituals are spacial habits chosen for the purpose of cultivating the Emotional Body and awakening the Mental Body. In ceremonial rituals, every action, word and thought receives special attention and becomes elevated in beauty, power and clarity.

Customs are social practices that introduce the individual to accepted social graces and spaces. These range from the agreed-to distance between two individuals when they shake hands, to how a person of a certain social standing should relate to others in the public arena. Customs also serve the function of placing a person into an accepted flow of time. They include families gathering together for regular meal-times, marking the changes of seasons and celebrating yearly festivals.

Over the past fifty years, we have broken or abandoned many previously accepted traditions. Young people, in particular, have turned their backs on age-old traditions that they found pointless and even hypocritical. Finding your Social Space involves building a new understanding of the importance of customs, habits, rites of passage and cultural practices. These new rituals can introduce the individual to the feeling and spacial experience of being part of something greater. This can entail creating new practices as well as re-enlivening old ones. These rituals can give form, structure and rhythm to the lives of children and adults alike. Many, many children today have never experienced any vestige of healthy ritual. The epidemic of ADHD (attention deficit hyperactivity disorder) bears testimony to a society without supportive traditions. Children need to enter into social forms which help them learn to focus their attentiveness into spaces where the Emotional Body and Mental Body can experience themselves in the stillness.

Social Spaces can also be personal, healing spaces. We all need to create a quiet space and to go there at least once a day. You may designate an actual place in your home or it might be a location that you visit. (It might not be an actual place at all, but perhaps a route that you take on a daily walk, or even a chosen reflective routine.) A garden that you care for is an ideal space. Your ritual need not be complicated. In fact, there is beauty and strength in simplicity. It is the regularity of your ritual that will enhance your ability to have a positive influence over your time and space.

Modern physiological research studying quiet meditative and sacred spaces indicates that the body reacts positively to ritual. Some of the documented physiological effects of meditative movements include the slowing down of metabolic rates, the stabilization of the breath and a corresponding quieting of the fight-or-flight responses that produce stress hormones like cortisol. As the Physical Body finds such rhythms, it creates an enveloping space that draws the Emotional Body around it. The Emotional Body can then become a dance partner for the Physical Body.

SUPRAPERSONAL SPACE

The **Suprapersonal Space** is the term for the state of being present in the physical body and in the surrounding space simultaneously. It is a feeling of "I am in the body" and "I am one with my surroundings." As an example, imagine the feeling you have when you stand on a hillside on a summer evening with the dome of the heavens overhead—you experience a unity and direct connection with every star.

This is a religious experience in the original sense of the word "religion," namely to *religare* or re-connect the individual with the realm of nature. The Suprapersonal Space transcends the moment and provides experience of timelessness: the past, the present and the future merge into one. These are the moments in which athletes perform at their peak, in which artists receive inspiration, in which pure communication and understanding occur; on the thinking level, these are the moments of breakthrough, of "understanding," in which you are "standing under" everything that you were attempting to grasp.

All of the movement exercises help you to experience Suprapersonal Space, particularly those in which the arms are led peripherally, from the outside. For example, if you see a hawk, you naturally point to the hawk. As the bird dips and soars, your hand will also have to move in order to follow it. You do not initiate this motion from within; instead, your hand follows the motion peripherally. The hawk in the distant sky determines the movement of your hand.

In a larger sense, we experience or recognize our destiny outside of ourselves and then follow it. We cannot push this process; rather, the opportunities present themselves to us for us to follow. When we follow our destiny in this way, rather than forcing it through an effort of will, we are engaging the Suprapersonal Space.

THE THREE PLANES

When we move, we actually sculpt all our bodies. The tool we use is space. The Physical Body is three-dimensional and can be divided by three planes. The plane that divides the body vertically into two symmetrical halves is called the Sagittal or **Symmetry Plane**. This plane gives the basis for concentration, focus and clarity; indeed it could be called the Judgment Plane. Here one weighs both sides of an argument before coming to a middle ground. When a judge signifies her decision with a tap of a hammer, or a king announces his decree with the downward motion of his sword, they are making a gesture that defines the Symmetry or Judgment Plane. When the communication between left and right sides of the body is poor, we can't "keep it together;" we are "beside ourselves."

The vertical plane that runs down the sides of our bodies, dividing the front from the back, is called the **Frontal Plane**. This plane divides the past—what you

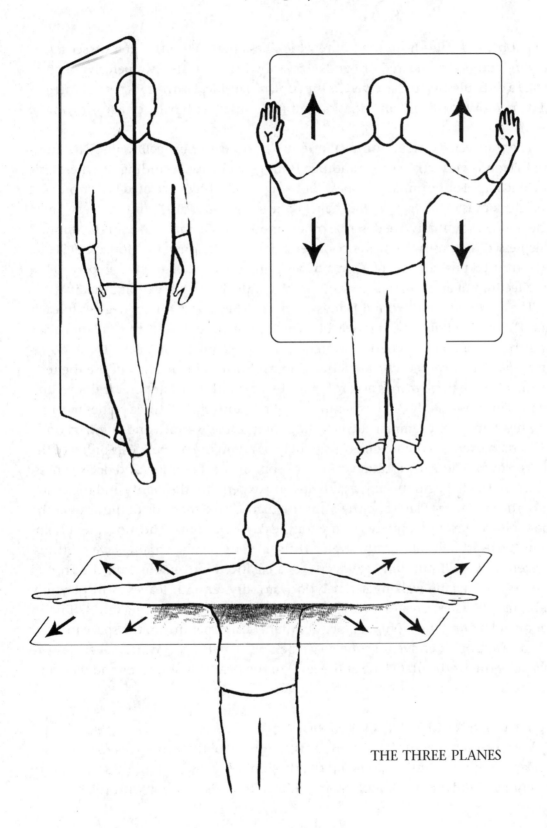

THE THREE PLANES

have put behind you—from the future which lies ahead of you. When we see a person who is stoop-shouldered or bends forward when he walks, we perceive that he has had a difficult life; his past weighs him down. The ideal carriage is perfect integration of memory (past) and anticipation (future), poised with balanced bearing in the present.

The transverse or **Horizontal Plane** has to do with our feeling life. The Horizontal Plane is very changeable and our feelings will vary according to where this plane ends up. For example, we speak of being "up," "high," "elated" or "on cloud nine." Rock musicians "get down," ballet dancers "go on point," and waltzers "meet in the middle." Similarly, we describe other emotions as being "down in the dumps" or "depressed" because we experience our emotions in relation to the Horizontal Plane. The horizontal position, such as swimming, lying on a beach, or even experiencing strong feelings of anger or aggression, can be conducive to a dreamlike quality.

The Symmetry and Frontal Planes are fixed. They are at ninety degrees to each other. The Horizontal Plane is moveable. The intersection of these three planes gives a single point, a focus of energy, awareness and possibility. Each activity we do requires a particular center. With practice you can learn to move and choose the relationship of these three planes according to the demands of what you are doing, and how the Emotional Body can best support that relationship. All three planes meeting in the heart area, for example, elicits feelings of interest, warmth and compassion.

Certain exercises or movements can help us attain the proper positioning of the various planes. The Tides creates gestures of composure, openness and decisiveness. It is a great way to begin the day, as it helps you experience the clarity and the exactness of the Symmetry Plane and the infinite expanse on either side of the arms at the same time—a most appropriate gesture for the daylight hours. The movement helps to slow the heart rate and breath, stretch the spine and regulate brain-wave rhythms. The exercise we call Autumn Leaves creates a balanced movement with the Frontal Plane. As we imagine walking serenely forward, dry autumn leaves swirl playfully behind us. The Crest creates a rhythmical juxtaposition of hovering and falling in front of and behind the Frontal Plane, simultaneously opening up the space in front while awakening or enlivening the space behind. Finally, the Water Level Gesture helps place the Horizontal Plane at the level of the heart. Descriptions and diagrams for these movements are given in Appendix C.

THREE DIFFERENT CENTERS OF THE BODY

We have seen that the Physical Body is composed of three interwoven systems—the head system, the limb system and the rhythmic system. Each of these has a very different spacial dynamic. Rudolf Steiner illustrated this concept with the drawing below, suggesting three "centers."

1. The head, pictured here like a crystal sphere has a resting dynamic. This point-centered form allows for focus, concentration and reflection. The head has a resting dynamic.

2. In direct contrast, the dynamic of the limbs is ever changing and comes about through the activities of the limbs, such as walking, sweeping and working. The opposite form of the point-centered head is an inverted infinite sphere, a point turned inside out. The limbs, then, have a peripheral orientation.

3. Lastly, the torso alternates between the qualities of point-centeredness and orientation on the peripheral. The chest has the dynamic of a moveable center, beating a dynamic rhythm between these two polar gestures.

Maintaining stillness inside the head is particularly difficult in this age of media mania. Advertisements, in particular, designed to titillate and stimulate, pull unwary viewers away from their centers and towards particular products. We are often unaware of the loss of inner quiet in the inside space of the head until we lie down and

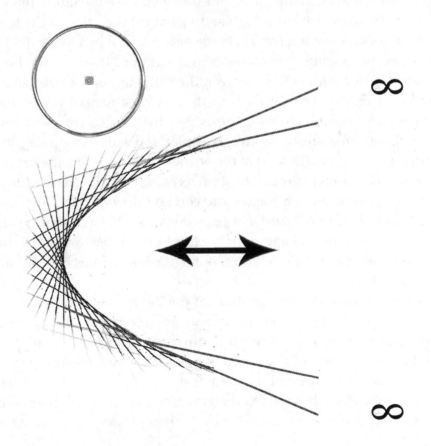

attempt to sleep. Only then do we notice how we are bombarded with unwanted thoughts and feelings. Superfluous feelings are disturbances in the pond of your reflections and if not checked will muddy the spaces you build for yourself.

A head that is not still does not give a basis for a clear connection to the world "out there." In extreme cases of isolation, as in the autistic child, the head will constantly move back and forth, preventing contact and calm reflection. In severe cases of mental illness, the patients will actually bang their heads on hard objects in a pathological attempt to make contact with the outside world.

In contrast to the head, whose space and gesture is a still point within, the limbs are linear and radial in character. The form and function of the limbs are *peripheral* in nature. The dynamics of the limbs are governed by the work or activity that they do. If the work is sewing, the movements will be small and precise. If the work involves putting a basketball through a hoop ten feet up and fifteen yards away, the gesture will be up, out and away, almost as though the ball is guided from the fingertips to the hoop along an invisible path.

Third and finally, the trunk or torso has the quality of a parabola with its center being neither central like the head, nor peripheral like the limbs, but projected forward in space. After years of experimenting with this picture of the trunk, I suggest that the trunk's point is not fixed as in the head, nor is it peripheral like the limbs, but rather an ever-changing telescoping focus determined by the individual's interest.

The trunk or torso swings between the still point of the head and the limitless terrain of the limbs. Like the heartbeat, the torso maintains a steady, gentle rhythm: point-periphery-point-periphery. This is the rhythmical area, home of the beating heart and measured breath: systole, diastole, in-breath, out-breath. Its center is in front of itself, ideally at the level of the heart. Our limbs reflect the nature and type of work we do; our heads maintain the stillness required for concentration and thought. The movements of the torso allow the ebb and flow of human emotions. For example, laughter has an outward motion, while crying has a contracted motion. When the emotions cannot find appropriate expression in the gestures of the torso, they will be reflected pathologically in trembling, jerking or mechanical motions of the head and limbs.

Applying these ideas to the study of the human being in space revolutionized my understanding and approach to movement in relationship to health. Using this model, I began to see that those who were spacially organized with the qualities of these three centers located and functioning as Steiner suggested, exhibited and experienced greater ease. Those who had these centers displaced, or who exhibited inappropriate gestures for those areas, struggled more, experienced more pain and moved with less grace. Continued confusion or disorder of these centers may lead not only to a loss of ease, but to overt dis-ease.

You can learn to design your body and its surrounding space into a living continuum that supports your choices with optimum clarity and strength. It is necessary to study the unique spacial dynamics for each part of the body that allow for optimal functioning. Rudolf Steiner drew a fascinating picture which suggests that the spaces around the upper and lower bodies must be viewed and imbued with totally different dynamics. The suggested dynamic for the space around the head, for example, is from the outside in towards a center, as in Figure 1, the Continuous Lemniscate. Here we are open to sense impressions and we collect information, we "get the point." The head needs adequate space to see clearly and to reflect on the outside world. When the head does not have this buffer zone, we feel threatened.

The spacial dynamic of the activity in the abdominal, metabolic area is the opposite, that is, from the inside outward, toward the periphery. The lower torso is a hearth of heat that radiates potential and transformation. These two gestures are to be balanced by the diaphragm which breathes between the point and the periphery,

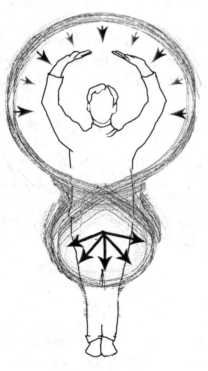

Figure 1
CONTINUOUS LEMNISCATE
Clarity above, power below

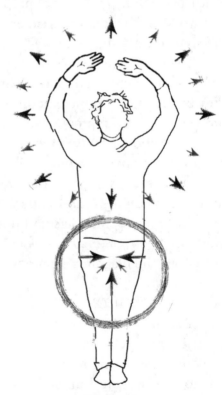

Figure 2
DISCONNECTED LEMNISCATE
"On send" above, constriction below

forming a figure-eight or lemniscate. In Figure 1 the lemniscate's transition is appropriately at the diaphragm.

On the other hand, if the space around the head expands or scatters, we feel confused. We are pushing against the input. If the gestures of an area of the body are directionally inverted or disjointed, as shown in Figure 2, the Disconnected Lemniscate, dis-ease will occur. Through selecting and practicing a more advantageous spacial dynamic, the gestures can be changed and healing can begin.

In a healthy body, governed by healthy emotions, the space around the head is wide and the proper dynamic is one of material coming in, as shown in the Continuous Lemniscate. The arrows coming toward the head represent the "stuff" of the outside world that we perceive calmly and deliberately. At the same time, the proper motion for the abdomen is down and out, with arrows radiating from a central point.

In the unhealthy body, in situations of pathology, the arrows are reversed. The head is not still but chaotic and muddied, so that it sends material out rather than receives what is coming in. This is the situation for the "estrogen dominant" or hysterical personality that cannot properly process and act on information from the outside world. Such individuals experience a chaotic character to their relationships and life-style. We say that they are "always on send."

The proper gesture for the energies of the abdomen is an outward flow, as in elimination, menstruation, birth and orgasm. If these energies are directed inward, they become trapped there, resulting in colitis, constipation, digestive disorders and problems with the reproductive organs.

The Silhouette Visualization, opposite, can help still the head and direct the gesture of the abdomen outward and away.

Other exercises for various areas of the body include the Spinal Stretch for the neck and spine; the Coat Hanger, Lowering the Sail, Shoulder Muscle Mapping and the Cowl for the shoulders and upper torso; the Abdominal Rhythm and Stomach Wave for the lower torso; and Foot Streaming and Knee Mapping for the lower limbs. Directions and diagrams are provided in Appendix C.

MOTION = EMOTION

To summarize, as you move, so will you be moved. Your movement patterns strongly affect your emotional state. Your emotional condition has a direct influence on your physical health. Similar ailments exhibit similar movement patterns that can lead to dis-ease. Long standing movement patterns can become locked in and chronic, weakening the effects of a healthy diet and appropriate therapies. Wear your Physical Body with ease, however, and you will not wear it down. Changing these movement patterns will enliven your Life-Force Body.

THE SILHOUETTE

The Silhouette gives a simultaneous experience of the form of the entire body. Remember, as a child, lying down, waving your arms and legs to make angels in the snow? Lie on the ground on a large piece of white paper and ask someone to trace the outline of your body with a crayon. Now stand up and step back from the outline and see the silhouette. This is a good exercise for people suffering from anorexia and other eating or body image disorders. It shows them the discrepancy between their perception of their Physical Body and objective reality. Alternately, you can create a silhouette made on a white sheet hung on a line with a light projected from behind your standing form. People find this phenomenon fascinating because the individual parts disappear while the entire form, the gestalt, appears as an entity in itself.

After having had visual experiences of your silhouette, ask a friend to stand behind you with both hands resting gently on the center of the top of your head. Then have them slowly "trace" or follow the contours of the body down—neck, shoulders, outside of the arms, hands, insides of hands and arms, rib cage, waist, hips, thighs, knees, calves, ankles and feet. You should have your eyes closed, and the motion should be done in a slow, flowing way so that it is possible to feel enveloped, encased, as a unit.

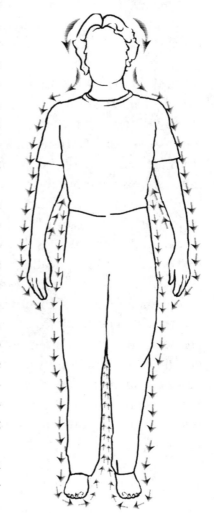

The Silhouette is a spacial dynamic that you can do at any time and in any place. With a bit of practice, it can be an effective aid to filling out and claiming your Body and Personal Spaces. As you imagine the silhouette, you will experience "gaps," one or more places that you skip over, or "holes" where the silhouette has sunken beneath the contours of the body. These are the places where disease is most likely to take hold. As you spacially fill in the silhouette, these "gaps" and "holes" will become "whole." The Silhouette is not only a healing exercise, but also a diagnostic tool that can be used prophylactically to prevent disease from manifesting.

The Silhouette fosters a sense of wholeness in the Emotional Body and is good for any disease condition.

By ennobling your motions, you ennoble your emotions and strengthen your Emotional Body. A healthy Emotional Body enables greater ease of movement, enhanced personal engagement, heightened *inter-esse* for others, and increases social response-ability. Through the process of choosing activity-specific spacial dynamics to re-form your Emotional Body, you have also practiced directing your own self-development. Having learned to differentiate and direct refined movements, you can apply this conscious discernment in all aspects of life. Having learned to free yourself from entrenched movement patterns, you are already on your way to integrating the Emotional Body with the Mental Body.

Six final exercises given in Appendix C—Letting Go, Bestowing, Rice Paper Walk, Victory Stretch, Sundial and Dipole—are designed to integrate the various movements that help us define our personal space, adjust the three planes and create appropriate gestures for the head, torso and limbs. In the chapters on specific disease, we will suggest one or more movements for each disease as a way of providing wholesome exercises and "innercize" for the Emotional Body.

BREAKING THE VICIOUS CIRCLE

Perhaps the movement pattern that best describes the gesture of chronic illness is the vicious circle. Here the Emotional Body is getting the "run around." It isn't going anywhere. Options have disappeared. There seems to be no way out. Addictions are examples of the vicious circle. The addict spins faster and faster but goes nowhere, except more and more out of control. The addict is controlled by the habit. Similarly, in a chronic illness, symptoms have taken on a life of their own, resulting in inappropriate gestures. These movements, if left unchecked, may become life-threatening. The exercises that we have provided can help break these vicious circles and open the door to healing on all levels.

We see that emotional healing does not come about from denying feelings or from trying to control them with a force of will. Emotional healing involves a free acknowledgment and acceptance of both wanted and unwanted feelings. This increases feelings of compassion and acceptance of self and the other. The process of emotional healing begins in the dynamic spaces created when we consciously embrace the interaction of conflicting emotions. Indeed, wholeness results in simultaneously experiencing the full spectrum of motion and emotions. Health is the rhythmical movement that creates balance from the extremes. Moving beautifully is an essential exercise for revitalizing the Emotional Body.

Maintenance Program

The movement exercises described in this chapter and in Appendix C help maintain good emotional and physical health when performed on a daily basis. A suggested maintenance program is as follows:

1. The Breathing Exercise for enhanced vitality and resiliency.

2. The Silhouette for the experience of the body as a whole.

3. The Victory Stretch for increased core stability and balance.

4. The Crest for suppleness of the spine and stimulating circulation in the head.

5. The Abdominal Massage and the Stomach Wave for healthier metabolism, digestion and elimination.

6. The Sundial for increased presence and peripheral awareness.

7. The Tides for the rhythm between concentration and relaxation.

8. The Dipole for integration of the cerebral with the metabolic poles.

9. The Rice Paper Walk for the circulation in the feet and enhanced balance.

10. Bestowing for enhanced calm, tranquility and undisturbed sleep.

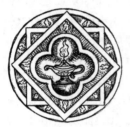

Chapter 4
Meditation: Healing the Mental Body

Any physician who has practiced medicine for many years knows that a patient's attitude plays a large role in determining the outcome of his illness. In fact, the connection between the attitude of a patient—what we might call his thought life—and his state of health has been the subject of much scientific enquiry. Some research indicates that driven, Type A personalities are prone to heart disease, for example, and that people who have difficulty expressing their feelings are more susceptible to cancer.

It is not my intention to debate the validity of these findings, however interesting they may be, but to reframe the question of whether our outlook has anything to do with our health. My experience has convinced me that it does, but not as usually presented in the many self-help books on the market. In spite of the enormous interest in meditation and the mind-body connection, and the hundreds of books that have been written on these subjects, it seems to me that few of us have yet learned to cultivate a healthy attitude or outlook on life; we do not think about our lives and our circumstances correctly, and it is the failure to think correctly that is one of the root causes of the diseases that afflict us today.

Before we go further we need to establish some definitions. The general view of meditation is that it is a state in which we allow the mind to become blank. In meditation we are supposed to assume an attitude of detachment about the world in which we live. The implication is that through meditation we can mitigate stress, forget our problems and remain aloof from the cares of the world. But the root of the word meditation is the Latin *meditatus,* which means "to think, to reflect upon, to revolve in one's mind." True meditation is engagement in focused *thinking,* and the sense of detachment that accompanies meditation should not be an attitude of insouciance but of objectivity.

We also need to establish the difference between thinking and feeling. When we think, our goal is to come to an understanding of what are called universal truths. In the field of mathematics this is relatively easy. We can think about the properties of numbers and come to an understanding that 2 + 2 = 4, or that the sum of the angles of a triangle is 180 degrees.

The truths of mathematics are universal—the same for every person in every culture. They are derived from pure thinking and not colored by opinions or emotions. Regardless of your feelings or your philosophy of life, 2 + 2 still equals 4.

Philosophy, which can be called the science of thinking, concerns itself with discovering universal truths in other areas besides mathematics. In these other areas there is far less agreement about what, if anything, is universal truth. Out of these disagreements arise different philosophical viewpoints about basic questions, such as the existence of God, the purpose of suffering, the nature of evil, the reasons for human existence, the characteristics of the human soul and so forth. The goal of philosophy is to consider these fundamental questions in a manner that is completely objective, untinged by emotion.

In contrast, our feelings are subjective. Our feelings are unique, highly individual reactions to specific persons, events or circumstances. In the realm of feelings we relate the events of the world to ourselves; in the realm of thinking, we relate ourselves to the objective world "out there."

According to Rudolf Steiner, the activity of thinking belongs to the Ego or Mental Body because it is the highest function of the human being. It is a uniquely human task to understand, to search for the truth. Those beings below us in the chain of existence, the animals, live and die and experience emotions like fear and affection, just as we do. They may know things intuitively but they do not think. Beings in higher realms experience knowledge through direct perception. But thinking is the unique faculty of human beings on earth, and it is through thinking that man reclaims the perfect health that is his birthright.

Most readers will be surprised at the notion that thinking defines what it is to be human. Most would say that it is feelings that define the human being and confer his uniqueness. But lacking self-reflection or objective thinking—which is what we mean by meditation—we would not even be aware of our feelings. And if we think properly, in a careful and objective manner, we will develop the kind of outlook that leads to true healing.

An event that occurred several years ago demonstrated to me the importance of objective thinking in the healing process. On the same day, two children were brought by their mothers to my office. Both patients were about two years old and both suffered from fever, stuffy nose and ear infection, both with a red, congested ear drum on the right side. Each child suffered some distress but neither was gravely sick. In both cases I prescribed my usual treatment for *otitis media* which consists of cod liver oil, milk of magnesia to clear the bowels, echinacea and two homeopathic remedies for ear infections, Erysidoron 1 and Levistecum-D3. In addition, I prescribed onion poultices over the ear for pain. In both cases I talked at length with the mothers about my experience and rationale for using this treatment instead of the usual course of antibiotics. As is my habit, I asked both to call me back the next day and to return the child for a checkup one week later.

But one of the mothers called me that evening. She was frantic that something dire would happen to her child if we didn't start antibiotics immediately. The child was no worse than she had been earlier in the day, but the mother had been talking to friends who urged her to give the child orthodox treatment. She was clearly frightened. We talked for a while and she finally agreed—with reluctance—to defer the decision to give antibiotics until the next day.

Both mothers did call me the next day, as instructed. The mother who had called the night before reported "a terrible night," but the other mother said calmly that her child was comfortable and doing well. As far as I could tell, both children were without fever or pain. The nervous mother agreed to wait out the week before trying antibiotics. When the children were brought to my office a week later, I found to my surprise that the child with the calm mother no longer had any sign of ear infection, but the other still had a red, fluid-filled middle ear.

This story is a good illustration of why it is so important for thinking to remain dominant over feelings. Now I'm not suggesting that we shouldn't have feelings or that our feelings shouldn't be powerful, passionate, varied and colorful. I am sure that the mother who remained calm and objective had just as much love and concern for her child as the mother who panicked. Her sense of detachment was not due to the fact that she didn't care, but derived from her ability to think objectively. But the story of the two mothers showed me that an attitude of objectivity is needed for healing to take place.

It is important to have emotions and express them for many reasons, but principally because emotions provide our thinking with powerful, vivid interactions with the world outside ourselves.

We all recognize that excessive fear or worry can have a negative impact on healing. But, paradoxically, I have observed that patients with a casual, jocular or Pollyanna approach to life often have equal difficulties with their health.

Successful healing requires the cultivation of the objective, thinking observer that lives in each one of us. This is what we mean by meditation. Meditation serves to strengthen the inner observer. If we can accept the notion that the purpose of meditation is to help people lead healthier lives, we can see that the founders of the various meditative religions and philosophies have reached the same conclusion, namely, that we do not achieve health through the cultivation of a certain feeling, such as optimism or happiness. Nor do anger, fear or worry cause illness or impede healing more than any other emotion. Rather it is the over-identification with the whole emotional realm—the lack of detachment—that makes us sick.

A patient who indulges in over-identification of the emotional realm will say: "I am depressed" or "I am optimistic." A patient in the habit of thinking objectively will say "I have a feeling of depression," or "I have a feeling of lethargy," or even "I have a feeling of happiness."

Consider how the poet Rumi analyzes his feelings in the following poem:

THE GUEST HOUSE

This being human is a guest house.
Every morning a new arrival.

A joy, a depression, a meanness.
Some momentary awareness comes
As an unexpected visitor.

Welcome and entertain them all!
Even if they're a crowd of sorrows,
Who violently sweep your house
Empty of its furniture,
Still, treat each guest honorably.
He may be clearing you out
For some new delight.

The dark thought, the shame, the malice,
Meet them at the door laughing,
And invite them in.

Be grateful for whoever comes,
Because each has been sent
As a guide from beyond.

All of my feelings tell me—the real me, my core or essential being—about my life. They can teach me what is working for me and what is not. My feelings can guide me toward needed change. If I feel pain or despair over my job, my feelings can lead me to find other work and a new, more fulfilling life. If I feel smothered by my domestic situation, my feelings can lead me to assert my independence or move on to a situation that is less stifling. The road to healing begins with the act of strengthening the observer, the thinking mind, while still remaining open to all the emotions that we can experience during our lifetimes. We need to greet our feelings at the door with delight and analyze them objectively.

The calm mother whose child got well successfully practiced objectivity or detachment. She had a sick child but accepted that sickness as an inevitable part of life. Although deeply concerned, she could still step back and dispassionately assess the child's condition. Along with the therapies that I suggested, she provided a quiet, warm atmosphere in which the child could rest. She lit candles, made tea and sang songs. Of course, she had worries and fears, but they did not prevent her from discussing the child's illness with me in a rational way. And, her objectivity allowed her to make changes in the treatment as needed.

We all have feelings of concern and anxiety when our loved ones get sick or when we get sick ourselves. When we feel this way, we employ our objective self, our Ego, Spirit or Mental Body. Our Mental Body uses objectivity or thinking, just as our Soul uses feelings. It is the Ego that has the clearest perspective on the totality of our life, including our goals, direction and purpose. Most of us neglect this Mental Body; we are not in the habit of clear thinking. We do not look carefully at our circumstances, our emotions, our experiences, we do not "revolve them in our minds" so that we see them from every angle.

When we are sick, the Ego literally cries out for objectivity because illness provokes such strong emotions. It is when we involve the thinking, objective Mental Body in our lives that we can unfurl our sails, so to speak, and move forward over the sea of emotions to achieve our purpose in life. Thus illness can be seen not as a misfortune, but as an opportunity to develop that objectivity we need to reach our goals. When tossed about in rough seas, or even mired in stagnant water, illness can actually be the means of putting wind in our sails and moving us forward.

How can we strengthen our capacity for thinking objectively? How can we experience our emotions without becoming a slave to fears, anxieties, passing feelings and conditioned responses? The technique that I have suggested to patients and have practiced myself for many years is one that Rudolf Steiner suggested as a basic and preliminary step in helping people find and maintain their center. He called it the *Rückschau* Meditation; *Rückschau* means reflection or contemplative review in German.

The meditation is a simple meditative device that takes five to fifteen minutes every evening. Ready yourself by sitting quietly in a chair, in a relaxed, comfortable position. Then carefully review the events of the day, starting with the most recent event and moving backwards to the events of the morning. Try to fashion a clear image of yourself as you worked, played sports, read the newspaper and interacted with your family and friends. Try to conjure in your mind the actual nature of each activity or encounter. At the same time, try to remember how you felt at the various moments that you recall. Resist all impulses to judge yourself, but rather cultivate a state of detached observation. Watch yourself as you live just as you would watch a good friend.

This may seem a simple exercise, but most will find it a challenge to make it all the way back to the morning. Inevitably, things will be left out or forgotten, but as time goes on this objective part of yourself will grow stronger and more confident. With its growing strength the Mental Body will be more available during normal waking moments, and it will provide you with a sure way to deal with both the stormy and becalming moments of life. Soon you will find that many activities which some would classify as drudgery—such as cooking, driving or gardening—are actually opportunities for focused meditation or objective thinking. Gradually this cultivated objectivity will help you understand yourself more thoroughly and deeply than any reliance on the emotions—whether they be the emotions of love or of fear.

Cultivation of the habit of thinking, of inner objectivity, may seem to have little to do with healing, but in fact it is crucial to its attainment. True health, in fact true freedom, is achieved when we can experience the full breadth and depth of the emotional realm while remaining objective about all that happens to us.

SUGGESTED READING
Non-Violent Communication by Marshall Rosenberg

Part 2:
The Art of Medicine

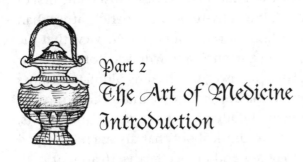

Part 2
The Art of Medicine
Introduction

About twenty years ago, I attended a lecture by a well-known professor of astronomy, Dr. Norman Davidson. Along with his impressive academic credentials, Dr. Davidson was a student of anthroposophy. The subject of his talk was the connection between astronomy and astrology.

He began his lecture by walking in front of the lectern, pointing his finger at the audience and, with a steely look in his eyes, making the following pronouncement: "If you want to have any idea about the connection between astronomy, that is the heavenly bodies themselves, and astrology, that is the influences of these structures on the human being, then you must understand that, in reality, the earth is still and flat, and the sun and the heavens circle around the earth—that is the soul's reality."

Naturally, we were shocked. But he explained further: we experience the heavens in relation to the earth as a moving panoply while we sit on fixed, flat, stable land; turning our gaze heavenwards, we see the sun rise and set; we see the moon wax and wane; we see Venus appear during those magical, romance-filled times of dusk and dawn; we see Mercury flitting across the sky on an erratic, seemingly chaotic course. We look out feeling like a child, in awe of the majesty that circles and moves around us. This is our soul's reality.

The intellectual reality is, of course, much different. Through study and observation, we have learned that we are not only hurtling through space but also spinning like a huge top. Dr. Davidson pointed out that this explanation simply makes no sense to our soul, and very few people can actually fathom the scientific explanation. We can only read about it and look at pictures. Astrology, he explained, is the soul's domain. The soul only experiences the reality that the earth is the center of the universe.

The intellectual mind has discovered that sunlight moving through the air at certain angles produces red and orange colors; and that the moon's light is due to photons bouncing off its surface. But when we experience the beauty of a sunset, or the magic of a moonlit night, we are not thinking of photons or refractive indices. The poetry of nature speaks, first and foremost, to the human soul.

A central thesis of this book is that the explanation of disease must come first of all from the level where the soul is honored. It will therefore be "poetic" rather than "factual." To orthodox medicine, this is tantamount to embracing the view that the earth is flat. But medicine is an art, rather than a science, and while doctors and their patients need to know about anatomy and biochemistry, true healing ultimately comes from a metaphorical, poetic perspective. Just as our emotions and feelings provide the material about which the spirit, the mental body, thinks and makes judgments, so the poetic image of each disease allows us to think about that disease in new and creative ways, ways that in the end lead to better and more effective treatment.

We may find that drugs or vitamins or an operation help us feel better, but these can only be partial cures, and unless our treatments address the soul's needs, the disease will be back next week or five years later.

We will begin each chapter, then, with the timeless, experiential, observable, poetic picture of the disease in an attempt to experience the world of the soul directly. Only then will we turn to our intellectual understanding of the known scientific factors about a particular condition. The goal is a marriage of the soul's emotional world with the analytical, thinking realm of the spirit. If we don't succeed in this marriage, we risk, on the one hand, remaining hopeless, dreaming primitives, out of touch with modern life; and, on the other hand, becoming caged, trapped robots, capable of building a computer or a rocket ship but unable to enjoy the language of the soul. The former leads to inertia and the latter to despair.

Treatment of each disease begins, however, on a very practical level with dietary changes for the physical body. The general principles of nutrition are outlined in Chapter 1 of Part I, but the emphasis will differ according to the condition. For blood sugar problems or weight loss, for example, I emphasize the careful measurement of the carbohydrate intake as crucial to success while for heart disease I stress the inclusion of liberal amounts of good fats. For some conditions the use of particular fats or lacto-fermented foods and beverages will be emphasized. Specific foods—such as butter, carrot juice, beet kvass, flax seed oil or millet—will be suggested as good sources of nutrients for specific problems. Basic recipes are included in Appendix A.

As part of the diet therapy, I encourage my patients to discontinue all nonfood-based supplements and synthetic vitamins. Instead, I suggest concentrated food extracts such as high-vitamin butter oil, cod liver oil, glandular concentrates or the Standard Process supplements developed by Dr. Royal Lee.

When the physical body is supported by a good diet, the medicines we take can help balance and energize the Life-Force Body. Usually the strategy involves identification of the organ or function (such as intestinal function) that needs support. I then give a specific Standard Process protomorphogen to relieve the organ from stress.

At the same time, herbal extracts chosen according to the principles of anthroposophical medicine help nourish the organ or system. Finally, I give homeopathic medicines, especially homeopathic preparations of the appropriate metals, to help readjust the picture or blueprint of the organ to one that is healthy in form and function. For certain conditions, adjunctive therapies such as bee venom therapy, castor oil packs, detoxification and mineral baths are particularly effective. Descriptions of various therapies are given in Appendix B. Sources for herbal and homeopathic medicines, as well as for various superfoods and supplements are given in Appendix D.

The Emotional Body is treated with specific movements for each disease, developed and described by Jaimen McMillan. Diagrams for each exercise are given in Appendix C.

The first three levels of treatment should give you strength and enthusiasm for the fourth category—meditation. The details of this work rest almost exclusively in the hands of the patient. All I can do is paint a picture of the disease for you and point you in a certain direction. It is in your daily meditative exercises that you will learn little by little to be completely objective about your feelings, situation and purpose while, at the same time, receptive to the voice of inspiration and instruction that always speaks to those ready to listen. In effect, your daily meditation teaches you to be the physician, the captain of your ship. When that happens, the family doctor merely plays the role of advisor, leaving you in control of your destiny.

Illness should be viewed not as a curse, but as a challenge to the human spirit, a stepping stone in the process of soul evolution, a crack in the door that, when opened, reveals inspiring vistas of the mysterious workings of the universe. The doctor can give potions and guidance, but each patient must make his or her own pilgrimage.

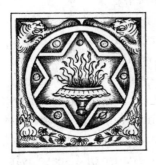

Chapter 1
Infectious Disease

Two things of opposite natures seem to depend
On one another, as a man depends
On a woman, day on night, the imagined

On the real. This is the origin of change.
Winter and spring, cold copulars, embrace
And forth the particulars of rapture come.

Wallace Stevens

The key to understanding the nature of infectious illness involves, paradoxically, an understanding of its counter-image, which is cancer. The poet understands that life emerges from the interplay of opposites. The scientist describes this phenomenon somewhat differently:

Rare events, properly interpreted, have been the source of much progress in science. The spontaneous regression of cancer is a case in point. Before the turn of the century, a few astute physicians observed that shrinkage of malignant tumors in patients sometimes coincided with the development of bacterial infections. They postulated that infectious agents or their products might somehow fight cancer. This notion and the later data that supported it prompted decades of search for a mechanism that could lead from infection to cancer regression. Some evidence suggested that the bacteria did not kill tumors directly but instead strengthened the activity of forces in the body that are capable of restraining cancer. In pursuit of the idea, my colleagues and I at the Memorial Sloan-Kettering Cancer Center some 15 years ago discovered a small polypeptide, or protein, that is produced by the body in the course of bacterial infections and that kills tumors in mice. We and others are now in the early stages of testing the substance, which we named tumor necrosis factor, as an anticancer treatment for human beings.

The scientist in this case is Dr. Lloyd Old, a former director of the Sloan-Kettering Cancer Center, and the phenomenon he describes is critical to the understanding of infectious illness, as well as of cancer. In fact, I have put the chapters on infectious illness and cancer back to back because in them can be found the whole conceptual framework of natural medicine. It is with these two diseases that we begin to understand our modern patterns of illness. In fact, in few other areas of medicine is it so crucial for us to examine the philosophical underpinnings of the cause of disease as it is with infectious or acute illness.

All of the major natural healing systems in the history of humanity have recognized that acute illness is the body's main mechanism for cleansing itself. Furthermore, whenever doctors have ignored this connection and rejected the therapeutic powers of acute illness, the incidence of chronic disease has increased.

Wise physicians have always made use of the "infectious" process. Hippocrates said, "Give me a medicine that will produce fever and I can cure any disease." James Coley, an oncology surgeon in the early part of this century, and to whom Dr. Old's remarks referred, cured many cancer patients by injecting them with attenuated forms of strep or staph organisms. By contrast, I know of a case of virulent cancer in a very young man who, before his diagnosis, had never been sick a day in his life, had never experienced infectious illness like a cold or the flu.

The true nature of acute illness presents a real challenge to orthodox therapies with their fever-reducing medicines, antibiotics and vaccines. Orthodox medicine is built on the notion that these illnesses are caused by various viruses or bacteria that invade our bodies, but this theory tells us only one side of the story. When we say that infection causes fevers, inflammation, colds, flu, earaches, mucus and cough, we are missing the point. Although it is true that microorganisms can infect us and make us ill, they can do so only under certain conditions. If we view the body as a kind of soil—or, as a "terrain"—we can easily grasp that it is in large part our soil or terrain that determines whether or not these infections will grow and flourish.

We all know both sides of this equation. The latest flu may be going around, with "everybody in the office getting sick" except the guy in the center office who never misses a day. Or, 80-year-old Aunt Nora never gets a cold but her grandchildren come down with them all the time. Some children suffer from constant ear infections, while their playmates never get them. Clearly, there are two factors at work here, the "germ" and the "terrain."

In general, conventional medicine has focused most of its attention on the germ, whereas the various systems of natural medicines have focused on the soil or terrain—the resistance. The explanation for each case of acute illness usually lies somewhere between these two paradigms.

Rudolf Steiner's concept of the three poles or systems in the human organism can shed light on the phenomenon of infectious disease. In his model, two opposing forces are held in balance by rhythm. One force is contraction, solidification or mineralization—called "sclerosis" in medical terminology. This force emanates from the nerve-sense or head pole. Opposing these is the force of dissolution, pus production, warmth and inflammation that finds its roots in the metabolic pole. When these two opposing forces are in harmony and balance, rhythm prevails and we are well. When one or the other force predominates, we become ill.

One of the central tenets of anthroposophical medicine and, in fact, of most successful natural healing systems throughout the history of mankind, is the precept that many diseases occur when an individual becomes too hardened or sclerotic too soon. We harden naturally and gradually as we age; the percentage of water in our tissues declines, our tissues become more calcified, our muscles gradually become less elastic. This is a normal and natural part of the life cycle and should not lead to illness, nor be a cause of concern—unless it happens too quickly.

In premature aging, the process of sclerosis accelerates. The causes are varied. Synthetic vitamin D, for example, can accelerate soft-tissue calcification; consumption of processed vegetable oils can lead to hardening of the arteries; and exposure to violence, hatred and cynicism in a child can lead to "hardening of the soul." In a sense, this hardening or sclerosis is the main enemy of a healthy life. On the physical level, hardening of the arteries is the dynamic behind every case of heart disease, calcification of the soft tissues in the joints is the root of every case of arthritis, and the mineralization of the affected organ is one of the dynamics underlying the disease of cancer. On an intellectual level close-mindedness or inflexibility in our thinking can create serious imbalances that eventually manifest in the physical body. On a soul level there is probably no greater illness than that of hard-heartedness or cynicism. Our bodies recognize this hardness on the intellectual and soul levels and respond by altering our physical soil or terrain in an unhealthy way.

On the physical level sclerosis seems to manifest as subtle changes in our body chemistry, leading to microbial growth. For example, the pH of our blood or saliva may subtly shift and we become more acidic. This then provides the environmental conditions for strep to proliferate and replace our usual beneficial mouth flora. Or, our consumption of antimicrobial fatty acids may be too low, leading to a reduction of healthy bacteria in our bowel. Soon after, we find ourselves with symptoms of gastroenteritis or stomach flu because the terrain in our gut lacks protective factors.

Our bodies' therapeutic response to excessive sclerosis is inflammation. Inflammation produces four major effects. The first is heat, bringing general or localized fever. Secondly, redness occurs as blood is brought in to "cleanse" the affected tissue. Then comes swelling as the body brings more lymph and white blood cells to the site of inflammation. Swelling is often accompanied by the production of pus or mucus to remove dead tissue and bacteria from the site. Finally, we experience pain as our consciousness is brought to bear on the phenomena of inflammation. We encounter pain to make us pay attention. As we will discuss in Chapter 12 on depression, pain makes us change our behavior. In the case of infectious illness, inflammation and fever make us take to our beds to rest the body.

Inflammation is the body's cleansing mechanism and the only possible response to sclerosis. Inflammation is the way we bring about balance. Thus, our therapy for inflammation and infectious disease should not suppress these conditions but guide them to their natural conclusion, which is the reestablishment of balance. And if we find ourselves getting sick too often, we should make an effort to avoid or eliminate those factors, whether they be physical, emotional, mental or spiritual, that are making us too hardened, too sclerotic. If we suppress our inflammatory response too vigorously, we actually push our biochemical balance more and more toward the sclerotic pole. That is one reason why, in a culture like our own where suppressive therapies are the main medical model, more and more people have become chronically ill.

As we shall see in the next chapter, the force that scientists such as Dr. Olds have been searching for, the force that is unleashed via acute inflammation like bacterial infections, is a model for cancer therapy. Bacterial infections can cleanse the body of the underlying sclerosis that leads to cancer.

A metaphor that relates to the treatment of acute illnesses and infection is that of the seasons of the year. As the ancient philosophers knew, we can gain an understanding of our inner processes by studying similar processes occurring in the outer world, in nature. In this case we can make a comparison between inflammation and sclerosis and the phenomena of summer and winter. Clearly, in a metaphorical sense, sclerosis can be likened to winter. Both represent the state of coldness, contraction and diminished exuberance. By contrast, summer, like inflammation, represents excessive exuberance, growth, movement of fluids and, above all, heat. We might say that during the summer heat, the earth is the most "inflamed." While summer is a beautiful season, we all would agree that it should not continue indefinitely. Winter must come so that this exuberant outer growth can be recycled back into the earth. Similarly, there is a time for our inflammation to end, for us to be restored to health and balance.

In nature the turning point in this seasonal transition from summer to winter occurs in mid-to-late August in the form of meteor showers. With this introduction of meteoric iron into the earth, the seasons begin to shift. The air changes, the leaves begin to turn, the earth becomes colder, the days get shorter, the light recedes. In myth, this event is depicted as the legend of Archangel Michael who wields his sword of iron to slay the sulfurous dragon that spews forth his flames. The dragon is clearly another symbol or metaphor for excessive heat, inflammation and sulfur of the metabolic pole. This wisdom is reflected in the Christian celebration of Michaelmas, occurring near the end of this transition, on September 29.

The remedy for inflammation is iron, represented by the sword of Michael. That iron is chosen as the "slayer of the dragon" should come as no surprise to those who study physiology or ecology, for iron is nature's detoxifier, the method employed by both nature and the human body to neutralize poisons. For example, if a stream contains life-threatening arsenic, nature binds the arsenic to iron, thereby producing a harmless arsenic salt. Whenever poison threatens, nature renders it harmless by binding it to iron. In our bodies the most toxic substance is free globin, the albuminous or protein part of the hemoglobin molecule that carries the oxygen in our blood. If this globulin is not bound to heme (iron), we develop a fatal disease called porphyria.

In our bodies as in nature, the antidote to inflammation is iron. One of the roles of fever is to act as a catalyst for the release of additional iron into the bloodstream. Thus, in treating inflammation, I often recommend homeopathic quantities of iron.

Next, we turn to one of the mysteries of "infections" that neither conventional nor alternative medicine has explored. One of the major roles of microorganisms in nature is to "biodegrade" and therefore "purify" or maintain ecosystems. For example, if a pond becomes polluted with waste products, eventually algae or other bacteria will emerge to "eat" the waste. This is nature's attempt to heal the pond. No one would suggest killing the algae to restore the pond to health. Similarly, when we become "unbalanced" in the sense of creating too many waste products or when we experience a poisoning from environmental causes such as poor food, chemicals or vaccines, the microorganisms will proliferate in our bodies in order to detoxify us. Infections are nothing more than a purification response, similar to that seen in nature. As in nature, sometimes infections in our bodies actually overwhelm the system. When this happens, the "infection" must be stopped, usually with antibiotics. But this is not healing, it is simply protection. When the protective measures have been accomplished, we face the still urgent need to "cleanse our pond."

Yeasts play a role similar to that of bacteria, which explains why those who live on high-carbohydrate diets, or diabetics with high sugar levels, get yeast infections. The yeast feed on sugars and biodegrade them. The common, so-called alternative strategy of killing the yeast does nothing more than leave the patient overburdened with sugar. Rather, the cause must be addressed and remedied, which in the case of yeast infections involves reducing sugar consumption; for diabetics it involves bringing down the level of sugar in the blood.

I have long suspected that the specific waste that bacteria are designed to clean up is nitrogenous waste, produced by the overconsumption of protein in comparison to fat. Traditional people were very careful not to overeat protein; and they took pains to consume protein foods with the accompanying or added fat. I believe this is a major reason they uniformly experienced resistance to "infectious" disease. The advice to consume lean meat, skinless chicken breasts, egg whites, skim milk and protein powders is very bad advice indeed as it overloads the system with protein that the body cannot absorb. Enter bacteria to clean up the waste.

A story from one of my patients demonstrates some of the underlying dynamics of "infectious" disease. Mr. D.W. was a 42-year-old man who "needed" to get a job to earn some money and went to work as a software engineer for a company in New England. It turns out the factory where he went to work was at the site of an old chemical factory that had been responsible for a number of leukemia deaths. According to management, the site had been "cleaned up." Soon after he began working at the factory he noticed that many of his co-workers were ill with "sinus infections." A few months later he felt ill himself and noticed green mucus coming from his nose. This resolved without treatment and he said to himself, "I need to get out of this place." He didn't listen to this inner voice, however, and kept working at the factory. A few months later the sick feeling and green mucus returned. This time it didn't clear so he went to his family doctor. Two months and three antibiotics later he came to me with a serious cough producing green sputum along with chronic hoarseness.

The diagnosis of "sinus infection" actually obscures the real cause of this man's problems. Upon exposure to noxious chemicals, his liver became burdened with toxins and his body tried to flush them out through his nose. Many traditional systems of medicine have identified a connection between the sinuses and the liver. In this patient, this dynamic played out right before our eyes. Unfortunately, his doctors did not understand this dynamic and tried to thwart this flushing process. After three attempts it "worked," only to leave him with a problem deeper in his body (in his lungs rather than his sinuses) and in a more precarious situation, that of retained chemical poisons that the body could not eliminate.

Two courses of action were necessary for him to resolve his problem. First, he needed to stop working at the factory, which he did. Second, he needed to treat the liver with bitter herbs which, according to traditional medicine, "drain the liver." I interpret this to mean that the bitter herbs help the liver to flush out its poisons. I suggested an herb called andrographis—king of the bitters—which helped him successfully flush out the mucus and restore him to health.

This example demonstrates that thickness and color of the mucus have nothing to do with bacteria or viruses, and everything to do with what is being flushed. If the body is attempting to get rid of nasty chemicals it will produce mucus that is green. If the body is attempting to flush out harmless stuff like dog hair or pollen, the mucus it produces will be clear. We call one condition sinusitis and the other hay fever, but both are actually the by-products of the body's housekeeping efforts, the attempt to get our organism free of unwanted and undigested foreign matter.

By the way, stress probably also played a role in this man's reaction to the toxins in his work environment. He actually had other interests he wished to pursue and working at the factory, only for money, exposed him to conflict and stress that almost surely contributed to his illness. The illness was actually a gift as it forced him to leave and follow his real dreams!

Again, the strategy for the treatment of infectious diseases begins with the recognition that the goal is not to suppress illness but to guide the inflammation to its natural conclusion, which is the restoration of health and balance. Following that, we can turn to simple remedies that gently help this process.

Nutrition

 At the first sign of any acute illness—fever, sore throat, congestion or diarrhea—avoid solid foods, particularly those high in sulfur, such as meat and eggs. (Actually, most people have an aversion to these foods during acute illness—a good example of the body's innate wisdom.) Adults should take only liquids, particularly homemade chicken broth mixed with whole coconut milk. The antimicrobial fats in coconut milk will neutralize pathogenic viruses, and the gelatin and minerals in chicken broth will facilitate healing. Homemade ice cream is a good source of vitamin A and is especially welcome to children with sore throats. Beet kvass, a lacto-fermented beverage made from fresh beets, is a good source of iron and beneficial microorganisms for the intestinal tract.

Once you begin improving, you may add cream of vegetable soup to the diet, along with some cooked vegetables and genuine whole-grain sourdough bread with cultured butter. Properly prepared oatmeal or other whole-grain cereal with plenty of butter and cream is appropriate for the convalescent period. Whole grains supply phosphorus, the light-bearing element.

Continue to consume coconut in the form of whole coconut milk (added to soups or sauces) or coconut oil used in cooking. A good way to ensure adequate intake of anti-microbial fatty acids is to consume 2 tablespoons melted coconut oil mixed with water, twice daily.

As vitamin A stores are depleted during fever, it is important to take cod liver oil. The normal dose of 10,000 IU vitamin A for adults and 5,000 IU for children can be doubled during this period. Finally, natural vitamin C complex from powdered acerola berries or amalaki (a vitamin-C-rich fruit from India) will help strengthen the white blood cells. The recommended dose is 1/4 teaspoon mixed with water, taken twice daily.

These dietary steps, taken during illness and continued after recovery, should help restore the proper acid/alkaline balance to the body. It is easy to test this balance using pH strips to determine the pH of the saliva. The saliva should be slightly alkaline, a condition that is maintained not by consuming lots of vegetables and fruits to the exclusion of animal foods, but by getting adequate minerals (notably calcium, but also phosphorus, magnesium and so forth), protein and fat-soluble vitamins in the diet. If you are subject to frequent bouts of infectious illness, I suggest you test regularly, noting any changes that occur before the flu sets in, and adjusting your diet to achieve the proper alkalinity. (For detailed instructions, see Appendix B.)

Therapeutics

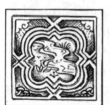 Medicines for acute illness should not suppress fever but bring it down gradually by strengthening the terrain. At the earliest symptom of infection, I recommend an anthroposophical preparation of meteoreisen/phosphor/quartz, produced by Uriel Pharmacy, a company that specializes in anthroposophical medicines. This medicine combines the detoxifying effect of meteoric iron with phosphorus and quartz. Why phosphorus and quartz? Once again, the answers come from nature herself. Phosphorus is the element in nature that bears light. It is used in match heads and light bulbs. The sparkle on ocean waves at night comes from phosphorus-bearing organisms in the water; and the glow of the glow worms comes from tiny bits of phosphorus in their skin. Phosphorus is mineral light or congealed light. When we use phosphorus homeopathically, we carry light into the human being. We all know that pathogenic microorganisms thrive best in darkness and are killed off by direct sunlight.

The quartz component of this medicine aids in the restoration of the nervous system. In nature, quartz represents clarity and precision. As our computers depend on quartz crystals, so quartz helps us think clearly. As a medicine, quartz helps clear the fog and mucus that accompany most colds and flu. This medicine is best given as a subcutaneous injection once per day, or as sublingual pillules 5-10 every two hours, until the illness resolves.

The next medicine given, especially if fever is present, is the anthroposophical preparation called Erysidoron 1, which consists of equal parts homeopathic apis (honeybee) and belladonna. The logic of this choice comes once again from the book of nature. In febrile illnesses, we can say that the patient is searching to regain the proper relationship to warmth. It is one of the many mysteries of bees that the temperature at the core of a beehive remains almost always exactly 98.6° F, the same temperature as the normal human body. Practitioners have used homeopathic apis for almost two hundred years to treat various states of fever. Perhaps the bee hive is showing us the way to achieve a normal temperature. Belladonna, another common homeopathic medicine for fevers, addresses the imbalance between the parasympathetic and sympathetic nervous systems. As such it softens the excessive destruction that can happen with high fevers. Erysidoron 1 is given orally at the dose of 10 drops hourly until the fever subsides.

Another medicine I have found very effective in treating a variety of acute illnesses is Congaplex from Standard Process. One of its main ingredients is thymus protomorphogen extract. In humans it is the thymus gland that produces antibodies. During acute illness, Congaplex may help the body produce the necessary antibodies needed to recover. The other main ingredients of Congaplex are vitamins A and C complex. Vitamin A complex helps fight off viral infections while vitamin C complex supports the leukocytes (white blood cells) in their destruction and elimination of microorganisms. Supplementing with these complexes often encourages the rapid resolution of the acute illness. Please notice that we are specifically referring to the A and C complexes and not their synthetic counterparts (retinal and ascorbic acid). One tablet of Congaplex, taken hourly, is the dose to use in combatting acute illness of any variety.

The above three measures can be used to treat virtually any acute illness. As for more specific acute conditions, such as tonsillitis, ear infections, bronchitis/pneumonia, or urinary tract infections, treatment involves giving the appropriate dose of the correct form of echinacea. Echinacea has been long used by traditional herbalists as the basis of their protocols for acute illness. When given properly it is truly a wonderful medicine for even fairly serious cases.

Scientists have delineated many of echinacea's biochemical and physiologic effects but it is the metaphor of echinacea that guides us to its use. In order to understand the metaphor of echinacea, we turn again to the work of Rudolf Steiner. According to Steiner the plant, like the human being, is a three-fold organism, but it is "upside-down" from the human being. In people, the round, still, clear structure that senses the world is the head. In plants, this activity is performed by the roots. Roots generally grow as a ball or sphere, they sense the nutritional environment of the plant and generally speaking they "should" be colorless. They are the nerve-sense pole of the plant.

In contrast, the flower-fruit realm is where the color, smell, taste and beauty "should" live. This is where reproduction and nourishment generally happen. This is the metabolic or warmth realm of the plant.

Finally, mediating between realms is the balancing or rhythmic aspect of the plant. This is the stem, corresponding to our circulation, and the leaves, which do the breathing for the plant.

Thus, it comes as no surprise that many roots "nourish" the senses (such as carrots for the eyes), leaves provide medicines for heart and lung problems (such as digitalis leaf for the heart) while flower medicines help the metabolic organs (such as chamomile flowers for intestinal cramps). As always, the book of nature provides our only reliable guide towards true healing.

As we have said, the root cause of all acute illnesses is an excessive inflammatory or metabolic process in the affected organ. To counteract this condition we need to bring a little more "hardness" or sclerosis into the metabolism, especially if the inflammation becomes overexuberant. The dominant feature of the echinacea plant is that its metabolic pole, the flower, has a hardened, purple "cone" (hence its common name "purple cone flower"). In short, it is a hard, rootlike flower. It is as though the hardening influences of this plant have escaped from the root into the metabolism or flower realm of the plant. This is exactly what we wish to do during acute illness, which is to temper the metabolic process thereby reducing inflammation.

Echinacea should always be used as an extract, which is the most concentrated form of an herbal medicine. Furthermore, the extract should have a "tongue-numbing" effect indicating the presence of the alkylamides, the active ingredients in the plant. An extract of echinacea that gives no oral sensation is unlikely to have any positive effect.

Finally, echinacea should be given in a relatively large dose, as prescribed by early, traditional herbalists and the Native Americans who pioneered its use. The form I use is Mediherb liquid, 1 teaspoon 4 times per day, until clear improvement occurs. For the patient who finds the extract too unpleasant, use the Mediherb tablets at a dose of 2 tablets 4 times per day until improvement occurs.

For the treatment of specific infections I will simply list the preparations I use most often. These are all concentrated herbal extracts from Mediherb, which in my experience have provided the most consistent results. More information about these treatments can be obtained by contacting Mediherb or Standard Process.

1. Cold/upper respiratory infection - Andrographis complex, which contains echinacea, 1 tablet hourly
2. Tonsillitis - Andrographis complex cold/upper respiratory infection plus gold-enseal, 1 tablet 4 times per day
3. Sinusitis - Echinacea plus euphrasia complex, 1 tablet 4-6 times per day
4. Bronchitis/pneumonia - Echinacea plus Bronchafect, 2 tablets 4 times per day
5. Urinary tract infection - Urico, which contains echinacea, 1 teaspoon 4 times per day plus cranberry complex, 1 tablet 4 times per day

Finally, during infection, we should aid the body in its detoxification process. This can be done by taking an enema, a Dulcolax suppository or milk of magnesia, all of which will clear the bowels and help us detoxify.

For patients with a temperature under 101, I recommend hydrotherapy. First drink two to three cups of tea made from elder or linden flowers. These teas encourage sweating and the elimination of toxins or poisons through the skin. Then take a 20-minute bath in plain hot water, or hot water to which is added 1 cup of Masada Dead Sea salts or 1 cup of Epsom salts. Continue to drink the teas or some beet kvass while in the bath. If you can stand it, take a cool or even cold shower for one minute after your bath. Then immediately wrap up and get into bed with a hot water bottle on your feet. Very shortly you will break into a profuse sweat. Most likely you will sleep well and wake up feeling completely refreshed.

Movement

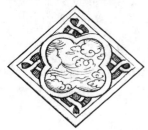

Fever is one of nature's most beautiful movements—it is an expansion of the body's space, a space that has become too cramped. Fever enlarges the body's space so the Life-Force Body can do its work. Children often have out-of-body experiences when they have a fever.

During a fever, enjoy the expansion and let it do its work by staying in bed. Extreme outward movement should be curtailed, while refined and imaginary movement can be enhanced. For the period of convalescence, honor the space of your bed. It is the unique space for giving oneself over to the horizontal plane, the plane of rhythm. We talk about a sea bed, ocean bed or stream bed. In the space of your bed and lying in the horizontal plane, you can strengthen the rhythmical processes of the metabolic pole.

For colds, it is important to activate the feet. Use socks, hot water bottles and foot baths to keep the feet warm. Stimulation of acupressure points in the feet can help create a movement to draw overactive or exaggerated movements down towards the feet so the body may remain in repose. This will allow the head to overcome the infectious process and regain its calm composure.

For infectious illness, the Breathing Exercise can be done sitting up in bed as you imagine waves coming in and out over the end of the bed; and the Silhouette can be done while lying down. Finally, the Tides can be very useful for infectious diseases as it encourages balance and provides alternating gestures of expansion and focus to help bring the expansiveness of inflammation and fever under control. The Rice Paper Walk and Bestowing help foster quiet and calm.

Meditation

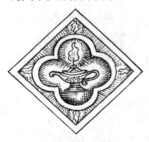

A bout of acute illness should be viewed not as a punishment, but as an exhilarating challenge to our thinking process. The onset of a cold or the flu is actually an opportunity to augment the body's cleansing process, one that we can accept with a genuine appreciation for the mysteries of nature and her infallible techniques for restoring balance to living organisms through the reconciliation of opposites.

As you do the *Rückschau* Meditation, allow the mental body to accept infectious illness for what it is—the body's demand for a chance to rest and detoxify. Infectious disease is actually illness that leads to health. It provides an interlude for contemplation, for reassessment of our life-style and goals and, above all, an opportunity to work in harmony—rather than in opposition—with the marvelous processes that occur within the human body.

RECOMMENDED READING
Principles and Practice of Phytotherapy by Kerry Bone and Simon Mills

Summary

Nutrition

* Avoid   Solid food
                 Foods high in sulfur, such as meat and eggs

* Emphasize   Bone broth or stock with coconut milk
                 Coconut oil, up to 4 tablespoons per day
                 Good quality butter
                 Cream of vegetable soup
                 Homemade ice cream
                 Properly prepared whole grain porridges
                 Beet kvass

* Supplements   Cod liver oil to provide 20,000 IU vitamin A for
                   adults and 10,000 IU for children
                 Acerola or amalaki powder, 1/4 teaspoon
                   2 times per day in water

Therapeutics

* Meteoreisen/phosphor/quartz by Uriel, 1 injection per day or 5-10 pillules under the tongue every 2 hours until better.
* Erysidoron 1 by Weleda, 10 drops orally as long as there is fever.
* Congaplex by Standard Process, 1 tablet hourly.
* Echinacea extract by Mediherb, 1 teaspoon 4 times per day, or 2 tablets 4 times per day.
* Echinacea protocols for specific acute illnesses:
  1. Cold/upper respiratory infection - Andrographis complex, which contains echinacea, 1 tablet hourly.
  2. Tonsillitis - Andrographis complex cold/upper respiratory infection plus goldenseal, 1 tablet 4 times per day.
  3. Sinusitis - Echinacea plus euphrasia complex, 1 tablet 4-6 times per day.
  4. Bronchitis/pneumonia - Echinacea plus Bronchafect, 2 tablets 4 times per day.

    5.   Urinary tract infection - Urico, which contains echinacea, 1 teaspoon 4 times per day plus cranberry complex, 1 tablet 4 times per day.

* Gentle bowel cleansing.
* Hydrotherapy.

Movement

* As much as possible, remain still and horizontal in the space of your bed, thus strengthening the rhythmical nature of the metabolic pole.
* The Breathing Exercise and the Silhouette while in bed.
* The Tides to foster balance and for alternating gestures of expansion and focus.
* The Rice Paper Walk and Bestowing to encourage quiet and calm.

Meditation

* Accept infectious disease as the road to health and an opportunity to restore balance to the body through the reconciliation of opposites.

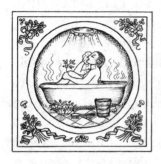

Chapter 2:
Cancer

I want to demonstrate to the world the architecture of a new and beautiful social commonwealth. The secret of my harmony? I alone know it. Each instrument in counterpoint, and as many contra puntal parts as there are instruments. It is the enlightened self-discipline of the various parts, each voluntarily imposing on itself the limits of its individual freedom for the well-being of the community. That is my message. Not the autocracy of a single stubborn melody on the one hand, nor the anarchy of the unchecked noise of the other. No, a delicate balance between the two; an enlightened freedom. The science of my art. The harmony of the stars in the heavens, the yearning for the brotherhood in the heart of man. This is the secret of my music.

Johann Sebastian Bach

. . . the pestilence that walketh in darkness.
Psalm 91:6

ince the events of September 11 in New York City and Washington, DC, the world has taken on a different hue. It is as though we Americans have collectively put on new glasses that allow us, or rather, force us to see the world in a different way.

To help us conceptualize this new threat, we have compared it to cancer, a kind of social cancer. We speak of violence spreading from "over there" and metastasizing to our shores. We speak of "cells" of "terrorists" that have migrated from their country of origin and now are found in virtually every country in the world. In our nation's response to these events, we speak of "surgical strikes" to rid regions of the suspected "terrorists." As America's first war of the 21st century has co-opted the language of this modern disease, we need to take a hard look at the reality behind this imagery in order to avoid a debacle similar the 30-year-plus war on cancer. Indeed, perhaps no other phenomenon is as important to understand as the phenomenon of cancer, unquestionably the dominant illness—and metaphor—of our time.

Like terrorism, cancer is surprisingly difficult to define. One usually thinks of cancer as a tumor (literally: new growth) that can be felt or seen on some sort of imaging device. However, not all cancers form themselves into tumors. Leukemia, for example, is one of several blood cancers where no tumors are formed. Cancer might also be defined as a pattern of accelerated cell growth. But cancers vary widely in their rate of growth. Some are highly aggressive and fast growing, others are more indolent and relatively harmless. Neither of these descriptions captures the essential nature of this illness. After all, harmless tumors, such as cysts and scars, happen all the time. Likewise, the body will often respond to a stimulus by turning on a rapid growth of cells. The replenishment of the blood cells after an episode of bleeding is one common example.

Cancer, while often characterized by tumor formation and cellular proliferation, actually has a different essence altogether. As I see it, cancer is actually a loss on the cellular level of the basic social impulse. Put another way, there is a kind of altruism that runs through the cells of a healthy body—the cells willingly submit themselves to participating in an endeavor larger than their own survival. This altruism is fundamentally a matter of social awareness, communication and the realization that for any cell to survive, all the cells, with their unique functions and attributes, must subjugate their own needs to the health of the whole organism.

In the human body there are billions of cells, each of which is assigned a tissue type and a mandate to participate in the healthy functioning of that tissue. Liver cells communicate and cooperate with other liver cells to do the work of the liver, brain cells form networks in the brain as they carry out the formidable task of doing the brain's work. For most people, this activity goes on for the lifetime of the individual without a hitch. For others, however, one of the cell types at some point goes into active rebellion and "decides" not to respect the form or the function of its tissue of origin. Instead of continuing to work as a liver cell, a cell in the liver reverts to a more primitive cell type and starts to grow on its own. Unless stopped by internal or external forces, this renegade cell will continue to grow until it turns virtually the whole body into its own type, ultimately leading to the death of the individual.

The war on cancer began with great fanfare in the early 1970s, during the Nixon Administration. The goal was to fully finance research into the causes and treatment of cancer in order to eradicate the disease within 10 to 15 years. Thirty years and hundreds of billions of dollars later, the percentage of the population that will get cancer has practically doubled, and for all the major types of cancer, the prognosis for survival has hardly budged. Furthermore, oncologists still have no idea what causes the cell to decide to go its own way. They know about risk factors—which often on further examination turn out not to be risk factors at all—but this is not the same as explaining or understanding how or why these antisocial cellular events occur. At best, current oncology theory only gives information about situations in which these events *may* happen, not *why* they happen.

What is the explanation for this state of affairs? Why, after all these years and all that money spent, can't we answer the simple question of why a cell decides to go its own way and actually kill its host, a host that, in fact, provides the cell with its sustenance?

Oncologists still cannot even explain whether the onset of cancer originates within the cell itself, for example, in an error in the DNA, or whether it is caused by some error in the host. These remain extremely important and practical questions, still begging for answers. We need to answer these questions because the answer determines the course of treatment. If the problem originates in the cell, which then grows into the tumor, then removing the tumor and all its cells should solve the problem. Alas, as all oncologists know and many, many patients have learned, removing all the known cancer cells does not usually solve the problem. We keep trying: we cut the cells out, we burn them with radiation (even though we know that radiation itself causes other cells to become cancerous), and finally we poison the cells with chemotherapy, hoping to kill the cancerous ones before we kill too many healthy cells and cause the death of the patient.

What can we conclude after over 30 years of a strategy that attempts to kill every last cancer cell in the body? In the case of the most common forms of solid tumors (breast, lung, pancreas, colon, prostate, etc.), when the tumor has spread (metastasized), this strategy never works. It never results in the permanent eradication of the cancer and the restoration of health. Never! In cases where the tumor is small and confined to its original site, it can work, and the person can be restored to health, but this occurs far less often than people realize. In fact, with small, confined tumors, it is difficult to determine whether this approach succeeds because of the treatment, or because the original tumor was slow-growing and relatively harmless in the first place.

In the previous chapter, I quoted Dr. Lloyd J. Old who suggested that the origins of cancer lie not within the cell but within the life-forces of its environment. If this is the case, then our full-scale assault on cells and tumors is misguided—even futile and dangerous. It's dangerous because attacking cells and tumors by weakening the organism just leaves the patient more defenseless than before treatment was started, and futile because spending all your energy and resources attacking the symptom of the problem will just leave you frustrated, angry and broke.

A growing movement in medicine attempts to frame cancer in terms of its terrain. However, we have very few words or ideas to characterize this phenomenon of host resistance, and very little understanding of what is it in the healthy human being that keeps the cells integrated into the life of the entire organism and disinclined to break away and assume a life of their own. What we can say is that in this model, it is not primarily the cell that is sick, and it is not the tumor that is the disease. They are simple manifestations of a disorder in the entire organism. To approach this problem more effectively, we must find the words and concepts to characterize the principles of form, order and social consciousness in the organism as a whole. When the principle of form breaks down, the liver cells grow into a form not proper to a healthy liver, or the brain cells grow into a form not proper to a healthy brain. When order dissolves into chaos, the cells begin to march ahead, unaware that they are marching to their own death. When the social consciousness of the organism breaks down, particularly in its communication channels, then a group of cells attempts to co-opt all the nourishment of the body for its own selfish aims. Again, this madness inevitably results in the death of the patient.

The part of the human being that accomplishes these integrating and harmonizing tasks is the Etheric or Life-Force Body. Without a true understanding and science of this body, of this principle of form in the world of nature, we are doomed to a futile and endless war on cancer.

Since September 11th, I have thought long and hard about why our nation found these events so shocking. There are obvious answers, such as the death of loved ones, the potential for it to have been much worse, and the fear that such an event might happen again. For those not personally connected to the tragedies, it is interesting to ponder why this event affected us so much more than, say, the cyanide gas leak in Bhopal, India, which killed at least twice as many people. While there are many possible answers to this question, I would like to suggest that the real horror for those of us not personally involved was that we suddenly were made to realize that the violence, despair and suicidal anger that we had heretofore accepted as being contained like a tumor in another part of the world, had, in fact, metastasized, and spread to our own nation. We are truly dealing with a cancer in our social body, in the body of humanity as a whole, and we all know from our experience of this disease during the past 30 years what it means to be diagnosed with metastasized cancer.

Our national reaction is eerily similar to that of a patient newly diagnosed with this disease. First there is shock and disbelief, as if to say, "This can't be happening to me." Often these emotions are followed by anger and even a sense of resolve "not to let this thing beat me." Next comes a sense akin to bravado as one searches for and decides on options for attacking the invader. Then the treatment starts. As with the war on cancer, our government is taking the approach used by oncologists, which is to define the enemy as cells of "terrorists" whom we must root out using whatever toxic means, and with whatever resources we have. We will use lethal force to kill these terrorists even if the use of this force results in the destruction of some of the good cells—in this case, innocent people—along the way.

Never mind that radiation and chemotherapy can create new and, in many cases, more virulent cancer cells. So, too, our national response to the attacks of September 11 will create only more bitterness, starvation, resentment and, ultimately, more "terrorists." When confronted with this probability, our leaders shrug and say "that's war," and then give some small relief, such as food aid, to the sufferers of our collateral damage, just as oncologists will mitigate the damage caused by their therapies with much-appreciated pain and anti-nausea medicines.

Meanwhile, the search goes on for more and more "terrorists" while we scratch our heads and wonder what the real definition of a terrorist is anyway. Are the members of the IRA terrorists, or are they fighting for national liberation? Is Hamas a terrorist group, or is it fighting to create a homeland for the Palestinian people? Are fundamentalist Christians who oppose our secular government terrorists? Are those who oppose our government's vaccination or nutrition policies terrorists? Can we even draw the line between terrorist and free-thinking citizen? Or, like the struggle against metastasized cancer, will there always be new cells to track down and destroy? Have we come to the age of war that never ends?

In the war on terrorism, as with orthodox cancer treatments, the toll on the host increases as "treatment" progresses. To combat terrorists, we have already passed laws that define any citizen who speaks out against governmental policies as a terrorist and that allow the security establishment unprecedented powers to deal with non-conformists. Ask any oncologist. He knows where this all leads. The patient will soon die, partly from the assault of the "terrorists," but also from the debilitating effects of the therapy.

As with the rise of terrorism, we can point to many reasons for the onslaught of cancer in the 20th century. The three most fundamental causes are bad food, social isolation and, perhaps most important, environmental destruction—the poisoning of every piece of earth, every drop of water and every breath of air with toxic, carcinogenic chemicals. Like hunger, isolation and injustice in human society, these factors lead to the breakdown of communication between our cells and ultimately to the malignancy we call cancer.

In order to solve the dilemma posed by cancer, we must alter our metaphors and transform our thinking. Rather than view cancer as something akin to terrorism, let us consider the idea that from the perspective of the natural world, cancer is a winter experience. It occurs in people with a lifelong history of low body temperature and it is antagonized by the warmth process of fever. As anyone who has ever felt a cancerous tumor knows, no other condition causes the normal soft, flexible tissue of our body to harden and mineralize so thoroughly. In medicine, sclerosis is the mineralizing, contracting, cold experience, likened to the season of winter. It stands in complete contrast to the inflammatory response with its heating, loosening qualities so often associated with summer.

Ancient people understood the characteristics of winter better than we do, living in heated, well lit houses. Winter is a time when the light and the sun recede into the heavens and, for the ancients, a time of starvation if one is not prepared. Cold winter is the time of inwardness and self-reflection, when all of nature seems dead. Think of a scene from the Arctic where it is almost always winter—desolate, lonely, foreboding.

Ancient people thought about winter in this way, but they also perceived another characteristic of the winter season, one that carried hope for a new birth, a fresh beginning. Inwardness is not only a condition of retrenchment, but also has within it the possibility for revelation and transformation. The traditional festivals of many religions have captured the essence of this winter mood. In Judaism, Hannukah is the winter festival, the festival of lights. Hannukah acknowledges the pervasiveness of the darkness at this time of the year, but also celebrates the possibility and the hope for renewal and the eternal nature of the light. One could not imagine celebrating the festival of the lights in the summer; its very essence belongs to the darkness of winter. Similarly, in the Christian tradition, the birth of the Christ child, the hope of mankind, is celebrated in this time of intense darkness. Again, one can hardly imagine celebrating the Christmas story at any other time of the year, with its message of redemption from darkness. In a very real sense Hanukkah and Christmas represent the essence of the winter mood and the possibility of redemption through the light during the darkest of times. These are the myths, found among all peoples, that give us hope that the true Prince of Peace will reign one day on this beleaguered planet.

These stories of Hanukkah, Christmas and other winter tales are no idle stories for religious dreamers. They are actually depictions of the therapy mankind must follow to overcome the twin scourges of terrorism and cancer. Deep contemplation of these myths can help us find a way to overcome the darkness that winter represents; another way makes use of the remarkable plant that provides us with the physical representation of these allegories. The plant is mistletoe. Mistletoe is the winter myth come to life.

Consider the life cycle of mistletoe: it is a semiparasitic plant, which means it can only obtain nourishment from other plants (in this case, trees) rather than from water and soil. Mistletoe grows all year round, liberated from the cycle of the seasons, which is so dominant in the life history of other plants. Mistletoe grows up, down, sideways, in all directions and with very undifferentiated tissues—there is very little distinction between its roots (called haustoria), stems and leaves. Because of this lack of differentiation, scientists describe mistletoe as having cells of a very primitive type. In short, mistletoe gives us a picture of cancer in nature: primitive cell type, undifferentiated, growing in all directions without regard to light, dark, seasons, and all the while obtaining its nourishment from the juices of its host.

But like the winter myths, mistletoe also provides a picture of redemption for, unlike practically any other plant, mistletoe flowers and bears fruit at midwinter, the darkest, coldest time of the year. Mistletoe seems to say, "I am the redeemer of the darkness, the promise that the fruits of the earth will come again. I am the hope for a new day." Mistletoe provides its berries not for simple nourishment; that is too pedestrian a task. Rather, their job is to heal the scourge of cancer, mankind's worst disease.

In many ways the science of mistletoe is even more fascinating than the myth. Given the two models of cancer etiology, two possible approaches to treatment present themselves. The first model considers cancer as a problem of errant cells that form tumors, which then spread to other organs of the body. According to this model, the sensible approach to cancer would be to eliminate these errant cells with as little damage as possible to the surrounding healthy tissue.

The second model considers the terrain or environment in which cancer grows, especially the health of the immune system. We must be careful that our model includes not only the physical cells of the immune system, but also that principle in us that maintains and restores form. This we call the Life-Force or Etheric Body. To treat cancer in this way, we would need a treatment that restores health and balance to our immune cells, increasing their numbers when they are depleted, strengthening their function when they are weak, and improving their ability to recognize and tag invaders. In our terrorism model, this would be akin to restoring the health and respect of the numerous impoverished societies across the world. It does not mean enforcing uniformity, but rather honoring diversity and fostering respect among and for all people. For as with cancer, uniform cells, like uniform cultures, are dangerous; true strength comes from respecting our differences.

Amazingly, while many substances can either kill cells (such as chemotherapy of all sorts), and many substances can alter the immune response (such as interferon), only mistletoe does both. On the one hand, mistletoe extracts selectively kill only cancer cells, leaving no collateral damage. On the other hand, mistletoe normalizes the immune response and helps restore healthy communication between the cells. Evidence for this twofold action has accumulated in more than 70 years of intensive research, which clearly shows that mistletoe extracts work in a more selec-

Suggested Daily Meals for Cancer Patients

BREAKFAST

Pasture-fed eggs and genuine whole grain sourdough bread with coconut butter or cultured butter; with some bacon or sausage made without additives, if available; or soaked and then cooked biodynamic oats with whole-milk yogurt, butter or raw cream, ground flax seeds and chopped "crispy" nuts. Either breakfast should include a lacto-fermented vegetable such as sauerkraut or lacto-fermented beet juice. You may also make a smoothie of raw egg yolks, molasses or honey, fruit and cultured milk (yoghurt, buttermilk or kefir).

SNACK

Homemade cream cheese (called "quark") mixed with 1 tablespoon of expeller-expressed flax seed oil; or a mixture of soaked or sprouted seeds and crispy nuts with raw cheese. Either snack should include a serving of lacto-fermented vegetables.

LUNCH

Homemade vegetable soup made with chicken or beef broth plus a large salad with chunks of pasture-fed meat or poultry; or a sandwich of natural meat and vegetables on genuine wholegrain sourdough or sprouted bread spread with raw or cultured butter. Include lacto-fermented vegetables, either on the sandwich or as a glass of lacto-fermented vegetable juice.

SNACK

Same as above.

DINNER

Include animal foods, properly prepared whole grains and vegetables, both cooked and raw. Vary nightly according to availability and taste. At least once a week, the animal food should be an organ meat, but only from a pasture-fed raised animal. If desired, include a dessert based on fresh seasonal fruit (raw or cooked) with raw cream (if available) a few times each week.

tive way than any other therapy known. Furthermore, misteltoe extract raises body temperature, bringing warmth to a winter condition. It is for these reasons that mistletoe extract is one of the most widely used medicines for cancer in the world today.

Although it is unclear which components of the plant are primarily responsible for the above actions, we are beginning to understand how mistletoe supports immune function. Research indicates that mistletoe affects the interleukin-2 (IL-2) "system." We know that when the IL-2 levels are low, mistletoe therapy will raise them, and when the levels are too high, mistletoe lowers them. We also know that many other natural medicines affect cancer and immunity via IL-2, and that IL-2 itself can be used as a cancer medicine. Mistletoe offers the best of these approaches because it guides the body to establish a new healthy level. It works on the principle of "give a man a fish and he eats for a day; teach him to fish and he will eat the rest of his life." This principle should be our therapeutic mantra: teach the body to restore health whenever possible, rather than just substituting for, or eliminating, what is wrong.

It should be clear that the goal of the cancer therapy, like all the therapies outlined in this book, is to restore harmony and balance in the patient. With cancer, we must provide optimal nutrition, encourage healthy movement and activate a healthy inward perspective through meditation and artistic activities. In addition we must provide specific therapies that accomplish a few goals. First, we must bring more light into the patient. In a sense, we need to use summer as a therapy for this condition of excessive winter. Second, we need to gently target the errant cells, eliminating them in as gentle a way as possible. Third, we need to restore the immune system. Fourth, we need to improve the patient's liver function, since it is the liver that organizes the Etheric body, hence, the form or blueprint of the organism. And finally, we need to bring more integration and communication between the cells, so that they function together as a healthy social organism rather than as an antisocial chaotic gang of cells.

Nutrition

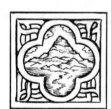

A diagnosis of cancer often accomplishes what good intentions and dozens of new years' resolutions have failed to do: ignite in the patient the will to make improvements in his or her diet. Usually this entails profound changes, a transition from a chaotic diet based on convenience foods or, in some cases, a strict lowfat vegetarian regimen to a healthy, satisfying diet consumed at well-established intervals throughout the day.

In addition to adopting the general dietary principles outlined in Chapter 1 of

Section I, the cancer patient needs to pay strict attention to the details of the diet program, avoiding pesticides by eating only organically or biodynamically grown food whenever possible; avoiding all processed and convenience foods containing sugar, white flour and vegetable oils; eating from the three major food groups (animal foods, whole grains and vegetables) three times each day, and in approximately equal proportions; consuming lacto-fermented foods and beverages every day; and making liberal use of soup broth. I also emphasize a few special foods that have proved their value in cancer treatment over the years. These include flax seeds and flax seed oil; beets, which have liver-strengthening properties, in the form of cooked beets, pickled beets, beet juice (available commercially under the Biotta label) or lacto-fermented beet kvass; whole coconut or coconut oil, with its immune-stimulating properties; and butterfat and the fat of grass-fed beef and lamb, which contain the proven anti-cancer nutrient CLA. Most cancer programs advise avoiding saturated fats in foods like coconut oil, butter and meat, but in fact, saturated fats are an important component of the biochemistry of cell communication, and thus are vital to the successful treatment of cancer.

The diet for cancer patients does not require deprivation. In fact, by using the menu suggestions provided on page 120, and with *Nourishing Traditions* as your guide, you can provide yourself with a variety of delicious meals, always remembering that the joy of eating should provide the foundations of any diet plan. Your diet should reflect balance—neither overindulgence nor deprivation. Above all, eat at regular intervals, never rushing through your meals.

Supplements include cod liver oil to provide at least 20,000 units of vitamin A per day; high-vitamin butter oil, 1/2 teaspoon per day; and Catalyn, the Standard Process multivitamin from whole-food sources, at a dosage of 6 per day.

Therapeutics

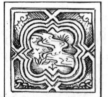
The cancer therapies I use are organized into three phases, depending on the course of the disease. Phase I treatment is given for at least six months, at which time we can usually judge its effectiveness. If the cancer spreads or fails to slow down, I usually proceed to Phase II and then, when necessary, to Phase III. These therapies must be undertaken with the help of a physician well versed in this form of treatment. Such practitioners can be found through the Weleda company, producers of Iscador, the extract of mistletoe.

PHASE I

A. Iscador

Treatment with Iscador, which is the extract of mistletoe, is the foundation of my cancer therapy. During Phase 1, I follow Weleda's recommended guidelines, starting with series 0 of the appropriate preparation and moving up through the series until the injection produces a temperature elevation over 100°F or a redness under the skin of more than 1 to 2 inches in diameter. Once the right dose for the patient is determined, I continue at this level for six months, giving injections three times per week. It is only after six months of treatment that I will change the type of Iscador used or the frequency of the injections.

B. Vitamin D

Over the past 30 years, numerous studies have documented the role natural vitamin D plays in the prevention and treatment of cancer. In fact, there are few types of cancer for which an association with vitamin D deficiency has not been found. This should not surprise anyone who contemplates the metaphor of cancer as winter, or a light-deficiency state. Vitamin D is the actual, physical product of sunlight, transformed in the bodies of all mammals. The chief role of vitamin D is the absorption of calcium and its deposition in the bones—without vitamin D our bones would be soft and weak, a disease we used to call rickets. But vitamin D is involved in many other functions including the development of muscle strength, health of the skin and nervous systems, and in the proper function of the immune system. When vitamin D is deficient, we not only lose our backbone but also our resistance to illness. It is not surprising that one of the illnesses this light-deficiency state provokes is cancer, the quintessential illness associated with lack of light.

Vitamin D therapy, like many other natural cancer therapies, has multiple benefits, affecting such processes as cell division, apoptosis (the regulation of cell death) and the immune system. Many authors, starting with Dr. Price, have made the case that vitamin D is in short supply in the typical American diet because vitamin D is a fat-soluble vitamin found only in certain animal fats that we now avoid. (We also obtain vitamin D by the action of sunlight on the skin but this happens only when UV-B light is present during the summer months.) Dr. Reinhold Veith has presented convincing evidence that the optimal range of vitamin D in the blood is between 60-80, as measured by the 25(OH)D test. For my cancer patients, I test this level at three-month intervals, and use Carlson's vitamin D capsules derived from cod liver oil, 1000 IU each, to maintain the level between 40-60. Usually I give 2 capsules per day, varying the dose depending on the outcome of the blood tests. (For detailed instructions, see Appendix B.) Whenever one uses vitamin D, extra calcium is required. In this case I prescribe calcium lactate from Standard Process, 6 tablets per day.

A word of caution: synthetic vitamin D in the form of D_2 has the opposite effect of natural vitamin D, composed mainly of D_3 isomers. Be sure to avoid all foods that have vitamin D_2 added, as well as supplements containing synthetic vitamin D.

C. Mushroom extracts

As with vitamin D, numerous references in the scientific literature reveal the effectiveness of medicinal mushrooms in the treatment of cancer. Mushrooms have been found to have mild cytotoxic effects, immune-strengthening properties and pronounced hepato (liver)-protective effects, all similar to the benefits of mistletoe.

Mushrooms are particularly relevant in connection to the theme of cancer as a light-deficiency illness. As all the great painters knew, one cannot really speak about light without a thorough understanding of its counterpart, darkness. Rembrandt was a master of the light, not because he painted light-filled pictures, but because he transformed the darkness, bringing light out of shadows. This is what the lowly mushroom does as well. Unlike most plants, mushrooms totally shun the light—some are even poisoned by exposure to light. They work their magic on shady forest floors where they "digest" dead matter so that it can be recycled back into the flow of nature. With their powerful enzymes they digest rotting wood and turn it into useful humus that serves as food for light-seeking plants. This is what needs to happen with our internal tumors. They need to be digested and brought back into the healthy cycle of life. There is nothing on earth better equipped to provide this transformation than the lowly and humble mushroom. I use the Mediherb preparation ganoderma/shiitake, 1 tablet 2-3 times per day, as part of my Phase I cancer treatment. This medicine also helps improve liver function, which must be an integral part of any cancer treatment.

D. Immune Support

In his early writings Dr. Royal Lee suggested that instead of *having* an immune system, we *are* an immune system. As such, there is no special organ or system that *is* the immune system and that requires specific support in cancer treatment; rather, the whole organism needs support. Traditional oncologists focus a lot of attention on the white blood cells and on liver function, but we are learning that many other biochemical systems are involved, including the endocrine system and the gastro-intestinal system with its crucial excretory function. Dr. Lee formulated an immune-support medicine called Immuplex, which has wide-ranging immune supportive effects. Immuplex is a mixture of protomorphogens (DNA extracts from homologous cell types) of all the systems that make up our immune system. In addition, Dr. Lee added specific nutrients, such as selenium, that in his time were not known to have any bearing on cancer, but whose relationship became clear in later years.

I use Immuplex at the dose of 1 capsule 3 times per day. In addition I add the specific protomorphogen of the tissue type from which the cancer originated. For example, with cancer originating from the breast, I use mammary PMG, 1 tablet 3 times per day. The specific protomorphogen helps restore the disturbed tissue to its proper form.

E. Individual Herbal Medicines

While focussing on the generalized process of cancer, we should not forget that each person with cancer is an individual, with an individual biography and needs. One patient may have a long history of insomnia, another of digestive or gall bladder complaints. These complaints should be addressed with a specific herbal mixture tailored to the patient's needs. Common themes emerge with many cancer patients, and often these can be treated with herbs that also have a known positive effect on cancer. For example, many cancer patients have digestive complaints and benefit from turmeric extract, burdock root and perhaps milk thistle, all herbs that benefit the liver-gall bladder system and that have a tradition of benefit in cancer. For cancers with hormonal implications, such as cancer of the breast and prostate, herbs like licorice and saw palmetto (which antagonize testosterone) are good choices. For many cancer patients I add poke root extract in the appropriate dose to help with lymphatic drainage. Usually, I prescribe a mixture of four to five herbs to be taken at the dose of 1-2 teaspoons 2 times per day.

One of the most remarkable patients I have encountered in my practice was a woman who came to me almost ten years ago. Ms. R.B. had recently found a lump in her breast. She felt well and had no other symptoms but she was sure the lump was cancer. Over the next few months we discussed whether she should have a biopsy to confirm the diagnosis; at one point she even went to a surgeon, but she ultimately refused this procedure. She knew it was cancer. I was reluctant to treat her without a solid diagnosis, but eventually we proceeded in a manner similar to that described as my Phase I treatment. She was very consistent and conscientious with the diet, medicines, Iscador and the mental and emotional aspects of the therapy. As time went on we talked more and more about her story. She had worked all her life as an environmental activist and a health writer and was quite well known in her field. During her work as an activist she was exposed to many pesticides and other toxins. She had also experienced a number of painful relationships and emotional events, but she always plugged on, doing much good and suffering much pain in her life. It was clear to her, partly through our discussions and her own inner work, that her tumor was a way to encapsulate all this "pain." As she put it, she separated the nastiness so she could experience the joy. This reminded me of a quote from one of my "heroes," which hangs in my office:

> *Yes, we suffer pain, we become ill, we die. But we also hope, laugh, celebrate; we know the joy of caring for one another, often we are healed and we recover by many means. We do not have to pursue the flattening out of human experience. I invite all to shift their gaze, their thoughts, from worrying about health care to cultivating the art of living. And, today with equal importance, the art of suffering, the art of dying.*
>
> Ivan Illich on the "Pursuit of Health"

This resilient patient had shifted her gaze from attacking the tumor to integrating it, understanding it and, at times, keeping it separate so that she could move on. Ten years later, I wish I could say the tumor is gone and she is well, but that is not the case. The tumor has grown to about the size of a ping-pong ball and threatens to break through the skin, but during this period, she has lived the most joyous years of her life. Now in her mid-80s she writes, takes photographs of ice crystals, eats a very careful traditional diet and makes her own lacto-fermented vegetables, vinegar, bread and most of her own food. She loves to eat game meat, ordering it from a specialty butchery in Chicago. She eats liberally of all the good fats, and radiates a peacefulness and glow that I rarely encounter. She has no pain, has no symptoms, and is otherwise in great health.

In many ways this is a remarkable outcome and demonstrates clearly that this "terrorist" tumor is better off as the subject of a dialogue, to be walled off and understood, rather than attacked. If one has the courage to walk this path, in spite of the way that the cancer establishment engenders fear in the cancer patient, then it is possible to live in a joyous, peaceful co-existence with our shadow side, which we call the tumor. As Illich points out, in our time we must cultivate the art of suffering, the art of dying. In truth, this art is nothing more or less than a joyful life, as this remarkable lady has shown me so beautifully.

PHASE II

I usually continue Phase I treatment for one to three years, with changes in the herbal prescription every one to two months. Sometimes, however, things do not go so smoothly and the cancer recurs or continues to grow. Phase II is appropriate, for example, when x-rays show progression of a pancreatic cancer or when a prostate cancer patient's PSA continues to rise. I will also use the Phase II treatment when there is a recurrence in spite of Phase I treatment, such as a breast cancer patient who has a recurrence after three years of being cancer-free.

The reason I don't begin with Phase II is that with each succeeding phase, I use medicines, albeit natural medicines, that tend to substitute for deficiencies rather than encourage balance. In other words, by going to Phase II, I have concluded that this patient not only needs to learn to fish, but also requires some fish to be provided, at least temporarily. I don't, however, abandon the Phase I approach, which is based on "healing" the light metabolism, rather, I just address it more directly.

Phase II includes the following additions:

F. Melatonin

The pineal gland, situated deep in our brains, is a curious organ. Traditional cultures have called it the third eye even though, as far as we know, it doesn't have anything to do with vision. We do know that the pineal gland participates in light metabolism and regulates sleep. Studies conducted some 20 years ago show that melatonin not only participates in the sleep response, but also has profound effects on our overall sense of well-being. When we go without sleep, or even when we sleep in rooms that are not totally dark, melatonin levels can fall and this decline can reduce immunity.

As with all our treatments, we should strive to understand the metaphor as well as the biochemistry. Consider the individual who, through years of sleep deprivation and chronic stress, gradually becomes deficient in the "light" hormone. In other words, winter sets in on a biochemical, hormonal basis. This situation is entirely analogous to hypothyroidism in which one gradually loses the ability to produce enough thyroid hormone to maintain good health.

Hypopinealism has profound consequences for our immunity, sense of well-being and level of inflammation. I suspect that Phase I treatment sometimes corrects this condition, although this is a difficult thing to test. When it doesn't, I give the patient 20 mg of melatonin one hour before bedtime, which I hope will be relatively early in the night. I also encourage these patients to sleep as much as possible, especially in a quiet and well darkened room. Often this intervention makes a huge difference in the patient's sense of well-being.

G. Digestive Enzymes

For the last 50 years, practitioners all over the world have used digestive enzymes to treat cancer. They became popularized as part of the Kelley Diet, a regimen developed by a dentist, William Kelley, that he used successfully to cure his own pancreatic cancer. Kelley postulated that tumors surround themselves with a protective "coating" that shields it from our immune system. The natural mechanism for breaking through this coating is our own digestive enzymes, a kind of internal digestive process. I use the formulation Wobenzym, which contains a broad spectrum of plant and animal enzymes, given at a dose of 3-10 tablets 3-4 times per day. The tablets are taken between meals, to encourage digestion of the coating, rather than the food we eat.

H. Essiac

Essiac is an herbal mixture based on an old Native American formula that is widely used in the treatment of cancer patients. Many studies have confirmed that each individual component of Essiac—rhubarb root, burdock, sheep sorrel and slippery elm—has its own anticancer effects. I use the formulation Burdock Complex from Mediherb, which contains these four herbs in the approximate ratios as are in the original formula. The dose is 2-4 tablets 2-3 times per day.

I. Specific Herbal Oncology Medicines

For cancers of the GI tract, including stomach, liver, colon and pancreatic cancers, aloe vera gel has been shown to have a beneficial effect. For cancers that have more of an immunologic basis, including melanoma and kidney cancer, the herbal medicine to add is echinacea, which seems to help the immune system identify aberrant cells. Another herbal medicine that helps with immune function is astragalus, which I will often add in this phase.

PHASE III
H. Iscador Special

If things still do not progress well in two to six months after beginning Phase II, I move on to Phase III. In this step I take advantage of a relatively new type of Iscador that has been standardized according to its lectin content. The mistletoe lectins are thought to be important contributors of both the immune-stimulating and cytotoxic properties of mistletoe. This type of Iscador is called Iscador Special and is derived from either oak tree mistletoe (Iscador Quercus) or apple tree mistletoe (Iscador Mali). For men, I replace the Iscador of Phase I with injections of Iscador Quercus Special, 3 times per week; for women, Iscador Mali Special is used. If these injections provoke a strong inflammatory reaction on the skin, the dose should be lowered to one well tolerated by the individual.

PHASE IV

I. Interleukin II Therapy

In this final phase I discontinue Iscador and other specific immune-enhancing herbs (such as echinacea) for at least one month and initiate low-dose subcutaneous Interleukin II therapy. This involves injecting 3 million units of IL-2, six out of seven days, for four consecutive weeks. As we discussed, our immune system depends on adequate levels of IL-2. In Phase IV we accept the fact that merely stimulating an immune response is failing to keep the cancer in check, so now we will *give* the immune response. Research on this therapy indicates that a 20-50 percent positive response can be expected. There are few side-effects, and it can be an effective and relatively gentle way to buy time before going back to Phase II. The literature is particularly positive about this therapy for cancers with a strong immunological basis, such as kidney cancer and melanoma.

Movement

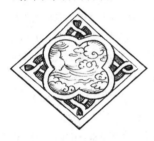

Much has been written about the "cancer personality." Studies have shown that people with cancer tend to internalize their emotions and have difficulty expressing themselves, in contrast to the "heart attack personality," which is characterized by lack of emotional control, over-reaction and even anger. Cancer patients are often apologetic, wanting to please others above all else.

As we discussed, our personal space should be neither too big nor too small. If the space is too big, we seem distant and cold-hearted. If it is too small, we are always affronted. In cancer patients, the personal space is often too small. People with cancer tend to take things too personally; those in the healing and nurturing professions often take on the illnesses of their patients subconsciously. They would profit from learning to meet their patients' illnesses where they are, not letting them invade their personal space.

Appropriate gestures and exercises can help the cancer patient claim a bigger space. The Personal Space Gesture and the Wrestling Stance can be very helpful and the Penguin exercise can help diffuse emotions by taking them away from the body. This exercise helps us to deflect forces that come towards our personal space and lead them out and away. Once the personal space has been defined, the patient can graduate to the Water Level Gesture and the Sundial, movements that create an expanse in the chest area, and help establish the Horizontal or Emotional plane at the level of the heart, where it should be.

Other useful movements for the cancer patient include the Grounding Exercise, Carriage Down and Carriage Up, the Cowl, Foot Streaming and the Victory Stretch, as well as the Breathing Exercise and the Silhouette. The Lemniscate Dynamic can help foster communication so crucial to the successful treatment of cancer.

Fever stimulates the immune system and it also helps the cancer patient in another way by enlarging the personal space around the body. The cancer patient should try to remember the feeling of having a fever and the fever-like extension around the body.

Meditation

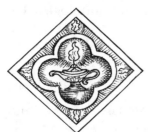

Numerous studies have attempted to document the beneficial effect of helping cancer patients with self-expression. Toward that end, engagement in artistic therapies can have good results. In fact, any therapy that fosters an encounter with one's true self can be helpful to cancer patients.

I would like to suggest another option, one that has actually been used to foster healing throughout the history of humankind, and that is the *contemplation* of great works of art. A theme of this chapter has been the achievement of dynamic and peaceful interchange between the cells of our bodies, as well as between individuals in human society, "the enlightened self-discipline of the various parts, each voluntarily imposing on itself the limits of its individual freedom for the well-being of the community," as Bach wrote so eloquently. We should all try to experience the reconciliation of freedom and self-discipline in the works of Bach and other great composers.

Contemplation of great paintings is especially appropriate for cancer patients because many painters worked with light as a predominant theme. The French impressionists caught the experience of summer light with great genius but the paintings of Raphael, Rembrandt and Turner can also be studied and used as sources of contemplation on the healing aspects of light.

Another source of meditation is a story by the great German philosopher, poet and scientist J.W. von Goethe. He called his "Fairy Tale of the Green Snake and the Beautiful Lily" a fairy tale for modern man, explaining that through deep contemplation of the images contained in this story, the reader could come to a "unification of the human self with the higher, spiritual being." Others have described this fairy tale as a description of the path of modern initiation. In other words, the path on which Goethe leads the reader in this tale mimics or reflects the path we each must take to transform our everyday existence into an experience laden with deeper meaning. It is the path of self-actualization described by psychologist Abraham Maslow, the Buddhist eightfold path, or the way of the cross in Christianity.

I encountered this tale about 20 years ago, and upon reading it I was moved to tears. It was as though this story satisfied some deep inner longing . Since then, I have reread the tale many times, wondering each time whether this story held the key to healing not only *the* illness of our time, cancer, but also our complex social ills. After the events of September 11, I reread "The Fairy Tale of the Green Snake and the Beautiful Lily" and was struck by the following passage:

> *"Where do you come from?"*
> *"From the subterranean passages where gold is found, "said the snake.*
> *"What is more precious than gold?" asked the king.*
> *"The Light," answered the snake.*
> *"What is more refreshing than light?" asked the king.*
> *"Conversation," said the snake.*

This passage distills the message of this chapter. More important than material wealth is the light, for in the absence of light comes first despair and depression (which affect the liver) and then a decline in physical health. More and more often in today's world, that decline results in cancer. All the riches in the world will not save one suffering from the absence of light. But there is something even more profound than light, says Goethe, and that is human conversation or, in today's parlance, communication. Isn't the lack of conversation the essence of both cancer and terrorism? In cancer the cells forget how to communicate, to converse with each other. They grow rampantly, out of control, unable to have any sort of conversation with the other cells or tissue types. The cancerous physiology could be likened to a group of individuals or nations shouting threats at each other, ultimately each going his own way, mindless of what happens to the whole. Isn't this also what happens when our world is gripped by terrorism? Each group shouts demands at each other, nobody is heard, the anger mounts and all ends in bloodshed. We think we can win this battle because we can shout louder than the others; in the case of cancer, we think can use more sophisticated radiation or surgical approaches. In either case, we are living an illusion. Eventually, our voice will tire, our resources will give out, and the world, or the patient, will be exhausted beyond repair. With this paradigm, there is no way out.

As you engage in the *Rückschau* Meditation each evening, call up those moments during your day when you engaged in communication with others at the border of your personal space and compare them to moments when you retreated from social contract, or were "on send," unable to take in communication from others.

Above all, we must seek understanding—of ourselves and of others. To treat cancer and other illnesses of our time, we must begin with the right metaphor. We cannot win cancer by doing battle, but only by shining light into the darkness and learning to communicate.

RECOMMENDED READING
 www.spiritworking.com for all Iscador research
 Principles and Practice of Phytotherapy by Kerry Bone and Simon Mills
 The Fairy Tale of the Green Snake and Beautiful Lily by Goethe

Summary

Nutrition

* Avoid   Processed and convenience foods

                      Non-organic foods, likely to be high in pesticides

                      Extreme diets, such as all-raw vegetarian

* Emphasize   Balanced meals containing animal foods, grains and vegetables

                      Lacto-fermented foods

                      Soup broths

                      Flax seeds and flax seed oil

                      Beets and lacto-fermented beet juice

                      Coconut oil and coconut products

                      Fat from grass-fed animals

* Supplements   Cod liver oil to provide 20,000 IU vitamin A per day

                      High-vitamin butter oil, 1/2 teaspoon per day

                      Catalyn by Standard Process, 6 per day

Therapeutics

* PHASE I (Basic Treatment)

     A. Iscador according to the recommended guidelines up to the dose that produces a redness greater that 1 to 2 inches or a temperature over 100F. In this phase the injections are given 3 times per week.

     B. First check the 25(OH)D level in the blood, then, using 1,000 IU increments, supplement with Carlson's vitamin D until the level in the blood is between 40-60. In conjunction, use calcium lactate, 6 tablets per day.

     C. Mediherb ganoderma/shiitake, 1 tablet 2-3 times per day.

    D. Immuplex by Standard Process, 1 capsule three times per day and the protomorphogen of the tissue of origin of the tumor, 1 tablet three times per day.

    E Individualized herbal therapy 1 teaspoon, two times per day.

* PHASE II

    F. Melatonin 20 mg, 1 hour before bedtime.

    G. Wobezym digestive enzymes, 3-10 tablets 3-4 times per day between meals.

    H. Burdock Complex (Essiac), 2-4 tablets 2-3 times per day.

    I. Specific medicines for specific cancer types.

        1. GI cancers - Aloe vera gel from Mediherb, 1 tablespoon 2 times per day.

        2. Melanoma and kidney cancer - Echinacea Premium from Mediherb, 1 tablet 3 times per day, or Astragalus Complex (Mediherb), 1 tablet 3 times per day.

* PHASE III

    H. Iscador Special, Mali for women, Quercus for men. The dose is still 3 times a week, but it is especially important to watch for excessive inflammatory reactions.

* PHASE IV

    I. IL-2 therapy is undertaken after stopping the Iscador. The dose is 3 million units a day, 6 out of 7 days for 4 weeks.

Movement

* Movement that widens the personal space, such as the Personal Space Gesture, the Wrestling Stance and Penguin Wrestling.

* The Water Level Gesture and the Sundial.

* Grounding, Carriage Down/Carriage Up, the Cowl, Foot Streaming and the Victory Stretch.

* Breathing, Silhouette and Lemniscate Dynamic.

Meditation

* Contemplation of great music (especially Baroque) and works of art (especially Impressionist).
* Contemplation of the "Fairy Tale of the Green Snake and the Beautiful Lily" by Goethe.
* Focus on moments of true communication during the *Rückschau* Meditation.

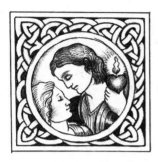

Chapter 3:
Heart Disease

i carry your heart with me
(I carry it in my heart)
i am never without it
(anywhere I go you go, my dear;
and whatever is done
by only me is your doing, my darling)

i fear not fate
(for you are my fate, my sweet)
i want no world
(for beautiful you are my world, my true)
and it's you who are whatever a moon has always meant
and whatever a sun will always sing is you

here is the deepest secret nobody knows
(here is the root of the root and the bud of the bud
and the sky of the sky of a tree called life;
which grows
higher than soul can hope or mind can hide)
and this is the wonder
that's keeping the stars apart

i carry your heart (i carry it in my heart)

e e cummings

In the latter part of his life Rudolf Steiner made several singular and provocative statements. When a student asked him what was needed in order for the proper development of humanity to occur in the future, he replied that mankind must

137

meet the following conditions:

1. He must understand that there is no difference between motor and sensory nerves.
2. He must no longer work for money.
3. He must understand that the heart is not a pump.

If any of us were asked the same question, we would probably give completely different answers—such as cleaning up environmental destruction or averting the threat of nuclear war. What are we to make of Steiner's astonishing reply?

We will discuss Steiner's first obstacle in Chapter 15 on neurological disorders. The second obstacle to overcome, that we must no longer work for money, seems logical. No emotional or spiritual progress can occur when people work for money. Of course, we need to be paid for what we do, but if our work is not interesting, challenging and meaningful, clearly the spirit will suffer. Only when our work responds to the deepest longing of the soul can we make emotional and spiritual progress in life.

The subject of this chapter is the third statement, the amazing suggestion that the heart is not a pump. We will discuss whether this statement is accurate, and then if it is, try to understand its significance for medicine, for the inner life of the human being, and for society in general. I have pondered this statement for over 20 years and only recently have I begun to understand its implications. In fact, Steiner's brilliant insight into the design of the heart and circulatory system has become my "unified field theory of medicine." What I mean is that in understanding the role of the heart, and how illnesses of the circulatory system can be healed, we can tie together many observations that otherwise remain obscure. We will see that this new understanding is crucial not only to the healing process but also to the forward evolution of humankind.

In a discussion as emotionally charged as this one, it is important to be as clear as possible with the words I am using. When I say "pump" I mean that part of the system that creates the force responsible for the movement of the fluid, in this case the blood. Normal science and medicine take it as a given that the organ or aspect of the circulatory system responsible for the movement of the blood is the heart. Specifically, we are taught that the muscular contraction of the heart walls provides the major impulse for the movement of the blood. Modern medicine accepts this assertion even though scientists do not understand how such a small and relatively weak organ can generate the amount of pressure needed to move a viscous fluid like blood through all the resistance presented by the miles and miles of blood vessels that make up the circulatory system. Nor do we really understand how the heart can perform this muscular activity minute after minute, day after day, year after year, for a whole lifetime.

Let's look at how the textbooks explain the modern view of the heart as a pump and how this viewpoint creeps into our everyday language. Arthur Guyton's *Textbook of Medical Physiology*, the "Bible" of human physiology, contains the following statement: "The heart can pump either a small or a large amount, depending on the amount that flows into it from the veins; and it automatically adapts to whatever this load might be as long as the total quantity of blood does not rise above the physiological limit that the heart can pump"

Credit for the discovery of the "pumping" action of the heart goes to William Harvey, the so-called father of modern cardiology. In 1628, Harvey claimed that the beating of the heart is the sole cause for the circulation of blood through living organisms. Another physiologist, Antoni, describes this succinctly when he claimed "The heart functions as the circulating pump that drives the blood through the vessels." This is the edifice upon which all modern cardiology is based. It is a distinctly modern, mechanistic view. Aristotle and Virgil taught that the heart rather than the brain was the seat of the mind, and a similar belief can be found in ancient Hindu scriptures and other Eastern philosophies.

Now let us look at the circulation as a whole as depicted in the diagram below:

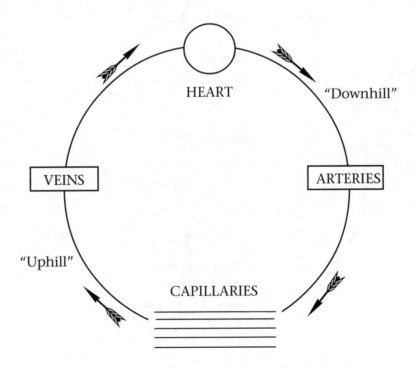

If we imagine the circulation as a closed loop, in which the blood is confined to the inside of the blood vessels, we can make some specific observations about the movement of the blood in this system. At the level of the heart, the cross sectional area is very small. In other words, the volume of the blood at the point of the heart is compressed into a small space. The blood travels through arteries that get progressively smaller until it reaches the tiny capillaries where a transfer of nutrients between the blood and the cells occurs. After this transfer, the blood enters the venous system, first the tiny venules and then the veins, which get progressively larger as they approach the heart. In contrast to the vessels going into and out of the heart, the cross sectional area at the level of the capillaries is very large. Indeed, some researchers have suggested that if all the capillaries were laid end to end, they would cover the area of three football fields.

Elementary hydraulics and common sense observation teach us that in a closed system in which fluid is moving, the velocity at any one point is inversely proportional to the cross sectional area. In other words, at the level of the heart, where the area is smallest, the velocity of the blood is the greatest while at the level of the capillaries, where the area is the greatest, the velocity is the smallest, as depicted in the diagram below:

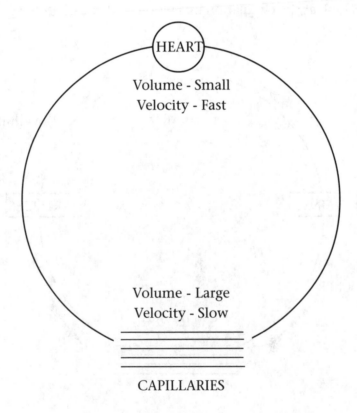

Actually, careful measurement of the speed of the blood shows that at the capillaries the blood actually stops, oscillates momentarily, and then proceeds. Another anomaly concerns the fact that the blood entering the heart does not actually go much faster than the blood exiting the heart. At these two points, before and after the heart, the blood moves at about the same rate. To visualize this more clearly, imagine a river that narrows down to a small width, and then widens into a pond. All of us would agree that the speed of the river is much faster at the narrowest point than it is at the pond. Consider further that except for the circulation to the head, a special exception which I will discuss later, the capillaries essentially lie downhill from the heart. By this I simply mean that the feet and legs are lower than the heart. The heart, relatively speaking, is near the top of the hill.

I have had numerous occasions over the past few years to present my views on nutrition and agriculture to farmers. I have often asked them the following question: If you had a narrow, fast-moving stream that went downhill into a pond and you needed to get that pond water back up to the level of the original stream, would you buy a pump from a man who told you he wanted to put the pump at the point of the original fast-moving stream and that this pump would not actually result in an appreciable increase in the velocity of the water? So far, I have had no takers. Instead, the farmer would put the pump at the bottom of the hill where the area is the greatest and the water has stopped. As anyone can see, putting the pump at the point in the system where the blood is moving the fastest is a serious design flaw! Of course, that suggestion is untenable—there are no design flaws in the human body, just flaws in our conception of it.

It is also problematic to consider the heart on its own as a pump. The diagram on page 142 shows the actual anatomy of the heart and its immediate vessels.

As you can see, the aorta or "outflow" tube leading away from the heart first goes up and then curves down again before it continues downward to the rest of the body. The vessels that lead up to the shoulders, neck and head come off the area of maximum bend. Another well-recognized fact is that during the time of maximum blood flow through the aorta—called the systole—the aorta actually bends more or, in engineering terms, "ascribes a more acute angle." Thus, when the heart is "pumping" at its maximum during the systole phase, the flexible outflow tube, the aorta, bends more than when the pumping is at a minimum. Anyone who has ever observed a pump at work knows that if you pump a fluid like water or blood very hard, in fact hard enough to overcome the tremendous resistance of the blood vessels, the outflow tube must straighten under this heavy pressure. But in the human system, it bends even more! Furthermore, the outflow tube faces uphill from the direction the blood eventually goes. Returning to our stream analogy, we are now asking a farmer to buy a pump, put it in at the top of the hill where the water is moving the fastest, a pump that has *no* effect on the speed of the water *and* we are going to face the pump backwards so that when the water goes out of the pipe it is going to bend the pipe even more. This is simply preposterous!

If the heart is a pump, it is like no other pump in the world. Given the facts about the design of the heart and circulatory system, we cannot accurately describe the heart as a pump. We must examine the situation anew and come up with a better explanation for these simple observations we have made.

From the simple image I outlined above it is easy to see that the "pump," that is the driving force for the movement of the blood, must begin at the level of the capillaries. But how can this be since there are no physical "pumps" located throughout the body? Let's skip this question for a moment and consider the dynamics of blood movement starting from the capillaries. As the blood returns to the heart and the cross sectional area in the veins progressively narrows, the blood moves faster and faster. The valves in the veins keep the blood moving "uphill" towards the heart, and contractions of the muscles in the legs help increase momentum. The blood builds up maximum speed as it enters the largest veins and meets the heart. The heart

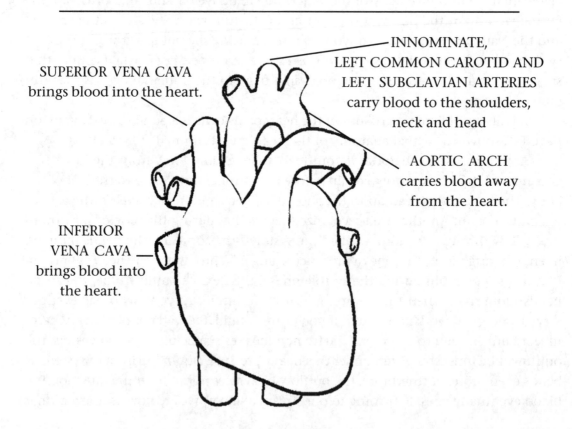

SUPERIOR VENA CAVA
brings blood into the heart.

INNOMINATE,
LEFT COMMON CAROTID AND
LEFT SUBCLAVIAN ARTERIES
carry blood to the shoulders,
neck and head

AORTIC ARCH
carries blood away
from the heart.

INFERIOR
VENA CAVA
brings blood into
the heart.

actually acts as a dam for this onrushing blood. It dams up the incoming blood and "traps" it in its four chambers, which can be likened to expandable holding tanks. When the chambers are filled to a maximum, the heart "gates" open up (we call the gates "valves") and the blood essentially falls down to the rest of the body due to the force of gravity. As it does so, it creates a kind of a suction that sucks or pulls the blood out of the heart, thereby creating a negative pressure, which bends the outflow tube during the point of maximum flow. Thus the heart is best described not as a pump, but as a hydraulic ram, a device engineers use to push fluids short distances up hills. This ingenious device is inserted into rapidly moving waters where it traps the "energy" of the water in an expandable tank; it has gates that open when the pressure builds in the tank and once the gates are opened, the water is essentially sucked out of the tank and the outflow tube bends, creating a kind of slingshot effect. The "pumping" is accomplished not by the walls of the tank, but by the trapped energy of the water. Typically, the outflow tube is put "backwards" to increase the suction. This model explains how the heart is able to do its job year after year, as it takes very little work to simply open the gates, and it puts no stress on the heart muscles. The electrical system of the heart helps to regulate the rhythmical opening of the gates, just as the hydraulic ram is attached to a power source to regulate the opening of its gates.

There *is* one area in this beautiful system that requires a nudge from the heart and that is the blood flow to the head, neck and and shoulders. As these are situated above the heart, the blood cannot get there via the force of gravity, but needs a little push. The blood to these areas goes through the innominate, left common carotid and left subclavier arteries, which as I said, come off the aortic arch. The amazing thing is that when the suction happens and the aorta curves more, this brings these arteries into an almost straight shot from the heart, facilitating this extra push. When understood properly, we can only marvel at this mastery of design, right down into the fine details involving the placement of the blood vessels.

We now return to the question of how the blood begins movement in the capillaries. Let us go back to our original drawing of the circulation, as shown on page 144.

If we imagine a certain fixed volume of blood, we can see that the amount of blood entering the capillaries should be the same as that exiting the capillaries through the venules or fine veins. However, this is not actually the case because inside the capillaries, the cells extract food and oxygen from the blood and put carbon dioxide and water into the venules. This increase in the volume of water on the vein side of the capillaries as opposed to the artery side creates a gradient of pressure, called osmotic pressure, which actually pushes the blood in the direction of the veins. The millions of cells acting independently and interdependently create enough osmotic pressure to get the blood moving, and then the narrowing of the vessels increases the flow. Clearly, it is the process of metabolism, or "eating" that provides the actual push for the movement of the blood. Osmotic pressure, in the form of the production of water from food and oxygen, is *the* pump.

One final point: The heart does not pump—what it does is *listen*. This amazing organ senses what is in the blood and then calls forth the necessary hormones so that homeostasis is maintained and the cells can function optimally. The heart serves the cells not by pushing blood towards them but by balancing and integrating the blood's chemistry. In fact, Steiner suggested that the heart also senses and integrates our thoughts, our emotions and our will to carry out tasks. The heart, then, is not a mechanical pump, but actually a sensitive integrator of all our experience.

But there is even more to this story, a fact well-known to poets throughout the ages and to the ancient cultures that viewed the Earth as the center of the universe, for the heart lies between Venus (the venous system) and Mars (the arterial system,

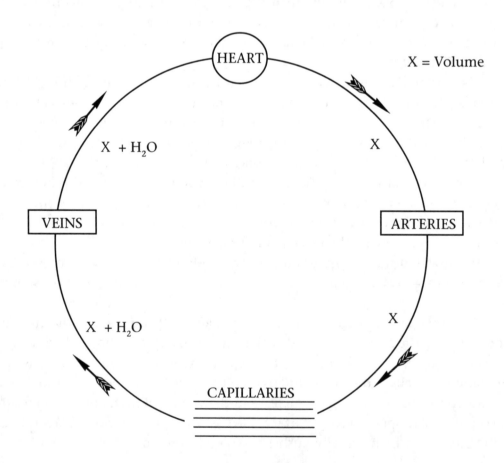

named after Ares or Mars), the namesakes of the basic male and female impulses. The heart, therefore, is the mediator between our male and female aspects, our *anima* and *animus*. In fact, the heart has a monumental task, acting as a kind of tireless therapist—integrating, sorting and processing all of our impressions, trying to create harmony and rhythm out of all that happens in our lives. It is no wonder that poets and sages have sung the praises of this indefatigable friend and clearly located the emotion of love in our hearts.

The repercussions of this model are legion. To begin with, any problem of the heart or circulation must first address the integrity of the "pump;" that is, the generation of osmotic pressure. Some of my patients on hearing about this model wonder whether they should drink more water in order to increase the efficiency of the pump. But that is the wrong approach. It is the gradient or *difference* of water pressure from the artery side to the vein side that provides the pump; in fact, increasing total volume in the system makes it harder to move the blood because the excess water volume makes it heavier. No, the only way to "pump" the blood is to increase the gradient. How can this be done? It is actually quite simple if we realize one important fact—that the amount of water liberated from the metabolism of fats, especially saturated fats, is much higher than the amount of water liberated from proteins or carbohydrates. According to the biochemistry textbooks, consumption of 10 grams of protein releases 4 grams of water; ten grams of carbohydrates release 6 grams of water. But consumption of 10 grams of fat releases a full 10 grams of water. This liberation only occurs, however, when sufficient oxygen is present in the blood. So, oxygen plus a metabolism in which the cells live predominately on fats instead of carbohydrates or protein results in the most efficient pump and the healthiest circulation.

Given this model, one would expect those people who do regular exercise and eat a diet consisting plentifully of healthy fats and low in carbohydrates to have the healthiest hearts and circulatory systems. This exactly fits Dr. Price's descriptions of the Swiss, Gaelics, Eskimos, African cattle herders and South Sea Islanders as well as modern observations of the French (the so-called French paradox). Finally, the confusing world of cardiology begins to make sense!

This simple model is the backbone of all my recommendations to those with problems of the heart and circulation: eat more fats and get more exercise. If possible, 80 percent of your caloric intake should be from fats, mostly saturated fats. Fortuitously, the high-fat diet will make you feel more like exercising. Metabolization of fats generates healthier circulation by making the osmotic gradient more pronounced. Besides, it is a wonderfully tasty therapy!

Here are a few points to remember as you begin to increase the fat content of your diet. The first is that signs of fat deficiency include the feeling of coldness; in his

Fundamentals of Therapy, Rudolf Steiner states that eating fats is *the* way to generate more warmth. This is because fats improve the circulation. Other signs of fat deficiency include craving for anything (from sugar to water), poor circulation, the feeling of dryness in any body part (such as eyes, skin and joints), or simply the feeling of tiredness. These are all signs of fat deficiency and you cannot solve them by drinking more water—this only makes the circulation more sluggish. You can only solve these problems by increasing the efficiency of the pump, that is by eating more good fats.

A sign of excess fat consumption is the feeling of nausea; if this happens reduce your fat intake temporarily and eat more bitters and fermented foods such as sauerkraut, beet kvass and dandelion greens, to help you digest the fats. If you undertake to increase the fat content of your diet along with a regimen of regular walking, your circulation will demonstrably inprove in a matter of weeks. Perhaps this requirement for regular walking was the reason Steiner said heart patients should never travel faster than their own two legs could carry them. He was encouraging people to walk!

This model also explains why there has been an "epidemic" of congestive heart failure in the recent era of lowfat diets. This phenomenon has also increased since the promotion of cholesterol-lowering regimes. Lowering the fat intake or level in the blood lowers the efficiency of the pump, the circulation gets sluggish, and eventually can hardly go forward. At that point the heart enlarges and weakens, a condition we call congestive heart failure. The basic cause of this condition is bad advice—the lowfat, cholesterol-lowering measures orthodox medicine promotes as gospel. Most cases of congestive heart failure can be reversed simply by increasing fat intake and engaging in regular walking.

It is not uncommon in the history of the world for philosophers or social scientists to look to the human being as a model for society at large. The alchemists summarized this way of thinking with the phrase "As above, so below." A famous example of this type of thinking was the use of social Darwinism to justify the mistreatment of the poor or the slaughter and repression of indigenous people. The Darwinian paradigm described these peoples as unfit, especially compared to the "more fit" peoples of European descent.

If we are to use the human being as a model for our social system, it is important to get the model correct. Survival of the fittest is no more an accurate description of human evolution than the model of the heart as a pump. Both models are inaccurate and inherently misleading. Recently, when I heard General Tommy Franks describe the US military as a system that functions like the circulatory system, where central command gives the orders (like the heart pumping blood) that are then transmitted to the soldiers who carry out these orders (like the blood to the cells), I knew another slaughter was in the offing. If the heart is not a pump, and the movement of the blood is initiated in the individual cells, then the orders should be given by the individual soldier; the role of central command, like the role of the heart, is simply to listen to the will of the people and the soldiers! A society that believes the heart is a pump is a society that accepts centralized control, planned economies, central banks, a national farm policy, government-dictated medical policy, chain stores for our clothing and one big company that makes everyone's shoes.

If the heart functions as a listener rather than as a pump, then the model for the state should not be one of central control, be it the socialist state or the Federal Reserve, but one of freedom and decentralization; of 10 million local farms each taking care of their own land and neighbors rather than a central farm policy; of thousands of artisans making shoes and clothes rather than a few large shoe companies and clothing produced in Third World sweatshops; of a billion religions, not three or five central dogmas; of a God that listens and reacts to our needs, just as the heart reacts to the circulation, not the other way around. The heart as a pump reflects itself onto society as control leading to slavery and the inability for mankind to progress, just as Rudolf Steiner suggested.

Nutrition

Using *Nourishing Traditions* as your guidebook, the strategy with any "disease" of the heart is to slowly increase the percentage of healthy fats in your diet. The target range is usually between 60-80 percent of total calories depending on your reaction to the food. Remember that fats contain twice as many calories as protein or carbohydrate foods and proteins and carbohydrates can contain as much as 85 percent water while fat contains none. Thus, a well-marbled steak contains about 80 percent of its calories as fat, even though fat comprises less than 25 percent of the volume or weight; whole milk contains 50 percent of calories as fat and cheese contains over 70 percent of calories as fat.

As I mentioned, let your body be your guide to the amount of fat that is right for you; watch for signs of cravings (too little fat), or nausea (too much fat). Most importantly, eat regularly of fermented and bitter foods, such as beet kvass, sauerkraut and bitter green vegetables, to help you digest and absorb the fats. These guidelines hold for any disease of the circulatory system, especially any feelings of coldness or fatigue (usually a result of poor circulation and deficient warmth).

The fats you eat should be largely animal fats, along with some olive oil, coconut oil and palm oil. Although the public rarely hears about them, many studies have implicated polyunsaturated vegetable oils, not animal fats, as a major cause of heart disease. In 1900, when heart attacks were unknown, the American diet was rich in saturated fat and cholesterol from butter, cream, lard, tallow, whole milk, cheese and meat. Today, most of our fat calories come from vegetable oils, a direct result of today's orthodox dietary advice! Modern commercial vegetable oils create imbalances at the cellular level that can lead to clots. And partially hydrogenated vegetable oils, the *trans* fatty acids, seem to disrupt the development of the cell membrane, making the cells stiffer and more inflexible, leading eventually to "hardening" of the blood vessels and a less efficient "pump." *Trans* fats also reduce the amount of energy available to the heart.

Furthermore, modern processing removes many important fat-soluble vitamins from our diet. Vitamin E is a natural antioxidant. It protects against clots and inflammation of the blood vessels. Vitamin E is removed or destroyed during the high-temperature processing of vegetable oils, as well as in the refinement of our grains. Vitamins A and D are needed for mineral assimilation and hence a host of processes that support optimal metabolism in the cells and the electrical system that regulates the heart. Dr. Price was able to demonstrate that deaths from heart disease went up during times of the year when the levels of fat-soluble vitamins in the local butter went down. These nutrients are found mostly in the fats and organ meats of animals that eat green grass and in seafood.

The food industry is aware that its processing methods destroy vitamin content. Its response has been to add synthetic vitamins to our foods. But synthetic vitamins are not as effective as those occurring naturally. In fact, synthetic vitamins may have an effect opposite to the natural form. Synthetic vitamin D_2, which was added to milk for many years, can cause softening of the hard tissues (such as the bone) and hardening of the soft tissues (such as the arteries). The dairy industry quietly dropped vitamin D_2 in favor of more natural vitamin D_3, but D_2 is now added to increasingly popular imitation milks made from soy, rice and oats.

The diet for heart disease should eliminate all processed foods containing sugar, white flour, additives, rancid vegetable oils and especially *trans* fatty acids from partially hydrogenated vegetable oils. It should be rich in fat soluble vitamins from grass-fed butter and cream (preferably raw), seafood, lard and liver. Liver is especially important because it supplies vitamin B_{12}, recently shown to be important for the cardiovascular function, and is the best dietary source of copper, a mineral that is vital for proper function of the artery lining. Bone broths for calcium and leafy green vegetables for magnesium should be included as these two minerals are also vital for cardiovascular health. Raw animal foods (raw milk and cheese, raw and marinated seafood, raw beef and lamb) supply vitamin B_6, another important nutrient for the heart. Finally, coconut oil supplies lauric acid, which has strong antimicrobial properties to combat viruses and other pathogens that can irritate the arteries.

Supplements should include cod liver oil to supply at least 10,000 IU vitamin A per day. The vitamin D content of cod liver oil is needed for the absorption of calcium and magnesium and the special fatty acids it contains have been shown in many studies to decrease platelet aggregation or clot formation leading to coronary thrombosis (blockage of the small coronary arteries). If you don't like liver, take 4-6 Carlson's desiccated liver capsules per day. Also, take 1/4 teaspoon of rose hip, acerola or amalaki powder mixed with water to supply vitamin C. Finally, I recommend Cataplex E2 by Standard Process for vitamin E. Many of us are familiar with the voluminous literature on the role of vitamin E in preventing heart disease. The Standard Process vitamin E formulation accentuates the particular nutrient that is responsible for prevention of thrombosis and should only be given to people diagnosed with coronary artery disease. The dose is 1-2 tablets 3 times per day.

Therapeutics

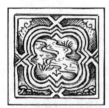 There are several medicines that are appropriate for virtually all patients with problems of the circulation, including coronary artery disease, cold hands and feet, varicose veins, and to a certain extent cardiac arrhythmias. All of these conditions, with the exception of arrythmias, are the result of "pump failure" in the way I have described above. They all respond quickly to the basic steps of a high-fat diet and regular walking.

The first medicine is Cardiodoron, a specially prepared mixture of three plants formulated by Rudolf Steiner. In creating this medicine his intention was to regulate or "harmonize" the "periphery" with the "middle." I understand this to mean that the combination helps the heart and the circulation work together, rather than oppose one another. Curiously, even though there are many folk remedies and plants that have been used for centures for heart conditions, none found its way into this medicine, which is composed of cowslip (*Primula veris*), Scotch thistle (*Onopordon acanthium*) and henbane (*Hyoscyamus niger*). In many ways, these three plants bring together the three possible strategies of a plant, the three roles that plants play in nature. Cowslip flowers as early as possible in spring, thistle flowers at midsummer and henbane reserves its flowering until almost autumn. Furthermore, these plants represent both the succulence and lightness of the primula and the darkness and heaviness of henbane, with thistle somewhere in the middle. This combination also gives us the nutritive qualities of primula plus the detoxification aspects of thistle, along with the outright poisonous qualities of henbane. In these we begin to get a picture of a medicine that is an integrator of much that lives in the world of nature, just as the heart is the integrator of the flow of blood.

An interesting research paper published in the German journal *Arzneimittelforschung*, 2000, sheds some light on the effects of the Cardiodoron combination. The researchers looked at the importance of what is called heart rate variability and noted that the healthier the heart, the greater the beat-to-beat variability. This is analogous to the difference between beat and rhythm. Beat can be mechanical, even done by a machine, as it keeps a constant, unchanging rhythm, a situation that is anathema to healthy, living organisms. A healthy circulatory system, requires a constantly changing, adapting rhythm, like the master drummer who uses changing rhythms to keep his band together. The heart's task of harmonizing and integration can never be accomplished by a mechanical beat. In the study, the researchers found that Cardiodoron increased heart rate variability after four weeks of use in healthy volunteers. In other words, Cardiodoron helps tune the heart so that it listens more closely and adapts to the rhythm of the pump, which is the metabolism. This is the very essence of cardiovascular health. The medicine is given in a rhythmical fashion, 20 drops in water 4 times per day for at least one full year.

Another important medicine is Cardioplus by Standard Process. It contains nutients that help the circulation, including coenzyme Q_{10} to strengthen the heart muscle, and magnesium, a nutrient that regulates cardiac rhythm, as well as the protomorphogen of the heart. It is clear from the writings of Royal Lee that while he may not have understood the true nature of the heart, he did suggest that treating the heart should be accomplished by improving the nourishment of the entire person and not just the heart. His developed a heart "test" called the acoustic cardiograph to listen to the heart as it adapts to the changing conditions of circulatory flow. Cardioplus is not designed to increase the pumping efficiency of the heart; rather it is a source of nourishment for the circulation. The dose is 2 tablets 3 times per day for virtually any circulatory imbalance.

The third general medicine for cardiovascular health is the herb hawthorn, which has been shown to improve virtually all conditions of the heart and circulation. Once again, this remedy is best thought of as food for the circulation. These flavonoid-rich leaves and berries help increase the integrity and tone of the blood vessels walls, facilitating the smooth circulation of the blood, thereby making it easier for our "pump" to work. I recommend hawthorn from Mediherb, 2 tablets 2 times per day for about 1 year.

In conjunction with these medicines, I often suggest a preparation made from homeopathic gold. Earlier, we presented the medieval philosophy of correspondences in the body, with each of the seven traditional metals linked to one of the seven planets in our solar system and to a human organ. Traditional cultures assigned qualities to each of the planets based on the length of their cycles and other properties. Then, invoking the philosophy of "as above, so below," they linked the qualities of each planet with the metals found in the earth, and with the organs of the human body, as summarized in the chart below:

Sun	Gold	Heart
Moon	Silver	Reproductive Organs and Brain (reflection)
Mercury	Mercury	Lungs, Large Intestine
Venus	Copper	Kidneys
Mars	Iron	Gall Bladder
Jupiter	Tin	Liver
Saturn	Lead	Spleen

It should come as no surpise that gold corresponds to the sun, which in turn relates to the organ of the heart. As the sun through its light and gravitational influence provides integration and harmony to the other six planets, so too does our heart provide integration and harmony to the other organs through its influence on the components of the blood. I give Aurum D10 as a subcutaneous injection 3 times per week in the left upper arm.

When heart arrhythmias accompany cardiovascular problems, I suggest an herbal combination of Tienchi ginseng 50%/ motherwort 20%/gingko leaves 30% from Mediherb. Arrhythmias involve the "electrical" system that controls the gating mechanism of the heart rather than the pump itself. They are often difficult to resolve and require proper diagnosis to assess the severity of the problem. While it is not entirely clear how this herbal combination works in combatting arrhythmias, each has both traditional and modern scientific evidence to support its use. My guess is that gingko increases the oxygen supply, thereby facilitating the conversion of food into available nutrients. Motherwort is a mild sedative for the autonomic nervous system. Tienchi ginseng, like gingko, works with oxygen, but in this case improving the efficiency of oxygen utilization. The dose is 1 teaspoon 2-3 times per day for 6 months.

By the way, excessive consumption of soy products can cause arrhythmias by disrupting potassium metabolism. Anyone suffering from this problem should cease all consumption of soy.

Movement

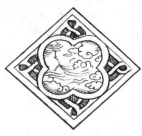

The heart is the place where the three spatial planes are balanced. In ideal conditions, there is a harmonious interplay between contraction and expansion. If the heart area has been locked in a gesture of contraction, or has been "boxed in," the blood vessels constrict and the heart muscle is deprived of the nutrients it needs for its integrating tasks. The result is strain rather than strength. The various exercises for defining the three planes can be helpful to the patient with heart disease, especially the Water Level Gesture and Autumn Leaves. Lowering the Sails can also help bring the horizontal plane down to the level of the heart and is especially helpful for angina. The Spinal Stretch is also recommended.

People with heart conditions tend to hold on to the past. Letting Go is an excellent gesture for removing constriction in the heart area. In addition, the Rice Paper Walk helps bring blood down from the head. In the Rice Paper Walk, we go forward without pushing from behind, but by releasing what is in the past. This is a serene, timeless walk that stimulates an "opening up," and is good for high blood pressure, menstrual problems and insomnia as well. Finally, the Wrestling Stance and Penguin Wrestling can be useful in mitigating aggressive tendencies.

Any exercise that is rhythmical can help the heart — dancing, swimming, walking or running in moderation. In a sport like tennis, emphasize graceful follow through rather than aggressive power.

Rudolf Steiner once remarked that high-speed travel can contribute to heart disease. If you are a very high-risk case, try to limit the amount of time spent in planes, trains and automobiles. However, it would be impractical to suggest that heart disease patients should never move faster than their own two legs can carry them. Try to do your errands either by walking or using a bicycle. Leisure activity involving hikes, nature walks and walking tours are especially appropriate. Jogging or running can be detrimental in serious cases. Wherever you travel, bring your own Personal Space with you and move with joy.

Meditation

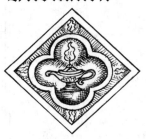

The meditation for the heart can be none other that the practical advice to "follow your heart," advice that is easy to give but often difficult to implement. I have found two ways that work for myself and my patients. First, since it is clear from this model that the "central" God listens, it is important that we talk to "Him." In other words "Ask, and it shall be given unto you." Explain your situation as though you were talking to your best friend, then ask for guidance. It is important that the image you carry is one of asking for help—no demands, no suggestions, just the heartfelt request for help.

The second approach is one I learned from the work of Marshall Rosenberg and described in his book *Non-Violent Communication*. Rosenberg suggests that you find the person in your life whom you consider the best listener, then sit down with him or her for 30 minutes and just tell your story in whatever way it comes out. Then have them ask you to answer the following question: "At this point, what would make your life more wonderful?" Then listen very carefully to your answer. If the answer makes you laugh or cry, it comes from your heart. Try to honor the answer you receive in the best way you know how. When you have finished this exercise try to do the same for at least three other people in your life. Continue this cycle until your heartfelt answer is, "Now my life is wonderful," and no more changes are needed. When that moment comes, your heart as well as your life will be whole.

RECOMMENDED READING

Non-Violent Communication by Marshall Rosenberg

Summary

Nutrition

*	Avoid	All processed foods, especially those containing *trans* fatty acids
*	Emphasize	Plenty of appropriate fats, up to 80 percent of calories
		Bitter and lacto-fermented foods
		Grass-fed butter and cream (preferably raw), seafood, lard and liver for fat-soluble vitamins
		Bone broths
		Leafy green vegetables
		Raw animal foods
		Coconut oil
*	Supplements	Cod liver oil to supply 10,000 IU vitamin A per day
		Desiccated liver capsules by Carlson's, 4-6 per day (if you don't like liver)
		1/4 teaspoon of acerola or amalaki powder mixed with water
		Cataplex E2 by Standard Process, 1-2 tablets 3 times per day

Therapeutics

* Cardiodoron from Weleda, 20 drops in water 4 times per day for at least 1 year.
* Cardio-Plus by Standard Process 2 tablets, 3 times per day for at least 1 year.
* Hawthorn tablets by Mediherb 2 tablets, 2 times per day for at least 1 year.
* Aurum D10 given as a subcutaneous injection 3 times per week in the left upper arm.

* For arrhythmias, Tienchi ginseng 50%/ motherwort 20%/gingko leaves 30% from Mediherb,1 teaspoon 2-3 times per day for 6 months.

Movement

* Exercises for balancing the intersection of the three planes, especially the Water Level Gesture and Autumn Leaves.
* Lowering the Sail for angina.
* The Spinal Stretch for increased circulation.
* Letting Go and the Rice Paper Walk.
* Wrestling Stance and Penguin Wrestling.
* Rhythmical exercise.
* Reduce time in planes, trains and automobiles as much as possible.
* Wherever you travel, bring your own Personal Space with you and move with joy.

Meditation

* Talk to "God" and ask for guidance so that you can "follow your heart."
* Tell your story to a friend who is a good listener and then have him or her ask the question, "What would make your life more wonderful?" and then honor the answer you receive.

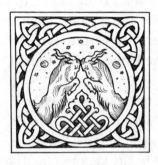

Chapter 4:
Hypertension

Ares, bane of all mankind,
crusted with blood, breacher of city walls . . .

He smiled at this, the father of gods and men,
and said to the pale-gold goddess Aphrodite:
"Warfare is not for you, child. Lend yourself
to the sighs of longing and the marriage bed."

Homer, The Illiad

Blood vessels come in two types, arteries and veins. Hypertension or high blood pressure is a condition in which the pressure in the arteries is too high. Medical literature enumerates dozens of different causes of high blood pressure, including narrowing of the arteries, mineral imbalances, kidney disease and water retention. Most of the drugs used to treat this condition, including diuretics (to induce water loss) and various enzyme inhibitors and blockers, have dangerous side effects.

In the previous chapter, we discussed a new model for heart disease, one that explains many other diverse medical phenomena including high blood pressure. It is easy to see that if the pump, that is the osmotic gradient, is weak, the body must increase the pressure in some other way. It does so, like any good engineer, by narrowing the outflow pipes, in this case the arteries, and making them less flexible (we call this arteriosclerosis). These are wonderful compensatory mechanisms, but it would be much better to simply increase the efficiency of the pump by changing the diet. Thus, the first step in treating high blood pressure is to adopt the diet and therapies for heart disease proposed in Chapter 3.

Another clue to the root cause of hypertension comes from the actual names of the blood vessels. The origin of the word "artery" is "Ares" or "Mars." From our earth-centered view, Mars is the symbol of all that is aggressive, active and warlike. Mars is the warrior image or the archetypal masculine force in nature. This picture seems to fit what we know about the active, forceful movement of the blood in the arterial circulation.

The venous system is quite different. Obviously, the word "vein" or "venous" shares a root with Venus, the goddess and the planet. In Greek mythology, Venus is known as Aphrodite, the nurturer, the giver of the harvest and archetypal feminine force. This also aptly describes the more passive flow of blood in the venous circulation.

High blood pressure often occurs when the fight-or-flight response of the sympathetic nervous system becomes excessive in the arteries, when the masculine qualities of aggressiveness, domination and anger become too strong and begin to overwhelm the more feminine and nurturing aspect of our nature. As we all know, neither force is bad, except when one overpowers the other. The masculine and the feminine need to work together, to nourish and support one another. Otherwise, the forceful tendencies of Mars win out, resulting in hypertension, a typically male disease; or the passive impulses of Venus predominate, resulting in varicose veins, a typically female disease. Varicose veins occur when the venous circulation is too sluggish, too passive, and the movement of the blood in the veins is unable to continue toward the heart. The blood becomes overly influenced by the force of gravity, and as it falls it creates the swollen, congested, painful veins that are the hallmark of this disease.

This model shows us the interconnection of the heart and circulation with the whole male-female polarity in particular, and with the reconciliation of opposites in general. The circulation is really the biological field where the soul lives out its life.

This model also helps explain the success I have had through the years in treating patients with diet and with homeopathic and herbal medicines based on copper, the metal that relates to the planet Venus and to the kidneys, the organs that regulate blood pressure. To understand the "gesture" of copper-containing herbs, we must examine how copper occurs in nature.

Globulins are oxygen-carrying proteins that occur in both animals and plants. They are similar in all respects except for the mineral that is found at the core. In mammals, the core mineral of globulin is iron or heme, hence the name hemoglobin (literally iron-globin). In plants, the analogous metal is magnesium. Chlorophyll is a magnesium globin, identical in every respect to hemoglobin except that it carries a magnesium molecule at its center instead of an iron molecule. In the mollusc family of bivalve shellfish, the mineral at the center of the globin is copper. The "blood" of molluscs has a bluish color, since this is the color of the copper-containing globin molecule.

Botticelli's painting of Venus standing on a clam shell as she arrives at the isle of Crete is full of hidden significance. Obviously this great master had access to esoteric teachings about Venus, the color blue, the mollusc family, and even the isle of Crete, which was the ancient world's richest supplier of copper.

An important copper-containing herb is chamomile. Although chamomile tea is yellow in color, the extract of chamomile has a bluish tinge, indicative of copper. Long valued for its ability to help release tension and spasms, gentle chamomile is the quintessential feminine medicine.

Rauwolfia serpentina is another valuable herb for the treatment of hypertension. Steiner wrote that rauwolfia gave the "gesture" of Venus and today we know that it is a copper-containing plant. Originally an Ayurvedic herb, it became popular in Western medicine as the source of Reserpine, a common hypertension medicine during the 1960s and 1970s. Rauwolfia seems to work by creating a release of tension in the central nervous system. As such, it was also used to treat various conditions of anxiety, and even mania. I have used rauwolfia extract for many years and found it to be a reliable, safe and effective medicine for bringing high blood pressure into the normal range.

Three case histories demonstrate how the problem of high blood pressure is related to an overemphasis on masculine characteristics. Mrs. G. L. was a 62-year-old woman with a five-year history of hypertension. Previously she had been treated with a lowfat, low-salt diet, as well as most of the normal medicines used for high blood pressure. She hated the diet and the side effects of the medicine. By the time she came to me, she had a dangerously high blood pressure of 220/130. She was adamant in her refusal to take more blood pressure medication. Her story was similar to that of many women who end up with hypertension. Her marriage was not good, and as the years went on and the hurts and disappointments built up, she increasingly armored herself. She assumed more "masculine" characteristics and suppressed her gentle, feminine side. Like so many women in her situation, she had no one who would accept her love and care. It was as though the warmth of her nurturing fell on stones instead of fertile soil. Even though her domestic situation did not change, her blood pressure gradually dropped to 160/80 with the appropriate diet, daily thirty-minute walks and copper-containing herbs.

Mr. D. F. was a 42-year-old man who complained of dizziness, ringing in his ears, frequent headaches and fatigue. He was a very high-strung person who worried because most of the male members of his family suffered from severe hypertension at an early age and died of coronary artery disease in their early forties. His blood pressure was in the range of 200/120, a level that is unsafe in both the short and long term. The rest of his examination was normal, and laboratory tests showed no evidence of organ damage or any other reasons for his high blood pressure. He was put on the same program as Mrs. L. and was able to bring his blood pressure down to about 160/90. He has generally felt well and never had to take conventional blood pressure medicines. Although he was not "cured" of his hypertension, he was able to lead a relatively symptom-free life.

Of particular note was the fact that the same medical problem occurred in virtually all the male members of his family, dating back at least two generations. In conventional medicine we might say that his hypertension and tendency to heart disease was genetic. I think "hereditary" is a better term because no one has ever isolated a gene or set of genes that causes hypertension so it cannot be said that the disease resides in the genes. But hypertension clearly resided in the male members of his clan.

One of Mr. F.'s primary struggles was to develop an identity and life-style different from that of his male relatives, a life-style that he perceived as a prison. Often when we try to break away from family patterns and search for new patterns or blueprints to help us model our lives, we experience uncertainty and even chaos in the soul. This struggle, like so many struggles, gets played out not only in the psyche but also in the body as well, as we all struggle for freedom from the bonds of our heredity.

In Mr. F.'s case, the struggle was clearly an attempt at liberation from the male dominance in his family life. Is it any wonder that the physical illness played itself out in the male part of his physiology, in his arteries, the domain of Mars? Many men are caught in this dilemma, as they struggle to find their inner feminine persona and liberate themselves from the confines of Mars aggression. This great life struggle has been immortalized in many of the myths that define our age, and to define it as a problem of genetics fails to honor the quest that many men must take and demeans the richness of the life of the soul.

Another case involved a 50-year-old woman who had suffered from hypertension for 20 years. She also had a severe case of psoriasis. At the time I saw her, red angry plaques covered well over a third of her entire skin surface. Her initial blood pressure, while on a beta-blocker (blood pressure medicine) was 210/120. Her impression was that the psoriasis skin lesions, were if not caused, at least exacerbated by the blood pressure medicine, which was also clearly not working. She had been following a lowfat diet for"health" reasons, along with the liberal use of protein supplements (which, by depleting vitamin A stores in the liver, can lead to skin conditions like psoriasis). Even though I was worried about the high level of her blood pressure, I decided to listen to her instincts, and stop the blood pressure medicine, use a high-fat diet as described in Chapter 3 and discontinue the protein powders.

I also suggested a four-week cleansing preparation consisting of about 15 different herbs formulated by Blessed Herb (See Appendix D). The herbal medicines are taken sequentially to increase the detoxification abilities of our bodies. In the first part of the cleanse, the herbs work on the bowels, resulting in three bowel movements per day. Then preparations are given in sequence for the liver, lungs, kidneys and finally the blood. This provides a thorough and gentle detoxificaiton program during which the patient eats normally. The cleanse restores good bacteria to the gut and often provides increased energy and vitality.

Three years later, her skin is completely clear and her blood pressure is below 130/90 most of the time. She also lost about 30 pounds as the increased fat content in her diet has mobilized and dissolved her fat stores as it has softened and moisturized her skin.

A note on the measurement of blood pressure: When I was in medical school, we were taught that normal blood pressure was anything under 140/90 or 100 plus the person's age over 90. Thus, for a 60-year-old patient, 160/90 is normal. However, today the values considered normal are considerably lower. Blood-pressure-lowering medicines are being used to bring blood pressure down to 120/70 or less, levels that for many people can actually be dangerously low. This situation is analogous to that of cholesterol, where the "risk" point, the number at which a person is said to be more at risk for heart disease, has been lowered from 240 to 200, with new guidelines implying that cholesterol levels should be below 180 mg/dL. By lowering the number at which the patient is said to be at risk, physicians can justify prescribing drugs to individuals who have nothing wrong with them. Blood pressure levels rise naturally and gradually with age; they may also go up under momentary stress—including the stress of having your blood pressure taken! If a patient has high blood pressure on the first reading, he should lie down and relax in a quiet room for about 15 minutes before a second reading is taken. Invariably this second reading is lower and often normal. Only when a second reading gives blood pressure numbers greater than the person's age plus 100 over 90, should the patient be diagnosed as hypertensive.

Nutrition

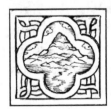

The usual treatment for high blood pressure restricts the patient to a low-salt, lowfat diet. Such a regimen may produce initial good results but this has nothing to do with the reduction of salt and fats because to achieve a low-salt, lowfat diet, it is necessary to avoid most processed foods. If a diet without salt is followed for any length of time, the patient will actually become weak, as salt is essential for digestion. And the right kinds of fats, as you now know, are absolutely essential for good health.

I do not restrict my hypertensive patients from salt. Rather, I suggest that they avoid all processed salt and use Celtic sea salt in liberal amounts. Celtic sea salt provides plentiful amounts of magnesium, which helps reduce high blood pressure. In addition, mineral-rich bone broth used in soups, stews and sauces will help with hypertensive conditions.

The patient should follow the general guidelines outlined in Chapter 3. Calves liver is a good source of copper and should be eaten once a week. Obviously, shellfish are another good choice.

Hypertensive patients should avoid consuming water, which can increase blood volume and edema (water retention); rather, liquids should be in the form of lacto-fermented beverages which hydrate the cells without upsetting the body's homeostasis. These beverages are also a good source of easily assimilated minerals.

Therapeutics

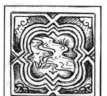
The basic therapy for high blood pressure is based on the use of copper-containing herbs. I prescribe a chamomile extract from Mediherb, 1-2 teaspoons per day, and rauwolfia extract from Herb Pharm at a dose of 4- 30 drops, 2 times per day.

I also prescribe hawthorn tablets from Mediherb, 1 tablet 3-4 times per day. As discussed in the previous chapter, hawthorn helps relax the walls of the arterial blood vessels and is a cardiotonic.

If the above dietary and medicinal interventions do not succeed in lowering the BP to the normal range, then the kidneys can be treated directly. The kidneys (and their adrenal glands) secrete two hormones that affect blood pressure levels. The first is angiotensin, the chemical in our bodies that determines the tone of our blood vessels, and hence our blood pressure. The second, aldosterone, is a mineralocorticoid, a hormone that determines salt and fluid balance. These hormonal systems can be influenced by conventional drugs, such as diuretics or ACE (angiotensin-converting enzyme) inhibitors that are commonly prescribed in conventional medicine to treat hypertension. In natural medicine we have access to safe medicines that cause diuresis and influence the kidney function. The first is Renafood from Standard Process, which contains the kidney protomorphogen and other kidney nutrients. This can be given at the dose of 1-2 tablets 3 times per day. The other medicine I use for hypertension is horsetail extract from Mediherb which has diuretic effects but is much safer than pharmaceutical diuretics. The dose is 1 teaspoon per day to help relieve edema and lower blood pressure.

The final therapy that should be mentioned is castor oil packs over the kidneys. They should be applied for one hour, at least 3-4 times per week. As we have discussed, castor oil relaxes the overaggressive sympathetic nervous system. Properly used, castor oil packs can bring about a physiological calming and subsequent lowering of blood pressure.

As for varicose veins, this condition requires extra amounts of flavonoids to increase the tone of the veins and thus facilitate our "pump." I recommend hawthorn tablets by Mediherb, at a dose of 2 tablets 2 times per day and horse chestnut complex by Mediherb, at a dose of 2 tablets 2 times per day for at least one year.

For skin conditions like psoriasis accompanying high blood pressure, I suggest the Blessed Herb cleanse.

Movement

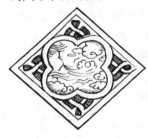

The gestures of hypertension are an upward contraction and a "water level" that is too high. Together—the rising of the water level plus contraction of the space in the upper body— these gestures constrict the personal space to a point above the heart. The relationship of gravity and levity is disturbed. Those suffering from high blood pressure have too much levity and not enough gravity; they do not let gravity work in their bodies. The best movers in the world have gravity—but that does not mean they are heavy.

Any exercises that help bring down the upward gesture and contraction of hypertension can be helpful, starting with the Water Level Gesture and also including Downright-Upright, Grounding, Pulley, Carriage Down/Carriage Up, Lowering the Sails and Shoulder Muscle Mapping. The serene Rice Paper Walk and Bestowing both help bring blood down from the head. The Lemniscate Dynamic is also excellent.

Chopping wood helps bring down blood pressure if done correctly by consciously lowering the center of gravity with every stroke. Similarly, Latin dancing can be very helpful as it helps shift the center of gravity lower to the ground, in contrast to ballet, which emphasizes levity.

Meditation

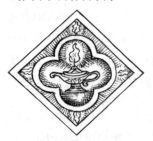

Male and female aspects of our being exist on both the soul and physical levels. To balance these polarities, represented by the arteries and Mars (aggression and dominance) and the veins and Venus (nurturing and receptivity), is the meditative content of your soul work. As you engage in your daily *Rückschau* Meditation, try to identify those activities, emotions and actions that are Mars-like and those that are Venus-like. If you suffer from hypertension, you will probably find a preponderance of the former. Your task, then, is to redress the balance, bringing the masculine qualities of your life more in harmony with those that are feminine.

The mental image that is most potent for working on the problem of hypertension is that of the reconciliation of opposites. Interestingly, this illness often occurs in those who aggressively and dogmatically believe in the truth of their position. I often suggest, just as an old history professor of mine once did, that you take a subject about which you feel passionate and argue in writing or verbally for the other side. Not only does this increase one's flexibility, a trait often lacking in patients with hypertension, but it also teaches that the truth lies not in absolutes, but in the reconciliation of opposites. This exercise will help you understand how to live comfortably with opposite polarities and to overcome the fundamental dynamic of this disease.

Summary

Nutrition

*	Avoid	Processed food
		Commercial salt
		Water
*	Emphasize	High-fat diet described in Chapter 3
		Celtic sea salt
		Bone broths
		Liver and shell fish
		Lacto-fermented beverages

Therapeutics

* Chamomile extract by Mediherb, 1-2 teaspoons per day.
* Rauwolfia extract by Herb Pharm, 4-30 drops in water 2 times per day, titrated to the needed dose.
* Hawthorn tablets by Mediherb, 1 tablet 3-4 times per day.
* Renafood from Standard Process, 1-2 tablets 3 times per day.
* Horsetail extract from Mediherb, 1 teaspoon per day.
* Castor oil packs three times a week over the adrenal glands.
* For varicose veins, horse chestnut complex by Mediherb, 2 tablets 2 times per day.
* For skin conditions, the Blessed Herb cleanse.

Movement

* Any exercises that help bring down the upward gesture and contraction of hypertension, especially the Water Level Gesture.
* Downright-Upright, Grounding, Pulley, Carriage Down/Carriage Up, Lowering the Sail and Shoulder Muscle Mapping.
* Rice Paper Walk and Bestowing.
* The Lemniscate Dynamic.
* Chopping Wood.
* Latin Dancing.

Meditation

* Identify masculine and feminine activities during your daily meditation.
* For a subject you feel passionate about, argue verbally or in writing for the other side.

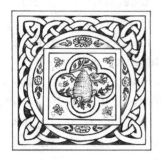

Chapter 5:
Diabetes

So sweet was ne'er so fatal.
Shakespeare's Othello

Diabetes is so common in America and other western countries that its presence in any human group has become a marker for civilization. Ironically, in no other field of western medicine has the promise of scientific breakthrough failed so poignantly as in that of diabetes.

Diabetes is characterized by abnormally high levels of sugar or glucose in the blood, which spills into the urine, causing it to be sweet. The disease was first described by the Greeks who called it *diabetes mellitus* or "honey passing through." Today there are at least 20 million diabetics in America, six million of whom must take shots of insulin daily. Scientists hailed the discovery of insulin in the 1920s as one of medicine's greatest achievements—as, in fact, it was. Insulin is a pancreatic hormone needed for the transfer of glucose from the blood to the cells. When this system fails—when the pancreas does not produce enough insulin or the insulin cannot get the glucose into the cells—then the sugar level in the blood remains abnormally high. This is the disease we call diabetes.

Originally, doctors thought that diabetes was simply a disease of insulin deficiency, a disease in which the pancreas was unable to produce enough insulin to meet the body's demands, and that it could be successfully managed once the right knowledge and technology were in place. Over time, researchers have produced better delivery systems for insulin, and ways to produce more purified and effective types of insulin—from porcine insulin to human insulin produced through genetic engineering. The medical profession has learned that giving insulin orally was unsuccessful, that subcutaneous injections were better, and that delivering it through a pump was best. Yet with all the improvements that have been made since 1920, diabetes remains one of the leading causes of death and disability in the western world. Complications of diabetes include heart disease and circulation problems, kidney disease, degeneration of the retina leading to blindness, neuropathy resulting in numbness, tingling, pain and burning in the extremities, foot ulcers leading to gangrene and high risk of infection.

Today, doctors realize that diabetes is a much more complicated condition than one of simple insulin deficiency. They have also discovered that there are two types of diabetes. Type I diabetes, which is also called insulin-dependent or childhood diabetes, usually develops before the age of 30, and involves a malfunction of the pancreas. Type I diabetes is thought of as autoimmune disease in which some trigger causes the body's immune system to attack its own insulin-producing cells (called the islets of Langerhans) in the pancreas. In time, the pancreas loses its ability to produce insulin, blood sugar rises, and serious adverse consequences, including death, can occur if the person is not supplied with insulin. As yet, there is no consensus as to what the autoimmune trigger for Type I diabetes might be. Some evidence points to early feeding of pasteurized cow's milk, soy products and grains, or the use of vaccines, as likely triggers. Type I diabetes is often very difficult to control and, if not successfully controlled, can lead to the early onset of many of the complications listed above.

Type II diabetes, which is much more common that Type I diabetes, has a different etiology. It is the form of diabetes that is literally crying out for a new perspective from the one currently offered by the medical profession.

In order to understand the diabetes epidemic in the Western world, and why the conventional treatment for this scourge has made almost no dent in its long-term impact on those who suffer from it, we must understand some basic biochemistry. The control of the blood sugar is one of the most fundamental requirements for a healthy life. Blood sugar levels can become abnormal in one of two ways: they can become too low, which we define as a blood sugar less than 80 and call hypoglycemia; or they can become too high, defined as a blood sugar over 110, which is called hyperglycemia. While neither hypoglycemia, nor hyperglycemia is good for your health, they appear to call forth very different reactions in the human being. For example, if your blood sugar drops below 40, you will become disoriented, confused, and if the situation persists, slip into a coma and die. This situation is a true medical emergency. When blood sugar is between 40-60, you feel shaky, jittery, anxious, sweaty, confused and irritable. When blood sugar is between 60-80 these same symptoms occur, but they are less severe.

The body reacts to the emergency situation of low blood sugar in many ways. When blood sugar even begins to drop below 80, the body produces a number of hormones, principally adrenaline and glucagon. The main effect of adrenaline is to make more sugar available to the cells. It is the production of adrenaline that accounts for the familiar shaky, jittery feeling that many have experienced during these hypoglycemic episodes. Glucagon helps raise blood sugar levels by increasing fat breakdown and stimulates the conversion of fat into sugar.

There may be as many as 10 or more hormonal or biochemical reactions that occur during the early stages of hypoglycemia. One is the release of growth hormone, which has also been found to increase blood sugar in times of stress. As you can see, the body is well prepared to ward off this potential emergency. It has multiple overlapping mechanisms to prevent a precipitous fall in blood sugar, and many of these reactions produce clear symptoms that provoke us into action. Severe hypoglycemia is clearly a situation our adaptive physiology has learned to avoid.

The situation is much different with respect to hyperglycemia. Many times during my practice I have asked a new diabetic patient how they felt and heard them reply, "A little tired, but not bad." Yet routine screening blood tests tell me that some of these unsuspecting patients have blood sugar levels as high as 400, almost 4 times the normal level. These people are at strong risk for all the major complications of diabetes including coronary artery disease and neurological disease, yet they feel nothing, their bodies give them little warning. Why is this?

Some have conjectured that the body has a hard time dealing with hyperglycemia because the conditions that cause it—namely overeating—are a relatively new phenomenon in human history. On the other hand, hypoglycemia induced by lack of food has been a frequent occurrence to which the body has adapted with a variety of mechanisms. Compared to dozens of hormones that are activated when our blood sugar drops too low, the body has only two mechanisms to deal with blood sugar that goes too high. One is exercise—any muscular activity drives the sugar from the blood into the muscle cells where it is used as fuel. The second is the production of insulin. Insulin production is the body's way of saying that the sugar level is too high, that the body is overfed with sugar. Insulin helps remove sugar from the blood into the cells where it is stored as fat. (It is interesting to note that the type of fat that is made by the body under the guidance of insulin is saturated fat.)

Understanding this basic physiology leads to some interesting conclusions. One is that controlling the level of insulin produced is the key to controlling obesity. For without insulin there can be no weight gain. People who lose the ability to make insulin (Type I diabetics) will never gain weight no matter how much food they eat unless they are supplemented with insulin. In fact, without insulin they literally starve to death.

The second conclusion we can draw is that the cause of Type II diabetes is actually quite simple. Type II diabetes occurs when for many years the consumption of foods that raise the blood sugar chronically exceeds the amount of sugar needed by the muscles for exercise. This forces the body to gradually make more and more insulin in order to bring this sugar level down. Eventually, the body cannot make enough insulin to lower the sugar level, the sugar level remains chronically high and the patient is diagnosed with diabetes.

Along the way a curious thing happens called insulin resistance. This means that as the blood sugars are chronically elevated, and the insulin levels are rising, the cells build a shield or wall around themselves to slow down this influx of excess sugar. Insulin resistance is a protective or adaptive response, it is the best the body can do to protect the cells from too much glucose. But as time goes on the sugar in the blood increases, more insulin is made by the pancreas to deal with this elevated sugar and the cells resist this sugar influx by becoming insulin resistant, in a sense by shutting the gates. This leads to the curious situation in which blood sugar levels are high but cellular sugar levels are low. The body perceives this as low blood sugar. The patient has low energy and feels hungry so he eats more, and the viscous cycle is under way.

Having a chronically elevated insulin level is detrimental for many other reasons. Not only do high insulin levels cause obesity (insulin tells your body to store fat), but they also signal that fluid should be retained, leading to edema and hypertension. Chronic high insulin provokes plaque development inside the arteries and also suppresses growth hormone needed for the regeneration of the tissues and many other physiological responses.

During the 1980s, researchers began to ask whether obesity, coronary artery disease, hypertension and other common medical problems that occur together are really separate diseases, or manifestations of one common physiological defect. The evidence now points to one defect and that is hyperinsulinemia, or excessive insulin levels in the blood. Hyperinsulinemia is the physiological event that links virtually all of our degenerative diseases. It is the biochemical corollary or marker of the events described in the previous chapter on heart disease.

The question we need to answer, then, is what causes hyperinsulinemia? In basic biochemistry we learn about the three basic food groups: fats, proteins and carbohydrates. Under normal circumstances it is the carbohydrates that are transformed into the sugar that goes into the blood. Fats are broken down into fatty acids and become the building blocks for hormones, prostaglandins and cell membranes. Proteins are broken down into amino acids which then are rebuilt into the various proteins in our bodies. Carbohydrates are used for one thing only and that is energy generation. This allows us to define a "balanced" diet, which is one where the energy used in movement and exercise equals the energy provided by the carbohydrates we consume.

For a person of a given size, protein and fat requirements are relatively fixed and can be controlled with the appetite. (It is actually difficult to overeat fats and proteins, as our bodies make us nauseous when we do.) However, carbohydrate intake should be intimately related to our level of activity. If we run a marathon every day, a balanced diet would probably include about 300 grams of carbohydrates per day, the amount contained in 20 potatoes or 6 brownies. If we sit on the couch all day, obviously our requirement for energy food will be less. In this case a balanced diet would include only about 65-70 grams of carbohydrates per day. Any more, and our bodies are forced to make more insulin and the whole vicious cycle begins.

The problem of diabetes can be summarized by saying that the western diet has us eating like marathon runners, when in fact most of us simply sit on the couch. When we regulate the carbohydrate intake to match our exercise level, Type II diabetes cannot develop; and, in fact, I have found that most cases of Type II diabetes respond well to treatment when these basic principles are kept in mind. Type I diabetes responds equally well to a high-fat, low-carbohydrate diet. In fact, before insulin was available, the only way to treat Type I diabetes was a high-fat diet from which carbohydrate foods were completely excluded as the body does not need insulin to assimilate proteins and fats.

Unless eaten to great excess, fats do not contribute to diabetes—with one exception. *Trans* fatty acids in partially hydrogenated vegetable oils can cause insulin resistance. When these man-made fats get built into the cell membrane, they interfere with the insulin receptors. In theory, this means that one could develop insulin resistance without eating lots of carbohydrates. But in practice, partially hydrogenated vegetable oils are always used in the very high-carbohydrate foods—french fries, cookies, crackers, donuts, and margarine on bread or potatoes—that flood the bloodstream with sugar. *Trans* fatty acids in modern processed foods present a double whammy for which the human species has developed no defenses.

Ms. G came to me about 2 years ago with a story that is sadly familiar in today's internal medicine clinics. She had a strong family history of diabetes, and one of her strongest and most fearful memories was watching her mother die from complications of diabetes at her same age of 52. When I first saw her, she had been diagnosed with diabetes, hypertension, obesity, arthritis, GERD (reflux disease), restless leg syndrome and "edema" (fluid retention) in her legs. The medications she took included an oral hypoglycemic (diabetes) drug, Lasix (a diuretic), a beta-blocker (for hypertension, which also "causes" elevated blood sugar), quinine for her legs, Voltaren (for her arthritis, which "causes" kidney failure and stomach irritation), a reflux medicine for her stomach irritation, and potassium for the potassium deficiency caused by the diuretic. She also took Synthroid (a thyroid supplement) for her long-standing hypothyroidism. She ate a"normal" American diet and needless to say felt horrible! Her doctors had told her that all her illnesses were "well managed" yet she knew somewhere in her heart she was headed down the same path as her mother.

From the information presented in the chapters on heart disease and hypertension it is easy to conclude that first of all her "pump" was broken due to her poor diet, hence the hypertension, stiff joints (arthritis), edema, hypothyroidism (excessive coldness) and restless legs. Furthermore, the preponderance of carbohydrates and *trans* fats in her diets had led directly to the elevated sugars in her blood, hence the diabetes.

There is, however, another aspect to her story that I would like to highlight. That is, there seems to be some "law" at work in people's lives that leads them to confront that which they fear the most. I call it the "law of freedom," freedom because living our lives afraid, in a subtle, energetic kind of way attracts us to that very thing we fear. Often people who have been imprisoned or sustained some horrible ordeal emerge with a sense of freedom that the rest of us can only envy. Perhaps this is the basis of many of the initiation rites practiced by native peoples as they intentionally allowed their young people to confront their fears. This crisis in this woman's life, coming when she felt so miserable, was so burderned by the weight of her poor health, and so worried about her future, transformed her medical appointments into a venue to confront her life. Luckily, she took up the challenge.

Two years later and with the simple approach outlined in these chapters, her only medicines consist of a very small dose of Armour Thyroid (30 mg per day) and gymnema, 1 tablet two times per day. Her weight is down, her blood pressure is normal, her legs feel good, her reflux is gone and and she feels well overall. Her blood sugar still runs high and when it goes higher she tends to get yeast infections. We let these run their course because the yeast seems to "biodegrade" the sugar and after every course of yeast "infection" her blood sugar declines to normal.

Nutrition

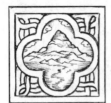

Studies of indigenous peoples by Weston Price and many others reveal the wisdom of native diets and life-style. For not only did so-called primitive peoples follow the "perfect" anti-diabetes life-style program, but their diets incorporated specific foods only recently discovered to play an important role in the prevention and treatment of this disease. In general, indigenous peoples had a low carbohydrate intake coupled with a lot of physical activity. In fact, those peoples especially prone to diabetes today, such as Native Americans and Inuits, consumed virtually no carbohydrate foods. In warmer climates, where tubers and fruits were more abundant, these foods were usually fermented and consumed with adequate protein and fat. It is only in the change to Western habits that their so-called "genetic" tendency to diabetes manifests.

There are three other nutritional factors in indigenous diets that are helpful for diabetics. First, the diets were rich in trace minerals. Modern science has shown us that trace mineral deficiencies—particularly deficiencies in zinc, vanadium and chromium—inhibit insulin production and absorption. Without vanadium, sugar in the blood cannot be driven into the cells and chromium is necessary for carbohydrate metabolism and the proper functioning of the insulin receptors. Zinc is a co-factor in the production of insulin. Traditional foods were grown in mineral-rich soil, contained mineral-rich bone broth and salt, and included mineral-rich water or beverages made with such water. In the modern diet, the best sources of zinc are red meats and shell fish, particularly oysters. Extra virgin unfiltered olive oil supplies vanadium, and chromium is found in nutritional yeast, molasses and organ meats like liver.

Second, indigenous peoples ate a portion of their animal foods, such as fish, milk or meat, uncooked—either raw or fermented. This strategy conserves vitamin B_6, which is easily destroyed by heat. Vitamin B_6 is essential for carbohydrate metabolism; it is often the rate-limiting vitamin of the B vitamin complex because it is one of the most difficult to obtain in the diet. Indigenous peoples intuitively understood the need to eat a portion of their animal foods completely raw.

Third, traditional peoples consumed foods rich in fat-soluble vitamins, including butterfat from grass-fed animals, organ meats, shellfish, fish liver oils and the fats of certain animals like bear and pig. High levels of vitamin A are absolutely essential for the diabetic because diabetics are unable to convert the carotenes in plant foods into true vitamin A. Vitamin A and vitamin D also protect against the complications of diabetes, such as retina and kidney problems. And vitamin D is necessary for the production of insulin.

Putting all these rules together, we find that the general diet recommended in this book and in *Nourishing Traditions* fits all the requirements for the prevention and treatment of diabetes. The diet should include sufficient trace minerals from organic and biodynamic foods, Celtic sea salt, bone broths, shellfish, red meat, organ meats, unfiltered olive oil and nutritional yeast. High levels of vitamins A and D are essential, as are raw animal foods to provide vitamin B_6.

Most importantly, diabetics must strictly limit their daily carbohydrate intake. While the optimum amount of carbohydrate foods depends somewhat on activity levels, most diabetics need to start on a 60-gram-per-day carbohydrate regimen until their sugars normalize. I recommend *The Schwarzbein Principle* as guide to carbohydrate consumption. The book contains easy-to-use charts that allow you to assess carbohydrate values. During the initial period of treatment, which can take up to a year, average blood sugar levels should be determined by a blood test that measures HgbA1c, a compound that indicates average blood sugar levels over a period of about 6 weeks. Carbohydrate restriction will also help with weight loss.

For Type II diabetics, this diet should help both blood sugar levels and weight to normalize, after which the daily carbohydrate intake can be liberalized to about 72 grams per day. This level should be maintained throughout the life of the diabetic. The same approach applies to the Type I diabetic, although it may not allow him to get off insulin. However, disciplined carbohydrate restriction should reduce insulin requirements, help keep blood sugar stable and, most importantly, prevent the many side effects associated with diabetes.

Please note that in this approach there are no restrictions on total food intake, nor do we pay attention to the so-called glycemic index of various carbohydrate foods. Fats consumed with any carbohydrate food will lower the glycemic index. Worrying about glycemic indices adds nothing to the therapy and only increases time spent calculating food values rather than enjoying its goodness. One should eat abundantly from good fats and proteins—only carbohydrate foods need to be restricted.

Supplements for the diabetic should include cod liver oil at a level that provides 20,000 IU vitamin A per day, and nutritional yeast for B vitamins and minerals. Another important supplement for the diabetic is evening primrose oil, borage oil or black currant oil, all of which supply a fatty acid called GLA, which the diabetic cannot make in sufficient quantities to be healthy.

Therapeutics

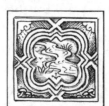 Plants speak to us of their properties in many ways. Plants like mistletoe show us their effects through the attributes of their life cycle. Others, like echinacea, reveal their inner nature through the attributes of their flowers. For diabetics, one plant that stands out above all others as the main medicine to use for therapy. That plant, *Gymnema sylvestre*, has been prescribed for diabetes in Ayruvedic medicine for thousands of years. In modern times, it has made its way into conventional therapy and shown its worth in numerous research papers. Ayruvedic practitioners referred to gymnema as the "sugar-buster." If you chew some leaves of this inauspicious plant, you eliminate the ability of your taste buds to perceive the sweet taste. If you eat a piece of candy or even some honey ten minutes later, it will taste like chalk. One can almost hear a slight chuckle emanating from the plant as if to say

"I truly am the sugar buster."

Gymnema also helps reduce blood sugar levels. It does this by lowering insulin resistance, much like conventional oral diabetic drugs, and also by increasing the secretion of insulin from the pancreas. Furthermore, gymnema is currently the only medicine we know of that actually helps regenerate destroyed pancreatic islet cells in Type I diabetics. Use of gymnema may not completely reverse Type I diabetes, but I have found that it always improves glucose control. Thus, gymnema addresses within itself the multifactorial etiology of diabetes in that it helps your body make more insulin, if that is needed, and it makes the insulin more effective.

I prescribe Mediherb gymnema tablets for all my diabetic patients and not once has it failed to improve the glycemic control and lower the HgbA1c levels. The dose used is 1 tablet 2-3 times per day. With gymnema there is no risk of provoking the dangerous hypoglycemic reactions so common with the conventional oral diabetic medication.

The other medicines I use for diabetes include Diaplex, the Standard Process diabetes preparation at a dose of 2-3 capsules 3 times per day, Organic Minerals by Standard Process, 1 tablet 3 times per day, and Pancreatrophin, the protomorphogen for the pancreas, 1-2 tablets 3 times per day. These preparations of organically grown food contain abundant trace minerals as well as vitamin B$_6$ from raw animal extracts.

Movement

The main gesture in diabetes is the body turning against itself; Type I diabetes involves an autoimmune reaction where the movements are turned inward to such an extent that they actually destroy the islets of the pancreas. In Type II diabetes, the gesture is one of heaviness, even if the patient is not physically heavy. Both types of diabetics need to learn that there is a direct connection between what we do with our limbs and our inner processes. We literally "organ"-ize the inner processes with rhythm, proportion and measure expressed in the limbs. The diabetic needs to spread out from the torso, the metabolic area.

Diabetics, especially those with Type I diabetes, may have trouble dealing with everyday situations; they often panic at small things or are unable to give a proper or adequate social response. Thus, they need to learn to meet these situations on the border of their personal space. The Personal Space Gesture, the Wrestling Stance and Penguin Wrestling can all be very helpful to the diabetic.

For all the diseases, it is helpful to create the space around the organs so that the natural rhythms of the organs can take their proper role again. With the diabetic especially, the space of the organs, particularly the pancreas, has become congested; the organs have taken on frightened, cramped, constricted gestures.

Any movement that involves the limbs, that emphasizes "up and out," is helpful to the diabetic, such as Abdominal Massage, Knee Mapping, the Victory Stretch, the Crest, the Sundial and the Dipole.

Rhythmic, joyful exercise in the out-of-doors is essential for the diabetic, exercise such as walking, gardening, swimming and sports. Diabetics should aim for 30 minutes per day, with one or two days per week spent largely outdoors participating in some gentle, enjoyable physical exertion.

It is not only exercise that the diabetic needs, it is levity, levity that transforms the body and its surrounding space into uplifting gestures. Thus dance, or even jump-roping, would be more appropriate than lumbering exercise on a treadmill.

Meditation

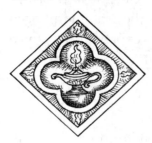

The dietary, therapeutic and exercise guidelines for diabetics are effective only if they are followed to the letter. Often my patients have difficulty adhering to these suggestions because food has too many other meanings for them—food may be the primary source of emotional comfort or even the primary relief from boredom. Thus for diabetics, the soul force most urgently required is that of resolve, and meditation exercises to strengthen one's ego are a necessity. For some, this may mean looking at the source of emotional wounds in one's life; for others moving forward into a program of meditation alone can be effective. The *Rückschau* Meditation can serve as the primary means to developing the objective consciousness that is the basis of a strong ego. This exercise will strengthen the thinking and sharpen the will, thereby giving the diet and movement approach a chance to work.

RECOMMENDED READING

    The Schwarzbein Principle by Dianna Schwarzbein
    Life without Bread by Wolfgang Lutz and Christian Allan

Summary

Nutrition

* Avoid Excess carbohydrates and all processed carbohydrates (sugar and white flour)

  Foods containing hydrogenated fats (*trans* fatty acids)

* Emphasize Carbohydrate restriction to 60 grams per day until blood sugar and HgbA1c are normal. Thereafter, about 70 grams per day depending on activity level

  Raw meat, fish and milk products for vitamin B_6

  Fats and organ meats rich in vitamins A and D

  Unfiltered olive oil for vanadium

  Red meat and oysters for zinc

  Organic and biodynamic foods, bone broths, Celtic sea salt and other sources of trace minerals

* Supplements Cod liver oil to provide 20,000 IU vitamin A for adults and 10,000 IU for children

  Acerola or amalaki powder, 1/4 teaspoon 2 times per day in water

  Evening primrose, borage or black currant oil, 1000 mg per day

Therapeutics

* Gymnema by Mediherb, 1 tablet 2-3 times per day.
* Diaplex by Standard Process, 2-3 capsules 3 times per day.
* Organic Minerals by Standard Process, 1 tablet 3 times per day.
* Pancreatrophin PMG, 1 tablet 3 times per day.

Movement

* The Personal Space Gesture, the Wrestling Stance and Penguin Wrestling to create space around the organs.
* Abdominal Massage, Knee Mapping, the Victory Stretch, the Crest, the Sundial and the Dipole to emphasize "up and out."
* Rhythmic, joyful exercise in the out-of-doors at least 30 minutes each day.
* Dance, or even jump-roping, to encourage levity.

Meditation

* *Rückschau* Meditation to strengthen the will.

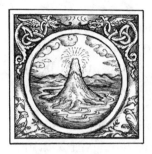

Chapter 6:
Diseases of Adrenal Cortex Insufficiency - Asthma, Allergies, Eczema

Turning and turning in the widening gyre
The falcon cannot hear the falconer;
Things fall apart; the center cannot hold;
Mere anarchy is loosed upon the world,
The blood-dimmed tide is loosed, and everywhere
The ceremony of innocence is drowned;
The best lack all convictions, while the worst
Are full of passionate intensity.

W.B. Yeats
The Second Coming

One of the most curious phenomena of modern medicine concerns the use of cortisone in its many forms. As anyone who has ever been a patient knows, doctors prescribe cortisone and its derivatives for practically all of our modern medical conditions: prednisone for poison ivy; cortisone inhalers for asthma; cortisone ointments for eczema, psoriasis and many other skin rashes; prednisone for ulcerative colitis and other inflammatory bowel diseases; cortisone for arthritis, bursitis and tendonitis; injectable steroids for severe allergic reactions; and even prednisone as a component of many cancer therapies.

Since cortisone and its derivatives are all hormonal products made by our adrenal gland, specifically the adrenal cortex, we are justified in asking whether in all these diverse illnesses, the underlying cause involves a problem with the adrenal gland. After all, if we give thyroid hormone to a patient, we would expect therapeutic benefits only for patients with thyroid disorders. A treatment with thyroid hormone extract will not help a person with constipation or dry skin unless the cause of these problems is a thyroid disorder. According to the same logic, a treatment with corti-

sone will help a person with some sort of inflammation (skin inflammation as eczema, lung inflammation as asthma, bowel inflammation as colitis) only if the cause
of these problems is an adrenal cortex disorder.

To fully understand the origins of the various inflammatory diseases, we must
examine more deeply the functions of the adrenal gland. In so doing, we will again
see the importance of achieving balance between the various systems in the body.

The adrenal gland is a small organ that sits like a hat on top of our kidneys,
hence its old name of suprarenal gland (above the kidney). About the size of a large
walnut and encased in fat, the gland has two distinct sections, the adrenal medulla
(middle), which makes adrenaline and its derivatives; and the adrenal cortex, which
makes cortisone and its relatives—glucocorticoids, which regulate sugar metabolism
and inflammation; mineralocorticoids, which regulate salt balance; precursors to the
sex hormones like testosterone and estrogen; and many other regulatory hormones.
Until about the 1930s, the function of this gland was unknown, or at least not ac-
knowledged by the mainstream medical profession. Occasionally surgeons removed
both adrenal glands, which always resulted in the rapid demise of the patient. Later,
after the discovery of cortisone, the crucial regulatory functions of the adrenal gland
gained recognition.

The adrenal cortex, like all of our glands, works via a feedback control mechanism connected to our central nervous system. The pituitary gland secretes a hormone called ACTH in response to the lowering of adrenal hormone concentrations in
the blood, or as part of a variety of biorhythms that govern the rhythmic nature of
hormonal secretions. In other words, when the concentration of adrenal cortex products like cortisone in the blood stream goes down, the pituitary, located in our brain,
senses this drop and secretes ACTH into the blood stream. This in turn stimulates the
adrenal cortex to raise the blood level of cortisone. When cortisone levels normalize,
ACTH secretion shuts off and cortisone production ceases. Under normal circumstances, this regulation occurs in a rhythmical fashion with ACTH levels peaking
every day at 7:00 in the morning.

Hormone secretions comprise the essence of mind-body phenomena with the
mind (brain) and body (glands) working together to create a proper rhythmic functioning of our physiology. While it is difficult to pinpoint where and how this remarkable system breaks down, in most cases glandular dysfunction occurs when the
gland in question becomes unable to respond effectively to the brain's messages. In
the case of adrenal cortex insufficiency, the levels of ACTH from the pituitary may be
sufficient but the adrenal response is weak, and the gland cannot produce sufficient
quantities of adrenal hormones. If the deficient hormone is a glucocorticoid, the
body will experience a disruption of blood sugar levels, leading most likely to hy-

poglycemia (low blood sugar) with symptoms such as sugar cravings, light-headedness, weakness, jitters and fatigue, as well as chronic inflammation manifesting as allergies, asthma or rashes. If the deficient hormone is a mineralocorticoid, then a salt imbalance will occur with the resultant edema (water retention). If the deficient hormones are precursors to the sex hormones, then abnormal sexual symptoms such as hirsutism (excessive hair growth), irregular menses, osteoporosis or a decline in libido will occur. These problems stem not so much from a simple hormone defect as from a mixture of imbalance and deficiency.

Another aspect of optimal adrenal function involves the balance between the adrenal medulla, which makes adrenaline, and the adrenal cortex which makes the corticoid or steroid hormones. Adrenaline is *the* central chemical of the sympathetic nervous system. It revs up the body to make the fight-or-flight response when we find ourselves under stress or in danger. In contrast, the adrenal cortex products help regulate metabolism, fluids and chemical balances, and therefore stimulate the nutritive parasympathetic nervous system. Thus the adrenal gland plays a key role in regulating the balance of the sympathetic and parasympathetic nervous system, so important to Cayce's thinking. From the viewpoint of Steiner's philosophy, the medulla with its outpourings of adrenaline represents the active, more aggressive nature of the Nerve-Sense pole while the adrenal cortex, with its outpourings of "chill out" corticoid products, represents the healing nature of the Metabolic pole.

As we have seen, the sympathetic nervous system refers to the regulation of the more active functions. Whenever a situation occurs in which our bodies become primed for intense physical activity, the adrenal glands release adrenaline which dilates the pupils, makes more glucose available to the muscles and raises the heart rate, and it is the sympathetic nervous system that accomplishes these tasks. By contrast, when the body requires nutritive or rebuilding activities, such as storage of fat or relaxation of muscles, then the parasympathetic system comes into play. In other words, the sympathetic nervous system responds to short-term stress, whereas the parasympathetic system supports long-term adaptation. Adrenal insufficiency results from a combination of insufficient raw materials to allow for adequate production of adrenal cortex hormones coupled with chronic stress that calls for constant outpourings of adreneline.

As we all know, modern people live with a constant barrage of stressful, challenging events, at levels most likely unequaled in human history. These events require a flight-or-fight response, but in most cases fight or flight cannot be carried out. Consider a drive home in noisy rush-hour traffic after a day of fighting with manufacturers or insurance companies on the phone; or the act of watching television in which one is continually presented with active, even aggressive images; or the experiences of vulnerable children living with abusive parents. In situations such as these, the body wants to fight or flee—but such responses are socially inappropriate.

As both Steiner and Cayce pointed out, a series of intense emotional challenges or shocks throws our system out of balance. Specifically, the adrenal medulla becomes overactive, and our ability to balance the outpourings of adrenaline with the nurturing and healing activity of the adrenal cortex grows weak.

Today, something like half our population suffers from conditions that require adrenal cortex support. The initial reaction of patients to the use of these medicines is usually nothing short of miraculous—pains vanish, bloody diarrhea clears up and difficult skin problems melt away. Unfortunately, for most people this is the classic Faustian bargain, for within a short time, not only do the original symptoms return, necessitating higher doses, but the side effects of cortisone begin to show up.

The side effects of cortisone, prednisone and similar drugs are legendary. They include diabetes, osteoporosis, edema of the face, mood swings, stomach ulcers and, very importantly, adrenal suppression. In other words, your own adrenal glands shut off their production of these valuable hormones. Why not, since the prednisone has essentially "told" them they are no longer needed. This bargain, then, becomes a nightmare as the effectiveness of the drugs wears off, side effects become more serious and the patient is unable to stop taking the medication.

True relief from asthma, allergies and other symptoms of adrenal insufficiency can only be achieved by rebuilding the gland with proper nutrition and by re-establishing the balance of the adrenal/pituitary system through various activities that heal the Emotional Body.

Diseases of adrenal cortex insufficiencey may involve other glands besides the adrenals. The "pituitary-endocrine" axis refers to the group of endocrine organs controlled by secretions of the pituitary gland including not only the adrenals (controlled through the secretion of ACTH) but also the thyroid gland (controlled through secretions of TSH, thyroid stimulating hormone), the ovaries (controlled through LH or leutinizing hormone) and the testicles (also controlled through secretion of LH). This axis lies deep at the heart of the brain-body or mind-body connection and responds best to treatment of the entire group, rather than of isolated organs. Treatments outlined for thyroid insufficiency (in Chapter 8 on chronic fatigue) and for diseases involving the reproductive system (Chapters 9 and 10) should accompany those outlined here for the adrenal glands.

According to Dr. Broda Barnes, a researcher who looked carefully at thyroid disorders during the 1950s, the condition called hypothyroidism or underactive thyroid is more frequent than commonly recognized. Dr. Barnes believed that blood tests do not accurately determine thyroid function—often people with underactive thyroid glands have normal results on blood tests. He believed that body temperature taken immediately upon awakening best determined thyroid function. The thermometer is held in the armpit for about 10 minutes. A reading of 98.0 or below for several days in a row indicates low thyroid function, especially when accompanied by other symptoms of hypothyroidism such as lack of energy, weight gain, thinning hair, dental caries, difficulty in concentrating and frequent allergies.

Another organ that seems to participate in allergic diseases is the spleen. In fact, in Europe during the 1930s and 1940s, the most widespread therapy for allergic diseases was desiccated spleen extract. The mythology behind this therapy is fascinating. The common thread of all allergic diseases is that the tissue involved becomes swollen, weepy and expanded. Another aspect is that these imbalances have a rhythmical quality. Hay fever, for example, comes with a change of season and asthma worsens at night. How does the spleen relate with these phenomena?

Rudolf Steiner revived the medieval notion that the spleen is associated with the planet Saturn, the god or force depicted as Kronos, popularly known as Father Time. Saturn lies at the outermost limit of the planetary system that we can experience with our naked eye, so it functions as a kind of shell or border to our consciousness or awareness. Kronos also has the task of timekeeper for our solar system. In these two aspects we can see clear associations with what we know about the function of the spleen; for the spleen also performs these two functions of timekeeper and limit-setter on overexuberant life forces. The main function of the spleen is to remove the cellular elements of the blood—like red blood cells, which carry oxygen, and white blood cells, which confer immunity—when their appointed time is up. After a red blood cell has been in circulation 120 days—often to the very day—the spleen digests and recycles it. Likewise, it keeps time for all the cellular elements of our blood, According to Chinese medicine, the spleen also regulates the rhythm of our digestion. Truly, this Wise Old Man living inside us not only keeps time for us and conserves our resources, but also keeps our blood and our metabolism within bounds—exactly those properties that are weak in an illness like hay fever, where we become swollen and weepy on a rhythmical basis and our metabolism or fluid element seems to know no boundaries.

Traditional peoples associated Kronos and his organ, the spleen, with the metal lead, which can also be clearly seen to dampen the metabolism, destroy excessive red blood cells and function as an impenetrable barrier. The symptoms of lead poisoning are abdominal pains, rupture of the red blood cells, anemia and eventual neurological degeneration. Containers or vessels are made of lead when the contents require protection from outside influences such as X-rays, as lead is the best of the known substances for forming an impassable boundary. We can use these principles of the spleen and its metal lead to create balance when the metabolism is too lively, the rhythm is off, and things are weepy, swollen and without boundary, as happens with allergies.

About 5 years ago Mr. D.W., a 35-year-old school teacher, came to my office wondering whether there was any way to get off the steroid inhalers, bronchodilators and occasional doses of prednisone that he took for his severe allergies to animals, dust and other environmental agents. When he was under stress at school or at home, he often had full-blown asthma-allergy attacks with flu-like symptoms. He normally ate a lowfat diet to try to "stay in shape," and he drank a lot of water, a common practice among people who weight train. As discussed in Chapter 3 on heart disease, the healthy water in our bodies is the water we make from fats. That is the "water" that gets our pump going, that enlivens us and keeps us warm as it stimulates a healthy circulation. When we are fat-deficient we become dehydrated so that thirst "forces" us to drink a lot of water. Then we become water-logged and swollen. This can show up as inflammation (excessive wateriness) in the lungs and other mucus membranes and manifest as hay fever and asthma. Upon starting an appropriate high-fat diet with lots of nourishment for his adrenal glands, he was gradually able to wean himself off all his asthma medicines. For the last few years he has taken only Drenamin, a Standard Process remedy, to support adrenal function, desiccated spleen for the "allergies" and, on the really high-pollen days, an herb called euphrasia for congestion. He has taken no prednisone in over 5 years. He drinks much less water now on his new diet, and is more fit than ever, in spite of less time spent on weight training.

The following suggestions form the basis for treatment of all allergic diseases including, but not limited to, hay fever, eczema, asthma, colitis and many other conditions.

Nutrition

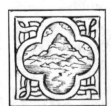 The pituitary-adrenal axis, like all of the body's systems, requires nourishment for optimal performance. When the raw materials used by a gland to produce its end product are in short supply, or are themselves "distorted," then imbalance will result. The nutrients most relevant to adrenal function are cholesterol, vitamin B_6, vitamin C complex, sodium and, of course, the fat-soluble nutrients A and D.

It is important to remember that all adrenal cortex products are derived from cholesterol. I can count literally hundreds of patients I have seen throughout the years who followed a strict lowfat or vegan diet and were thrilled because their total cholesterol dropped below 150; but far too often these same patients suffered from the characteristic symptoms of adrenal insufficiency—allergies, hay fever, eczema, menstrual irregularities, hypoglycemia, sugar cravings and fatigue. I can only wonder whether these cases were largely a result of the adrenal gland lacking sufficient raw materials with which to make its regulatory products. My suspicions have often been confirmed when a dramatic resolution of these symptoms has occurred after the patient makes the recommended dietary changes.

It should be noted that the enzyme system used by the body to produce the various steroid hormones (the P450 cytochrome enzyme system) is inhibited by *trans* fatty acids from partially hydrogenated vegetable oils—the kind of fats found in margarines, shortenings and almost all commercially prepared snack foods, french fries and salad dressings. Thus, avoidance of these foods is key to restoration of adrenal function.

Another critical nutrient for adrenal function is vitamin B_6, which participates in carbohydrate metabolism and glucocorticoid regulation. Animal products are the richest source of vitamin B_6. This water-soluble nutrient is very heat sensitive and thus is primarily available through *unheated* animal foods. It is therefore logical to conclude that one factor contributing to an increase in allergic and inflammatory illnesses this century is our abandonment of raw milk and other unheated animal products in the diet.

Vitamin C is also crucial to adrenal function, and here I specifically mean the complex of substances that occur naturally with vitamin C, and not just plain ascorbic acid. Some of these substances, such as quercetin, are well known for their anti-allergic effects, while other cofactors such as bioflavonoids, manganese and copper are also in short supply in the modern diet. Vitamin C complex is mostly found is unheated food from many sources such as fresh, organically grown fruits and vegetables eaten raw or lightly steamed, sprouted seeds and fermented foods—raw sauerkraut is an especially rich source of vitamin C. It is interesting to note that Native Americans included small amounts of foods such as pine needles and raw buffalo adrenal glands in their diets in order to protect themselves from illnesses similar to those of adrenal cortex insufficiency; and until the mid-20th century, the basic source of vitamin C complex for Americans was raw cow's milk.

The disappearance of raw milk, which supplies in abundance the nutrients vital to adrenal function—cholesterol, B_6 and vitamin C, along with the fat-soluble activators necessary for their utilization—is probably the single fundamental reason that allergies and chronic inflammatory diseases have steadily increased during the past few decades. With all the stress that modern life puts on the adrenal gland, perhaps the greatest stress of all has been a dietary one, in which hormone-treated, pasteurized skim milk from unhealthy cows kept in barns and given inappropriate feed has replaced fresh, raw, whole milk from healthy pasture-fed cows.

The fat-soluble nutrients, so important to the findings of Dr. Weston Price, also play a key role in the function of the pituitary and adrenal glands. Every step of the conversion of cholesterol into the various adrenal cortex hormones requires vitamin A. Vitamin A along with vitamin D are also key to assimilation of minerals needed by the entire endocrine system.

Another nutrient needed for healthy adrenal function is sodium. This is one reason that salt-free diets cause fatigue. Those with depleted adrenal function need liberal amounts of salt in their diets, and by this I mean unrefined Celtic sea salt. Thus, all store-bought foods should be avoided, but it is important to add unrefined Celtic sea salt to the food you prepare—in fact, use as much of this high-quality salt as you like. Zucchini is an excellent source of naturally occurring sodium and should be eaten on a daily basis in soups and salads, or lightly cooked as a vegetable.

In addition to inclusion of liberal amounts of nutrient-dense foods, the dietary treatment for allergic diseases should be based on the fact that the glucocorticoid hormones that control blood sugar also regulate the inflammatory condition. Therefore, the diet to combat allergies should be similar to the diet for hypoglycemia (low blood sugar) and diabetes; that is, a diet in which the use of refined carbohydrates, pasta, white flour, sugar and other sweeteners is strictly avoided. Even whole grains and potatoes should be limited to 25 percent or less of the diet until the symptoms are largely resolved.

Another substance that puts a great deal of stress on the adrenal gland is caffeine. Caffeine stimulates the production of adrenaline—that's why a cup of coffee makes us more alert. But continued reliance on caffeine in the form of coffee, tea, cocoa and soft drinks leads to the same kind of imbalance that occurs when a person is under constant stress—the adrenal medulla is constantly secreting adrenaline while the adrenal cortex becomes exhausted in the effort to balance these secretions with healing (corticoid) products. Giving up coffee and tea is a difficult but extremely important step in the process of overcoming inflammatory diseases. How much better to achieve steady, unlimited energy and alertness through a diet of nutrient-dense foods than to suffer the vicious cycle of the coffee drinker—bursts of nervous energy followed by periods of let-down and exhaustion.

A key component of the healing diet is high-quality butter and cultured cream. There is no need to skimp on these beneficial fats. Whole, raw dairy products from local pasture-fed cows can be beneficial, not only because such products will be rich in nutrients, but also because milk from cows that eat local grasses, pollens and weeds actually introduces these plant antibodies into the milk, thereby partly "immunizing" the consumer against these allergens. An old remedy for hay fever and asthma was colostrum (first milk) from cows that eat local grasses and weeds. (Incidentally, since cows enjoy eating poison ivy this colostrum treatment also helps people who suffer from poison ivy dermatitis.)

If you cannot obtain raw local dairy products, you should make a habit of consuming raw meat or fish several times a week, prepared according to the recipes in *Nourishing Traditions.*

The only sugar in the diet should be locally collected, really raw honey. Patients who tolerate fresh bee pollen without exacerbation of their allergic symptoms can add about 1 tablespoon to their honey. Pollen occurring in locally produced honey encourages the production of antibodies by the lymph tissue around the intestines (called Peyer's patches), which is a process of food-based immunization against pollen allergies.

Finally, it should be mentioned that overeating even the best quality food can in itself be a source of stress. People with a tendency to overweight should avoid all snacks but consume nutrient-dense food only at regular mealtimes. If hypoglycemia is a problem, a few high-protein, high-fat snacks such as properly prepared crispy nuts, raw whole cheeses or whole yoghurt can be eaten between meals. In time the hypoglycemia should improve and the snacks can be eliminated.

Supplements of natural vitamin C complex and cod liver oil to supply 20,000 IU vitamin A daily are often helpful. In addition small amounts of flax oil, in capsule form or added to salad dressings, as well as evening primrose oil in capsule form, supply the precursors the body needs to produce anti-inflammatory prostaglandins on the cellular level.

Therapeutics

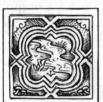

First and foremost among therapies for problems of adrenal insufficiency are glandular extracts that strengthen the adrenal cortex. In fact, use of glandular extracts to alleviate symptoms and correct imbalances is one of the oldest and most successful forms of medicine. Few doctors or patients need convincing of the success of thyroid extracts for treatment of the myriad symptoms of hypothyroidism, or of insulin to treat diabetes. Likewise, the treatment of allergic diseases with adrenal cortex extract and spleen extract can help restore balance when no other therapy is successful.

Adrenal cortical extract therapy dates to the late 1800s and was further refined by Drs. John Tintera and Francis Pottenger in the 1940s and 1950s. Dr. Tintera originally used adrenal cortex extract to treat patients with hypoglycemia and alcoholism.

He recognized that sugar and alcohol cravings were a sign of hypoadrenalism. He treated hundreds of patients successfully with a diet similar to the one I have described, and with intravenous injections of 10 cc whole adrenal cortical extract plus 100 mg vitamin B_6, 1-5 times per week for a period of six to ten weeks. He was able to show that his therapy, rather than suppressing adrenal function as does prednisone, actually improves adrenal function so that the symptoms lessened even after the therapy was completed. Today, I still follow this basic protocol, but instead of using raw adrenal extract I use the adrenal protomorphogen Drenatrophin PMG by Standard Process, 1-2 tablets three times per day. For more difficult cases, especially for those trying to wean themselves from prednisone and other steroid drugs, I suggest an adrenal cortex extract from American Biologics. For some, it is the only thing that works. Usually 2-3 drops per day is enough, but often we need to double this amount. I usually keep this going for 6 weeks after the prednisone has been stopped to avoid relapses. All the time during this treatment the diet and Standard Process supplements should continue.

As discussed earlier, the protomorphogens act as a kind of blueprint for the regeneration and rebuilding of a distressed organ. In a sense, this therapy imitates the practice of the Plains Indians who ate raw buffalo adrenal gland to maintain their health during stressful times.

I also recommend Symplex F (for women) or Symplex M (for men), both from Standard Process. These medicines are composed of the protomorphogens of the pituitary gland, thyroid gland, adrenal gland and ovaries for women, testicles for men. Using these as a group one helps put the "axis" in balance rather than simply focusing on the most obviously disordered gland.

In certain cases when digestive symptoms predominate and sex hormone symptoms are absent (as in women with poor digestion but no menstrual complaints) I will substitute Paraplex for Symplex F (or Symplex M). This changes the ovary component to pancreatrophin, thereby supporting pancreatic function, especially enzyme production.

When hypothyroidism is indicated, I recommend Thytrophin PMG, a protomorphogen complex specifically formulated for the thyroid gland. I have consistently found this group approach to treatment more satisfactory than simply singling out one organ for treatment. This seems much more in line with how the body actually functions, rather than how we conceptualize illness.

The usual dose for all protomorphogens is 1-2 tablets 3 times per day, often for 6 months or until normal functioning is restored.

In addition to these protomorphogens, I recommend licorice root extract to all patients except those who suffer from high blood pressure. Our bodies are able to synthesize adrenal cortical hormones from the substances contained in licorice root extract. This undoubtedly accounts for the wide utility of licorice for many allergic and stress-related illnesses. My favorite preparation is Withania Complex by Mediherb because it combines licorice extract with other adaptogenic herbs that also boost adrenal cortical function. The dose is 1 tablet 3-4 times per day.

Adaptogenic herbs—herbs that help the body deal with stress—are widely used herbal medicines in virtually all traditional healing systems. Korean ginseng, Siberian ginseng, withania (ashwaganda) and licorice are some of the better known adaptogenic herbs. The research on these and many other adaptogenic herbs shows that they all improve adrenal cortical function. Such herbs provide the backbone of traditional herbal practice—they are even used as anti-aging medicines. In my experience, all patients with allergic disease or stress-related illness should be treated with these valuable herbal preparations.

As for treatment of the spleen, the first choice would be the mild homeopathic preparation of Plumbum (lead) D30 combined with Lien (spleen) D8, given as 10 pills under the tongue, 2 times per day, or as an injection over the spleen two times per week, given for about a year. A more direct option is desiccated spleen or spleen PMG extract given orally three times per day.

Another therapy that can be helpful to strengthen this boundary is calcium, which is the element often used in nature for borders, as in shells and tree bark. This remedy will be particularly helpful if the salivary pH is 6.6 or below. (See Appendix B.) I prefer to use calcium lactate by Standard Process, 9-12 42.5 mg tablets per day, along with cod liver oil to facilitate absorption.

Dr. Price's cod liver oil and high-vitamin butter oil treatment (Appendix B) is also a useful therapy for the many problems of adrenal insufficiency.

Finally, for asthma, homeopathic tobacco can be helpful. The medicine is called Nicotiana D6, 10 drops 3 times per day before meals.

Chiropractic adjustments occasionally give dramatic relief for asthma attacks.

Finally, for those who suffer allergies on heavy pollen days in spite of the above treatments I recommend Euphrasia Complex from Mediherb, at a dose of 4-8 tablets per day.

Movement

Problems of adrenal insufficiency occur because the adrenal gland is chronically revved up, producing adrenaline for fight or flight. Exercises for adrenal insufficiency are designed to accomplish a grounding of energies, specifically through pressure on the heel and through harmonious breathing.

Every part of the body has areas that correspond to the head, the limbs and the torso. In the foot, the toes represent the head and central nervous system, the ticklish instep represents the torso, and the heel represents the limbs and bottom. Patients who suffer from symptoms of adrenal insufficiency—allergies, asthma and so forth—literally and figuratively need to sit down, to be grounded, to have their feet on the ground.

An excellent way to accomplish this and to strengthen the adrenal gland is to walk in place on a rebounder (small trampoline), putting pressure on the heel with each step. Walking uphill and hiking up mountains is another way to achieve the necessary grounding, as it puts more pressure on the heels than the toes. (We use our toes more when we walk in the sand.) In addition, when we climb high hills and mountains, we must take deeper breaths of air than we do at sea level. This forces us to deepen our breathing and quiet the whole metabolism, stimulated to frenzied activity by outpourings of adrenaline.

Many of the movement exercises we describe can be helpful for problems of adrenal insufficiency, including the Grounding Exercise and Carriage Down/Carriage Up; Autumn Leaves, the Crest and the Water Level Gesture; the Silhouette and the Lemniscate Dynamic; Coat Hanger, the Spinal Stretch and the Cowl; and Rice Paper Walk, Bestowing and the Sundial. For asthma, the Pulley, Lowering the Sail, Foot Streaming and the Victory Stretch can be very helpful.

Those suffering from asthma need to direct particular attention to breathing. We have said that the Emotional Body has a strong connection to the element of air. We know that our breathing is strongly affected by our feelings. We say that something "took my breath away." A change in breathing is one of the primary signs of sexual arousal. We are told to take a few deep breaths when we are faced with stage fright. Looking at breathing as a movement, we see that it is a dynamic process of interacting with the inside and outside spaces. We are not separate from our surroundings. We draw the outside atmosphere inside our physical bodies, transform it and give it back.

Nor is breathing an activity that is localized solely in the lungs. It is something that happens soul-ly in every cell of our bodies. In the early stages of embryological development, there is a family of cells that is designated to take on the role of respiration. Some of the sister cells turn inside to become the lungs, while some brother cells encase the entire body to become skin. The lungs are our skin turned outside in, our skin is a lung turned inside out. We breathe then with our entire body—and with all our Bodies. Including the surface of our skin in the process of respiration allows for an expanded space which encourages the calming of emotions. This fuller space can slow hasty breathing patterns, allow for a more thorough out-breath for the asthma sufferer, and can give the adrenals some well-deserved rest.

When performing the Breathing Exercise, those with asthma should put particular emphasis on the moment of exhalation. As you imagine yourself on a beach looking out to sea, exhale at the moment the sea comes in and surrounds your feet with foam. The exhalation should be long and lightly audible, just as the incoming wave is audible as it lingers around you on the sand. Pause briefly as the ocean recalls the wave. Follow the dynamic of the ocean. Let the suction of the departing wave enlarge your chest and make an inbreath possible. This inbreath should be silent. Then pause again just as the ocean prepares for the next wave. When the wave breaks as it comes in, exhale again, audibly as the wave is now audible. Try to imagine the breathing process taking place through your skin as well as through your lungs. This exercise, performed calmly and rhythmically, can retrain the breathing of the asthma sufferer.

Meditation

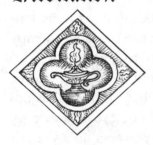

As we have seen, all of the allergic diseases involve an expansion or swelling of the tissue. In hay fever, the classic allergic illness, the eyes are swollen and weepy. The nose runs, the face seems swollen and it even feels as though one's brain is expanded or heavy. Everything feels waterlogged and drippy. In his medical writings, Rudolf Steiner described these "waterlogged" physical symptoms as a manifestation on a soul level of what he called hysteria. Today we prefer the words anxiety or fearfulness, which describe the same thing.

There is a "passionate intensity" in our lives, but it is directed toward its worst possible aspects—worry, fear, unthinking reaction—while the passionate conviction to achieve our life's work, a conviction that in healthy situations elicits clear thinking and the driving force of the adrenal hormones, is lacking. The result is a lack of "centeredness," a kind of anarchy loosed on the physical body that manifests as allergies, asthma and inflammation.

Many people with allergies are in fact anxious and fearful, and they tend to overreact on many levels. On the physical level, for example, a walk in the spring, in which one sees the beautiful lilac trees and breathes their sweet scent—an experience that should be peaceful and soothing—can provoke an almost violent reaction with sneezing, runny eyes and shortness of breath. For others, the ingestion of certain foods that provide nourishment and delight to most people can provoke life-threatening effects.

The usual treatment for these kinds of allergies—involving lists of foods to avoid, complicated rotation diets and expensive blood tests—actually serves to heighten our anxiety or fear. Consider the patient who is instructed to avoid a huge range of foods, some of which he may not tolerate, but others that he enjoys and can eat without suffering any ill-effects. It seems to me that this approach, rather than accomplishing much in the way of long-term benefit, increases the sense of powerlessness and despair in the patient. Instead, we should try to rebuild his physiology and at the same time work on a soul level to overcome his feeling of anxiety, fearfulness and powerlessness. After all, the goal is to return to a state in which we can enjoy our food, the trees and flowers, our pets and all aspects of our environment, not to foster a kind of hysteria or paranoia about the simple pleasures of life.

As I have pointed out, a fundamental cause of fear and anxiety is a shortness of vision or lack of perspective. Traditional people suffered from allergic diseases much less frequently, which I believe is related to the fact that native peoples took the long view. Rather than working for the bottom line this year or this month, the creed of some American Indian tribes was to consider the impact of each decision on the next seven generations. While such a great leap of perspective may be difficult for modern Americans, if we strive to lengthen our perspective, we undertake true soul therapy in the treatment of allergic diseases, one that forms the basis of true healing.

Taking the long view in life, as opposed to worrying about short-term effects, can be compared to the nutritional and remedial strategies I have outlined, as opposed to taking cortisone. The patient needs to ask himself: is it best to do a therapy that will make my symptoms better now but leave me more weakened in a year, or should I look for a slower but more long-lasting approach?

We can practice taking the long view in everything we do. When purchasing food, clothes or a car, for example, we can ask ourselves which choices are likely to satisfy our short-term wants and which are more likely to be pleasing, satisfying and useful in the long term. And we can consider each purchase, each activity, each decision on the basis of how it affects our friends, family and community as well as ourselves.

When practicing the *Rückschau* Meditation, take note of the difference between the events of the day—which may be quite stressful—and the way we perceive these events—which can and should be philosophical. This difference is crucial because it is the perception of the events in our lives that affects our physiology, not the actual events. Daily or frequent application of this kind of mental exercise can help us achieve balance in the physical performance of our adrenal glands.

Lengthening one's perspective and overcoming anxiety is partly a matter of practice. The more you exercise this faculty, the easier it becomes. In fact, you will soon find the practice of thinking in the long term a stimulating challenge and creative exercise in itself, one that leads us to see everything that happens in life as an adventure rather than an ordeal, as an experience to be savored rather than a hardship to be endured.

A final word. The adrenal gland is the processor of stress in our bodies. It is there to help us adapt. When we become exhausted by life, on a mental or physical level, our adrenal glands often fail to keep up, and illness ensues.

I define stress as anything that forces us to live contrary to what our inner guide is telling us is right for us. I want to emphasize that we need to follow our inner guide—not our parents, not the church, not our culture, not government nor anyone or anything else. So many people with adrenal illnesses live a life of "should." To me, that is stress. In our comprehensive approach to illness this aspect of our health must be considered as vitally important.

RECOMMENDED READING
   Waking the Tiger by Peter A. Levine
   Duck Soup for the Soul by Swami Beyondananda

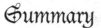

Summary

Nutrition

✳	Avoid	All processed foods
		Foods high in carbohydrates
		Foods containing hydrogenated fats
		Caffeine (coffee, tea, cocoa, chocolate, soft drinks)
✳	Emphasize	Best quality local raw dairy products
		Cultured butter and cream
		Raw meat and fish
		Fresh and fermented vegetables and fruits
		Zucchini
		Raw local honey
		Celtic Sea salt
✳	Supplements	Cataplex C by Standard Process, 2-3 tablets 3 times per day
		Cod liver oil to provide 10,000 IU vitamin A per day
		Flax oil, about 1 teaspoon per day
		Evening primrose oil, 2-4 capsules per day

Therapeutics

* Drenatrophin PMG by Standard Process, 1-2 tablet 3 times per day.
* Symplex F (for women) or Symplex M (for men) by Standard Process, 1-2 tablets 3 times per day, or, when digestive symptoms predominate, Paraplex by Standard Process, 1-2 tablets 3 times per day.
* For symptoms of underactive thyroid, Thytrophin PMG by Standard Process, 1-2 tablets 3 times per day.
* In difficult cases, adrenal cortex extract from Apothecure to wean off corticoid drugs, 2-3 drops per day or up to 6 drops per day.
* Withania complex by Mediherb, 1 tablet 3-4 times per day.

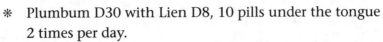

* Plumbum D30 with Lien D8, 10 pills under the tongue 2 times per day.
* Spleen, whole desiccated, 1 tablet 3 times per day for 6 months.
* Calcium lactate from Standard Process, 9-12 42.5 mg tablets per day.
* Nicotiana D6, 3 times per day for 10 days, taken before meals (for asthma).
* Chiropractic adjustments (for asthma).
* For heavy pollen days, euphrasia complex from Mediherb, at a dose of 4-8 tablets per day.

Movement

* Walk in place on a rebounder, with pressure on the heels for grounding.
* Walk up steep hills for stamina.
* Grounding Exercise and Carriage Down/Carriage Up.
* Autumn Leaves, the Crest and Water Level Gesture.
* The Silhouette and the Lemniscate Dynamic.
* Coat Hanger, the Spinal Stretch and the Cowl.
* Rice Paper Walk, Bestowing and the Sundial.
* For asthma, the Pulley, Lowering the Sail, Foot Streaming, the Victory Stretch and particular attention to the Breathing Exercise.

Meditation

* Practice the long view.
* Live according to your inner guide.

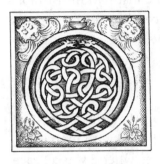

Chapter 7:
Digestive Disorders

And the earth was without form, and void; and darkness was upon the face of the deep. . .
                                                                 Genesis 1:1

"What is REAL?" asked the Rabbit one day when they were lying side by side near the nursery fender before Nana came to tidy the room. "Does it mean having things that buzz inside you and a stick-out hand?"

"Real isn't how you are made," said the Skin Horse. "It's a thing that happens to you. When a child loves you for a long, long time, not just to play with, but REALLY loves you, then you become real."

"Does it hurt?" asked the Rabbit.

"Sometimes," said the Skin Horse, for he was always truthful. "When you are real you don't mind being hurt."

"Does it happen all at once, like being wound up," he asked, "or bit by bit?"

"It doesn't happen all at once," said the Skin Horse. "You become. It takes a long time. That's why it doesn't often happen to people who break easily, or have sharp edges, or who have to be carefully kept. Generally, by the time you are real most of your hair has been loved off, and your eyes drop out and you get loose in the joints and very shabby. But these things don't matter at all because once you are real you can't be ugly, except to people who don't understand."

"I suppose you are real?" said the Rabbit. And then he wished he had not said it for he thought the Skin Horse might be sensitive. But the Skin Horse only smiled.

"The boy's uncle made me real," he said. "That was a great many years ago; but once you are real you can't become unreal again. It lasts for always."

> Margery Williams
> The Velveteen Rabbit

igestive diseases can be divided into two types, chronic and acute. Acute digestive disorders include dysentery, viral hepatitis and appendicitis.

Chronic digestive problems include recurrent heartburn or stomach pains, the inability to digest various foods or types of food, persistent constipation, irritable bowel syndrome, ulcerative colitis, loss of appetite, peptic ulcer disease and cancers of the digestive tract. In principle, the former resolve quickly, or they respond relatively well to drugs and surgery. But chronic digestive disorders continue to baffle the medical profession and cannot be successfully treated without a basic understanding of the digestive process.

Most of us have experienced an acute digestive problem. We drink some bad water while traveling and in less than 24 hours find ourselves in bed with high fever, shakes, chills and profuse watery diarrhea. This happened to me when I was a Peace Corps volunteer in southern Africa. I remember quite clearly the desperate two-mile walk home, my head ready to explode. I realized I was getting a taste of what old-fashioned, *bona fide* illness is all about. The rapidity of its onset was astonishing. Luckily I was escorted over a bumpy dirt road to a local clinic (which was actually 100 miles away) where medical workers made a diagnosis of amoebic dysentery. I took fluids, rested and soon regained my health.

Unfortunately, the kind of digestive disorders I usually hear about in my practice are not so easily cured. The typical patient complains of frequent constipation, with stools coming irregularly or not at all for two to four days, alternating with bouts of diarrhea—a sign that the bowel walls are getting weak as a result of the constipation. Symptoms include abdominal bloating, abdominal pains, a feeling of overall sluggishness or fatigue, frequent bouts of flu-like illness and—most embarrassing—leakage of stool. The diagnosis is irritable bowel syndrome, but the underlying condition is disturbed digestion.

To understand how to treat the chronic digestive disorders—and even some of the acute problems, such as appendicitis and hepatitis—we must look at the work of scientists who spent time in Africa, including Dennis Burkett, Albert Schweitzer and Weston Price. They noted that Africans on their native diets rarely suffered digestive or gastrointestinal diseases. Appendicitis, colitis, hepatitis, constipation, bowel problems and colon cancer were virtually nonexistent as long as the Africans continued with their tribal foodways.

Heartburn is another common chronic complaint. Consider Mr. R. W., a 45-year-old patient who had suffered from heartburn for more than twenty years. After eating, Mr. W. had a feeling of burning in his chest. No matter what he ate, the food would "just sit there, like a lead ball." He had tried many of the usual nostrums, including antacids, Tums and Tagamet, and at various times had submitted to X-rays and gastroscopes. He had even tried alternative medicines, such as slippery elm, and homeopathic remedies for stressed-out, executive types with recurrent stomach pains.

My prescription for Mr. W. was the following: Use Celtic sea salt instead of regular table salt and drink about one ounce of beet kvass or lacto-fermented ginger ale with each meal. (See Appendix A.) Ten days later, he reported that his lead ball was lifted and his lifelong symptoms were gone.

To understand why this simple intervention had such a positive effect, we need a fundamental understanding of the digestive process. According to Rudolf Steiner, digestion is the annihilation or breaking down of the outer world, which is food, into nothingness or chaos. Digestion begins when we take food into our mouth, chew it and mix it with enzyme-rich saliva. Then the partially digested food goes to our stomach where strong acids begin the breakdown of proteins. Next the mass goes through the duodenum where it is mixed with bile from the liver and digestive enzymes from the pancreas specifically tailored to the type of food ingested. This digestive system, with its thousands of enzymes and precise system of pH regulation, has one goal—to completely break down the food into nothingness or chaos.

In biology we learn about the breakdown of the proteins into constituent amino acids, the fats into fatty acids of various lengths and the carbohydrates into glucose and other sugars, but this is not the whole story, for these food stuffs must also have any traces of their origin "annihilated." This means that the carrot we eat is not only broken down into its constituent proteins, fats, carbohydrates, vitamins and minerals, but also that the "life" of the carrot is broken down or annihilated. Only when every trace of the outer world is removed from the carrot can we use it to effectively build our own body.

Good digestion transforms our foods, which are highly organized, into chaos. But chaos does not mean disorder or confusion. Rather, it is a void, pregnant with possibility, from which creation can now occur. This is the concept of chaos that is given to us in the first chapter of Genesis. The Greeks referred to chaos as a state of becoming, not a state of disarray. Science refers to chaos as a colloidal state out of which structure can be created. The entire physical universe was created out of chaos, and our physical bodies are created out of the product of our digestion—which is chaos, unorganized but fecund.

The problem underlying all modern digestive disturbances—and all cases of food allergies—is that the process of annihilation is weak and therefore incomplete. The food is not completely annihilated, the state of chaos is never reached. The result is that we absorb undigested components that sicken us and to which we have violent reactions, which we call allergies.

Why is the process of annihilation weak? The first reason is that most of what we put in our mouths today is not really food, does not represent food as it is supposed to be. Pasteurized, homogenized, skimmed or lowfat milk from hormone-treated, grain-fed cows, for example, is not really milk. Our digestive systems do not recognize it as a food, it cannot be properly broken down, and therefore we are allergic to it. The carrot grown in lifeless, chemically treated soil will itself lack life. Margarine and the other factory-made fats that permeate the food supply are dead. Leave some margarine on the counter and it will gather dust but will not attract microscopic or insect life. The bacteria and the insects know that it is not a food, that it is not real. Likewise, irradiated food will not sustain microscopic life—how can we expect it to sustain our own? Processed soups, sauces, imitation meats and frozen meals have a meat-like taste imparted by artificial flavorings and MSG. The tongue senses the meat-like taste and alerts the digestive tract to produce enzymes for meat or broth made from meat and bones, but these nourishing foods never arrive and the digestive apparatus is left unprepared to break down the chemicals in the imitation foods.

Almost every item available in the modern supermarket is, at best, only partially "real." The quality is missing.

For food to nourish us, for it to stimulate digestion, give us energy and build up our bodies, it must be real. The question here is, what is real? To be real, food must be grown with care, love and insight. Like the Velveteen Rabbit, real food must be respected for what it is. The cow must be allowed to live its life as a healthy, happy cow. The carrot must be grown in healthy soil. Then our foods must be prepared with knowledge and wisdom, and eaten with love and reverence. Only when the food is real will it stimulate our digestive juices and help us create healthy bodies.

Real food has aroma, it is properly flavored, it fills our houses with wonderful smells, it is the centerpiece of family conversation and good friendships. Real food is recognized by the digestive system, calls forth the forces of digestion and opens itself up to annihilation. Eating real food is the key to good digestion.

The second reason that digestion is weak is that our glands and organs are unable to supply a sufficient quantity of digestive enzymes. This may be because our digestive organs—the pancreas, liver and salivary glands—are weak and overloaded; or it may be because we lack certain trace minerals. Enzymes are complex proteins that act as catalysts, and each enzyme contains one molecule of a specific trace mineral.

The reason the treatment for Mr. W. worked so well is because the Celtic sea salt provided trace minerals and the fermented drinks provided enzymes to help his body digest his food. Unfortunately, most people in the West do not use unrefined salt and almost never consume lacto-fermented foods.

Undigested food provokes the body into secreting more hydrochloric acid, which leads to the symptoms of acid indigestion or heartburn. Undigested food or sluggish digestion often results in food "sitting like a lead weight in the stomach," or gastric reflux (GERD), commonly referred to as heartburn. Insufficient pancreatic and liver enzymes provoke sludging of the bile leading to gall bladder problems. Some practitioners believe that a shortage of digestive enzymes is even responsible for the sclerotic process leading to arthritis, because when plentiful, these enzymes show up in the blood and can help break down deposits of debris in the joints.

The third reason our digestion is weak has to do with the ecology of the digestive tract. The modern ecological movement began in the 1960s when Marjorie Spock, sister of the famous Dr. Spock and a student of Rudolf Steiner, spearheaded a lawsuit against the spraying of DDT on Long Island. This grass roots action was followed by the publication of *Silent Spring* by Rachel Carson and a reevaluation of how we treat our environment. But one aspect of the environmental movement that has not yet received much notice is the connection between the external environment and our inner environment, particularly the environment in our intestines. The content of our small and large intestines is actually an ecosystem, full of a wide variety of interdependent organisms. While these microorganisms live independent lives, they also interact with each other, they interact with their host, and they interact with the larger world around them.

Our intestinal microorganisms help digest our food and are nourished by our food. They synthesize vitamins, especially B vitamins, that are essential for our health. It is not fiber but dead microorganisms that supply bulk for our stools, without which we would suffer from painful constipation. They secrete antibiotic-type substances that protect us from infections. They interact with our intestinal wall, keeping it healthy and able to perform its role as a semipermeable barrier.

Dennis Burkett, a British physician, spent most of his career studying indigenous African populations. He confirmed what Weston Price and Albert Schweitzer had noted earlier, that the Africans enjoyed remarkable digestive health and a complete absence of constipation, irritable bowel syndrome, gall bladder disease, appendicitis, ulcerative colitis, Crohn's disease and bowel cancer. Burkett's conclusion—which has become the gospel of modern bowel health—is that the good health these people achieved was a direct result of the high fiber content of their diet. This led to the oat bran fad and the appearance of health claims on high fiber breakfast cereals.

Closer examination of Burkett's work, however, reveals that he ignored some conflicting evidence that might have given him a fuller picture and led him to different conclusions. For while many healthy African people do eat a high fiber diet, some, like the Masai, eat a low fiber diet and still have excellent intestinal health. The common thread in all the groups studied by Burkett, Schweitzer and Price is that they consumed large amounts of lacto-fermented foods, the kind that provide a steady supply of healthy bacteria to enrich the ecology of the bowels. Some groups ate fermented millet, or *ogi*; others drank sorghum beer, a lacto-fermented drink; others drank *emasi* or sour fermented milk. In all cases, as the cultures changed and the art of fermentation was lost, the people began to have bowel diseases just like westernized peoples.

When DDT or some other pesticide is introduced into an ecosystem like a pond, many beneficial microorganisms in the pond die out. These beneficial organisms, whose function is to oxygenate the pond, are replaced by algae, which further deplete the oxygen supply. It is as though the pond has an infection like the yeast infections I see so often in my patients. Next the flora dies, then the larger fish and finally mammalian life. Finally, the host itself succumbs. This is more than hypothetical. As a child, I often visited my grandparents at their summer cottage on Lake Erie. My early years were filled with the continuing tragedy of Lake Erie, which, after years of industrial pollution, could no longer support life.

We can see, then, what happens when we pollute the ecosystem of the bowel with antibiotics and other drugs, and with processed food. To regain health we must first stop polluting the ecosystem and then repopulate it with the beneficial flora provided by lacto-fermented foods.

One thing that pollutes the ecosystem of the bowel is large amounts of grains, either refined or whole. In both forms, grains encourage the proliferation of yeasts to break them down. In any case of yeast overgrowth or bowel problems, I recommend that grains be cut back sharply. Later they can be reintroduced, but only in fermented form. This was my recommendation for Mrs. T. C., a 28-year-old woman with a three-year history of Crohn's disease. She suffered from chronic diarrhea, malabsorption, weight loss, bloody stools and fatigue. Occasionally she had other symptoms, such as joint aches, irregular menses and depression. The accepted treatment is long-term oral antibiotics and steroids to suppress the inflammation. Mrs. C. had fairly severe flare-ups for which she took prednisone, but she found the side effects intolerable. I suggested a program that eliminated most of her carbohydrate intake and that included lacto-fermented foods and bone broth. She soon went into remission and began gaining weight. Her periods resumed and her joint pain resolved as she was able to absorb the nutrients in her food more thoroughly.

The treatment of stomach irritation (gastritis), reflux disease, and even stomach or duodenal ulcers is fairly straightforward and accentuates the above principles. That is, for a period of about 2 weeks the total carbohydrate content of the diet is kept very low, under 20 grams per day. During this period, no grains or fruit are eaten. The relief from this dietary intervention is profound and reliable. Usually the pain improves in 3-4 days, and is gone in 2 weeks. At that point fermented grains can be slowly added back to the diet.

Nutrition

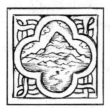

Digestive disorders represent nature's plea for us to return to real, whole foods, foods grown in healthy soil and from animals that graze on healthy pasture. When we eat processed and imitation foods, we are, in essence, polluting the finely tuned ecosystem of the gut. Fermented foods, such as sauerkraut and cultured milk, are vital to any treatment of digestive disorders. Grains—either refined or whole— should be kept to a minimum until the condition resolves and then eaten only after proper preparation—soaking, sprouting or sour leavening—so that they are easy to digest. Beet kvass, lacto-fermented ginger ale and other enzyme-rich beverages should accompany every meal. Bone broths make digestion easier, and Celtic sea salt provides trace minerals needed for enzyme structure.

For constipation and hemorrhoids, use 1 tablespoon of freshly ground flax seeds mixed into 1-2 cups of warm water every morning. This drink softens the stool in addition to providing valuable omega-3 fatty acids so beneficial to our overall health. Coconut oil, taken 2 tablespoons as melted oil mixed with a little water, twice daily, can have a very positive effect on constipation as the short- and medium-chain fatty acids promote beneficial flora in the gut and colon.

Finally, for all digestive orders, I have found Dr. Price's high-vitamin butter oil therapy to be useful, particularly for digestive tracts that have been badly damaged from celiac disease or treatment with chemotherapy and radiation. (See Appendix B.)

Therapeutics

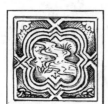

All digestive problems are aided by Zypan, a pancreatic enzyme formulation from Standard Process. The dose is 1-2 tablets 3 times per day.

For mild symptoms of reflux or upper GI distress, Bolus Alba complex from Weleda will often provide relief. This compound is a mixture of powdered herbs and herbs that have been processed into a kind of charcoal. Some of the herbs, like gentiana, are bitters that stimulate the production of digestive juices; others like chamomilla and anise are soothing to the GI mucosa. This powder of roasted herbs, like any orally ingested charcoal, absorbs toxins that are irritating to the lining of the stomach and intestines. The dose is 1/4 teaspoon in warm water 2-4 times per day.

For more chronic conditions, I have had great success with using a combination of homeopathic Stibium D6 along with the Standard Process medicines Okra-Pepsin and chlorophyll complex. Stibium is a homeopathic remedy which, according to Rudolf

Steiner, provides the image of proper protein formation. With chronic inflammation the inner structure of the GI tract becomes broken down. Stibium provides help in rebuilding a healthy GI lining. The dose is 1 pea-sized portion 3 times per day.

Okra-Pepsin combines pepsin, an enzyme that helps with protein digestion, with orka, a slimy, mucilagenous vegetable that adds a layer of protection to the GI lining. Chlorophyll complex aids in the binding of toxins liberated from the increased protein digestion arising from taking pepsin. The dose for both is 2 tablets 3 times per day.

For people with ulcerative colitis or Crohn's disease I add Zymex from Standard Process, which is a mixture of beneficial bacteria that restore our inner pond to its proper eco-balance. Zymex contains the same bacteria found in lacto-fermented foods, such as yoghurt and sauerkraut, in a base of substances known to help restore the health of the lining of the GI tract. The dose is 1-2 tablets 3 times per day.

Stomach problems such as ulcers respond well to licorice drops, which have mucosal healing properties. I use an extract from Mediherb at a dose of 10-20 drops 3-4 times per day. In addition, I suggest Gastrex tablets from Standard Process to help heal the irritated tissue. The dose is 2 tablets with meals.

For constipation I recommend Gastrofiber by Standard Process, 3 capsules 1-2 times per day.

These medicines work together to form a picture of healthy digestion. Some work on improving the breakdown of the food, others bind and help excrete unwanted by-products of digestion, others work on the rebuilding the structure of the intestinal lining. At the same time, we reintroduce healthy micro-organisms to fill the void. In this way, we point the way towards true healing, rather than merely a suppression of symptoms or removal of a diseased organ.

Castor oil packs over the abdominal area, one to two times per week, can also be helpful for all digestive problems.

Movement

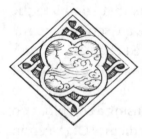

Most of us have experienced digestive difficulties when we are in the throes of negative emotions like anger, fear or anxiety. If the body is in the "fight or flight" mode that these emotions stimulate, the blood supply to the digestive organs is greatly affected. The initial symptoms are indigestion, diarrhea and loss of appetite. If we harbor these emotions for any length of time, these emotions may manifest as chronic problems like ulcers or colitis.

When the head is in turmoil from anger or fear, the still and fixed quality that should characterize the head is misappropriated to the abdomen. The appropriate gesture for the abdomen is down and out, not inward and fixed. When the stillness of the head becomes misplaced, constriction results—in the stomach as an ulcer, in the intestines as Crohn's disease, in the colon as constipation.

The Lemniscate Dynamic helps replace constriction in the abdomen with the gesture of down, release and out. The Body Space Imagination can also be useful. The Crest, the Spinal Stretch, Knee Mapping, Letting Go and the Rice Paper Walk are all excellent, along with the Breathing Exercise and the Silhouette for practicing releasing.

For ulcers, the Stomach Wave is excellent. The command of "chest-out, stomach-in," still required of children, models and military men, is actually a recipe for an ulcer, because it causes a constriction in the stomach. Proper muscle tone of the abdomen gives the stomach a gentle massage that aids in the kneading necessary in digestion. The Stomach Wave is a gesture that also strengthens and frees the abdominal area at the same time.

Constipation can be relieved with the clockwise Abdomen Massage.

Meditation

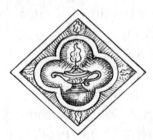

As many people know, and as many physicians have observed throughout the years, digestive troubles are strongly connected with the emotions. We now know that the same receptors for serotonin that are found in the brain and participate in the emotional responses in the brain are also found in the gut wall. We most definitely feel things in our guts, a concept that is easy to experience and, in fact, is part of our common language. Like any condition of emotional instability, this situation begs for the patient to learn to feel his or her emotions, but not to have their emotional life dominate their thinking life. Throughout the most intense emotional storms, the head should remain still.

GI troubles ask us to learn the basic principles of meditation, which are all about learning objectivity. Use the *Rückschau* Meditation every evening to cultivate the habit of objectivity. This can be the most profound therapy of all for anyone who suffers from problems with the gastrointestinal tract.

Summary

Nutrition

* Avoid   All processed food
       Refined grains
       Improperly processed whole grains
       Commercial dairy products

* Emphasize Whole foods grown in healthy soil, or from
        animals that graze on healthy pasture
       Fermented foods such as sauerkraut and cultured
        milk
       Beet kvass, lacto-fermented ginger ale and
        other fermented drinks with meals
       Bone broths
       Celtic sea salt
       Low-carbohydrate diet for rapid relief of acute
        GI conditions
       For constipation and hemorrhoids, 1 tablespoon
        freshly ground flax seeds mixed into 1-2 cups
        of warm water every morning.

Therapeutics

* Zypan from Standard Process, 1-2 tablets 3 times per day.
* For mild symptoms of reflux or upper GI distress, Bolus Alba complex from Weleda, 1/4 teaspoon in warm water 2-4 times per day.
* For chronic conditions, Stibium D6, 1 pea-sized portion 3 times per day.
* Okra-Pepsin from Standard Process, 2 tablets 3 times per day.
* Chlorophyll complex, 2 tablets 3 times per day.
* For ulcerative colitis or Crohn's disease, Zymex from Standard Process, 1-2 tablets 3 times per day.
* For stomach problems such as ulcers, licorice drops from Mediherb, 10-20 drops 3-4 times per day and Gastrex from Standard Process, 2 tablets with meals.

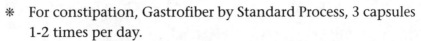

* For constipation, Gastrofiber by Standard Process, 3 capsules 1-2 times per day.
* Castor oil packs over the abdominal area, 1-2 times per week.

Movement

* The Lemniscate Dynamic helps replace constriction in the abdomen with the gestures of down, release and out.
* The Body Space Imagination.
* The Crest, the Spinal Stretch, Knee Mapping, Letting Go and the Rice Paper Walk for release.
* The Breathing Exercise and the Silhouette for expansion.
* The Stomach Wave for ulcers.
* The Abdomen Massage for constipation.

Meditation

* Practice stillness in the head.
* Cultivate objectivity with the *Rückschau* Meditation.

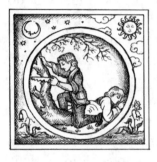

Chapter 8:
Chronic Fatigue

The world can only be grasped by action, not by contemplation. . .
The hand is the cutting edge of the mind.

Jacob Bronowski

And thus the native hue of resolution
Is sicklied o'er with the pale cast of thought,
And enterprises of great pith and moment
With this regard their currents turn awry,
And lose the name of action.

Shakespeare's Hamlet

*L*ike many physicians, I first met the baffling condition called chronic fatigue in the late 1980s. The typical patient was a previously healthy woman in her 20s or 30s who came to see me in extreme distress. The main symptom was profound fatigue along with a variety of other complaints, including muscle weakness, sore throat and frequent infections. In addition, the patients were often depressed. As a rule, laboratory tests revealed little that was helpful.

As the years went by, physicians developed a number of theories to shed light on this mysterious condition. Some said chronic fatigue was the result of a bad yeast overgrowth; others claimed that the problem was a chronic viral infection caused by the Epstein-Barr virus, the same virus that causes mononucleosis. Others believed that chronic fatigue was caused by magnesium deficiency, hormonal imbalances or a myriad of other organic defects.

I looked carefully for signs of these imbalances in my patients but rarely found any consistent pattern. In other words, I simply could not convince myself that the severe symptoms I was seeing were the result of any of the explanations in vogue.

Clues to the treatment of chronic fatigue came to me from two sources—the work of Rudolf Steiner and the folk traditions of the Eskimos. Once during a lecture

Rudolf Steiner was asked to explain why so many people, especially those with high ideals, often have so much difficulty translating their ideals into action. Why do modern people exhibit such a strong inertia? His answer surprised many in the audience. He said the lack of will to translate ideals into action was a problem of nutrition. Unfortunately, at the time he didn't elaborate on the particulars of nutrition, but in other situations he did discuss the connection between nutrition and fatigue.

What can the Eskimos teach us? According to the Eskimos, "We can feed our dogs raw fish and they can run for six hours, or we can feed them fermented fish and they can run all day." Clearly, they, too, were making the connection between nutrition and fatigue, or at least endurance. For the Eskimo, the key to avoiding fatigue and having plenty of stamina was fermented foods.

As I was pondering the problems of chronic fatigue, a new patient came to me. Mr. P. F. had suffered from severe tiredness for at least seven years. He was in his mid-forties and worked as chairman of the environmental science department at a local graduate school. He was happily married and in general seemed to have rich and fulfilling life. He was thin but not yet gaunt. The symptoms of profound fatigue, repeated sore throats and muscle weakness had become progressively worse over the seven-year period.

When he came for his first appointment, his activity level consisted of about two hours of work in the morning, followed by a prolonged rest period, then another two hours in the afternoon. This schedule was maintained for three days per week. During the rest of the week, he spent almost all his time in bed. Through the years he was forced to give up the recreational activities he enjoyed, such as hiking, biking and canoeing . He had seen many physicians who ran all the usual tests—and some that were unusual. As is common for these patients, his Epstein-Barr titer was somewhat high and he had a moderate elevation of *Candida albicans* yeast in his stool, but the rest of the conventional blood tests were normal. He had been through many therapies over the years including immune stimulation protocols, anti-virals, antidepressants, anti-yeast diets and treatment with various vitamin regimens. He had the impression that many of these were helpful for a short time but the symptoms were slowly getting worse through the years. He came to me for a new approach.

Mr. F. had suffered so many disappointments with both conventional and alternative medicine that he felt hopeless and defeated. In this situation, faced with a patient who had "done everything" and for whom there was no clear laboratory diagnosis, I had to take a deep breath and resolve to adhere to the protocol suggested by the two disparate sources—Rudolf Steiner and the Eskimos. Together they indicated that the body is a kind of self-enclosed system, which has a relatively fixed amount of energy. This energy is parceled out among the various functions that are needed to sustain life, such as digestion, muscular activity, thinking, wound repair, immune function and hormone synthesis. Based on this perspective, the problem of chronic fatigue can be explained by the fact that too much energy is being taken up with digestion and shunted away from the other functions. As the ongoing nourishment and repair of the muscles and organs begins to deteriorate, their ability to carry out their tasks grows weaker. After a time the other symptoms appear: muscle weakness as lactic acid, the by-product of muscular metabolism, builds up in the tissues; sore throats as the immune system breaks down; and depression as the brain becomes starved of nutrients.

The key therapeutic principle in this scenario is that the lack of nourishment or energy available to our muscles and organs is directly related to how much energy we put into digestion. That is, the more we need to use our own energy to digest our food, the less energy we have for other functions. The result is chronic fatigue.

The strategy that helped this patient recover from his chronic fatigue was built on a diet in which there was great emphasis on fermented foods. Fermentation is actually a "predigestion," and consumption of fermented foods allows the body to digest its meals with a minimum of energy, thereby freeing up more energy for other functions. Fermented foods supply enzymes and friendly bacteria that help the body in the complex process of breaking down the food that supplies its nourishment. In addition, fermentation makes many nutrients more immediately available to the body, thereby making it easier to maintain normal energy levels.

The strategy outlined below required considerable patience but the results were remarkable. The patient began feeling better by three months and by six months he was able to work three full days per week and participate more actively around the house. He no longer suffered from sore throats or other infections. After a year he was able to resume his recreational activities, such as hiking and canoeing. His muscle strength and endurance returned. At the end of two years he felt as though he had gotten his life back and his energy level was as strong as it had ever been.

At no point during the treatment did we resort to any of the accepted protocols for chronic fatigue syndrome. We simply stuck with the program.

Nutrition

The basic diet for chronic fatigue consists of 40 percent animal foods, 40 percent vegetables and only about 20 percent whole grains. Although grains provide energy and important nutrients, they are difficult to digest, even when prepared by soaking and fermenting. In cases of extreme fatigue, it is best to temporarily lower the proportion of grains to almost zero, even though the patient must put up with less variety in his food.

For the animal foods, the first rule is to completely avoid all pasteurized milk products as these call for great reserves of energy to digest them. In addition, cooked meat or fish is allowed only three times per week. The rest of the animal foods should be completely raw—such as raw milk, raw butter, raw cream or any of the raw meat and fish recipes given in *Nourishing Traditions*—or fermented, such as kefir, yoghurt or cheese. If fermented meats are available, such as the many cured meat products produced in Europe, they can be included liberally in the diet.

The other important meat product is bone broth. The gelatin it contains makes food much easier to digest and sauces or gravies made from bone broth make cooked meats much easier to digest. Soup based on bone broth at the beginning of a meal makes the whole meal more digestible.

For vegetable foods, a good rule is one-third cooked (steamed, blanched, baked or in soups); one-third raw (salads and sprouts); and one-third fermented (sauerkraut, kimchee, ginger-carrots, etc.). Fermented foods should be included with every meal. Seasonal fruits, both raw and cooked, may be included.

Nuts, another vegetable food, should be prepared as crispy nuts according to the recipes in *Nourishing Traditions*, to make them more digestible. Properly prepared nuts make an excellent between-meal snack that is easily digested.

Only grains that have been soaked, sprouted or prepared by the process of sour leavening are allowed. Cooked whole grains, such as brown rice, are first soaked and then steamed in bone broth. Rolled oats are soaked overnight, cooked well and then eaten with yoghurt or kefir. Only genuine sourdough or sprouted grain breads are allowed.

Naturally, all refined grains are forbidden, as are refined sweeteners, which require a great deal of energy to digest and which rob the body of nutrients. A small amount of raw honey may be used on cooked cereal and sourdough bread.

Refined and commercial vegetable oils are also forbidden. Raw butter can be used liberally. The other important fat for treatment of chronic fatigue is coconut oil. The fatty acids in coconut oil do not need to be acted upon by the bile; the body uses them directly for quick energy. In addition, they ward off yeasts and other infection-promoting pathogens in the gut. I recommend at least one-half can of whole coconut milk per day for chronic fatigue. Coconut oil can also be used in cooking and added to yoghurt-based smoothies or simply consumed melted and mixed with water. The recommended dose is 2 tablespoons with the morning and evening meals.

Patients with chronic fatigue must avoid all commercial salt. Unrefined Celtic sea salt, a good source of magnesium, may be used liberally.

Finally, the patient with chronic fatigue should consume large quantities of lacto-fermented beverages, both with and between meals. Recipes are given in Appendix A and in *Nourishing Traditions*. The most important of these is beet kvass, which should be consumed at least twice a day, four ounces in the morning and four ounces at night.

Cod liver oil is extremely important in the treatment of chronic fatigue. The fat-soluble vitamins it supplies are necessary for mineral absorption and the special fatty acids EPA and DHA help with depression. Most importantly, vitamin D is crucial for calcium metabolism and for the processes that clear lactic acid from the cells. The dose is one that supplies 20,000 IU vitamin A per day.

Therapeutics

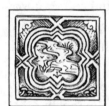

While it is always nice to be a purist and encourage people with chronic fatigue to use diet as their only therapy, in practice there are a number of medicines which have proven helpful. The main categories of these medicines include digestive tonics, particularly tonics for the liver, and adaptogenic/adrenal medicines that help the body adapt to stress, including the stress of a chronic illness. This category of medicines was discussed in Chapter 6.

The first medicine that should always be used with chronic fatigue patients is the Chinese herb schisandra. This is because much of the actual fatigue and muscle pain in chronic fatigue patients comes from the buildup of lactic acid in the cells and the lack of clearing that is the normal process of muscle metabolism. Chinese herbal tradition considers schisandra as both an adaptogen and a liver/digestive herb. Contemporary studies have shown that this adaptogenic effect may be due to the herb's ability to help the muscles metabolize and rid themselves of lactic acid. With the improved ability to clear lactic acid comes increased stamina and lessened pain. This allows for increased exercise and further improvement and the vicious cycle is broken. One can use schisandra extract on its own, or in the Mediherb tablet Livco, which also contains milk thistle, another liver herb, and rosemary which functions as an antioxidant in the tissues. In this case, the dose is 1 tablet 4 times per day.

For adrenal support with chronic fatigue patients, I usually choose the Mediherb tablet withania complex and the Standard Process protomorphogen Drenatrophin made from bovine adrenal gland, both discussed in Chapter 6.

Movement

Chronic fatigue is brought on when the activities of the lower body alternate between lack of warmth and momentary intensity. It is as though one's food is being digested by high flames that consume lots of energy and then burn out quickly, rather than by slowly burning embers that give out a steady, expansive heat. Movement exercises for chronic fatigue should be designed to stimulate a steady, even heat in the lower body, such as the Abdominal Massage and the Stomach Wave. These exercises will also provide a balance to the excess of thought without action that is the marker for chronic fatigue.

Rudolf Steiner taught that the Metabolic System, that is, the organs and processes of digestion and excretion, is intimately related to the soul force he refers to as the will. The will, according to Steiner, is the ability of the individual to go out of himself or herself to meet and change the world. Without the will, there is no action, no accomplishment and no transformation in the physical world. The will involves the realm of the deed and is a brother to the family of thinking and feeling.

It is helpful to consider chronic fatigue as the opposite disease to adrenal insufficiency (although the symptoms may be similar). In chronic fatigue, the mechanism for producing the right amount of stimulating adrenaline is compromised, making concentration difficult and the nervous system sluggish. Therefore, walking barefoot on the beach is recommended, as this gently massages the toes, that area of the feet that corresponds to the nervous system. An added benefit of walking along the shore is that we also breathe in air that has been suffused with iodine. As the thyroid gland is usually involved in chronic fatigue, the iodine-rich air of the beach can be a wonderful tonic.

Swimming is an excellent exercise for fatigue as water gestures strengthen the life-force body. The motions and feeling of swimming should be carried over into all other movements.

Chronic fatigue is often tied to thyroid insufficiency involving the neck and voice. People with underactive thyroid glands frequently speak in a hoarse or rasping voice and when they speak the tendons in the neck tense up and become prominent. When we speak correctly, the whole chest should vibrate. The Carriage Down/Carriage Up gestures, the Spinal Stretch and the Victory Stretch can all help stimulate a sluggish thyroid gland and remove constriction from the voice box.

The Cowl Gesture is therapeutic for those with an overactive thyroid gland. This moves tension down off the neck so that it can dissipate into the shoulders and torso. Many people, particularly those with an overactive thyroid gland, are figuratively "bottlenecked," lacking a connection between the neck and the torso. This exercise redefines the neck as a functional unit down to the ninth thoracic vertebra. The neck is not an isolated body part but actually an integral part of the chest. Many sculptures of antiquity were "busts" showing the head, neck and chest as a unity. Sculptures of just the head and neck seem disembodied and unnatural.

Other exercises for chronic fatigue include the Pulley, Autumn Leaves, Shoulder Muscle Mapping, Foot Streaming, Knee Mapping and Letting Go as they rhythmically transform a release into gravity into a readiness for activity.

Meditation

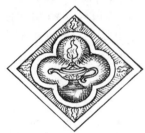

Steiner taught that we exercise our will forces when we eat food, for in this encounter with the outside world we muster our energies so as to meet and overcome this outside material that has entered into our bodies. If we do not become the master of this food, it makes us tired and causes allergies. We must annihilate the food as the first step in building up our own healthy organism.

Steiner often pointed out that eating raw or fermented food was a good temporary therapeutic diet because one's metabolic forces or will is strongly activated through the encounter with raw food. During the process of breaking down our food, the muscular system—which, according to Steiner, is intimately tied up with the metabolism—meets and interacts with the outside world though our deeds. That is, inwardly we meet and overcome our food with our inner will forces. Outwardly, we meet and interact with the world through our limbs. "By his deeds you shall know him." It is only by the deeds, the actions, that the true measure of a person can be taken. The man or woman who merely thinks accomplishes nothing.

The therapy outlined here is not only a treatment for Chronic Fatigue Syndrome, a specific illness, but also a therapy for our culture as a whole. Our culture is tremendously biased, and in a very unhealthy way, towards valuing the thinking pole first and foremost. Our whole educational system—which now even considers recess for elementary age children to be an unnecessary luxury—is geared almost exclusively to the education of the thinking or Nerve-Sense pole. The work that most of us do rarely involves actually creating something with our hands, but more and more has to do with manipulating images, numbers or concepts in our heads, or in the outer image of our head which is the computer. We sit all day before a computer screen or a television screen, our feelings occasionally aroused but our will sound asleep.

Chronic Fatigue Syndrome is therefore not only a disease, it is also a metaphor for our culture. It is related to a deadening of our ability to create in the physical world with our actions, rather than just formulate concepts. It is paralleled by our persistent encounter with lifeless food that calls forth nothing from our digestive organs while, at the same time, burdening our digestion and leaving our organs chronically undernourished. Chronic Fatigue Syndrome is a kind of individual encounter with this struggle that is ongoing in our culture. Where do we find the will forces to right our world?

It is not enough to think lofty thoughts or feel deep feelings. To be fully human, our thoughts must inspire us to take actions that can change our world. Therefore, during the *Rückschau* Meditation, we should consider carefully whether our ideals have inspired us to constructive action or whether their expression is blocked by inertia. Consider carefully which factors must be changed to allow the will to manifest. The first step is to embrace a diet that the body can easily digest. Only then will the forces of the will be able to overcome other blocks to lasting accomplishment.

Summary

Nutrition

* Avoid

All processed foods
Whole grains not properly prepared
Commercial salt

* Emphasize

Fermented foods
Raw animal foods
Vegetables
Lacto-fermented beverages, especially beet kvass

* Supplements

Cod liver oil to provide 20,000 IU vitamin A
per day

Therapeutics

* Schisandra extract by Mediherb, 1-2 teaspoons per day or
* Livco by Mediherb, 1 tablet 3-4 times per day.
* Withania tablets by Mediherb, 1 tablet 3-4 times per day.
* Drenatrophin by Standard Process, 1-2 tablets 3 times per day between meals.

Movement

* Abdominal Massage and Stomach Wave.
* Walking in the sand.
* Swimming.
* Carriage Up/Carriage Forward, Spinal Stretch and the Victory Stretch for underactive thyroid.
* Cowl Exercise for overactive thyroid.
* The Pulley, Autumn Leaves, Shoulder Muscle Mapping, Foot Streaming, Knee Mapping and Letting Go for "pulling one's self up by one's boot straps."

Meditation

*   Consider carefully whether your ideals have inspired you to constructive action.

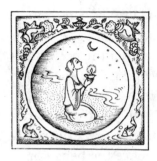

Chapter 9:
Women's Diseases

. . . Lo, the Moon's self!
Here in London, yonder late in Florence,
Still we find her face, the thrice-transfigured.
Curving on a sky imbued with colour,
Drifted over Fiesole by twilight,
Came she, our new crescent of a hair's-breadth.
Full she flared it, lamping Samminiato,
rounder 'twixt the cypresses and rounder,
Perfect till the nightingales applauded. . .

One Word More
Robert Browning

"Lady Moon, Lady Moon, where are you roving?"
    "Over the sea."
"Lady Moon, Lady Moon, whom are you loving?"
    "All that love me."

A Child's Song
Richard Monckton Milnes Houghton

As we have pointed out, ancient philosophers recognized a relationship between celestial bodies, various metals found on earth and the function of human organs. Modern students of medicine dismiss these correspondences as medieval superstition, having no real bearing on the question of health and disease.

Yet it is impossible to gain insight into women's diseases without an understanding of the relationship between menstruation and the lunar cycle. While many

219

of the medieval correspondences—such as the connection between lead, the spleen and the planet Saturn discussed in Chapter 3—seem far-fetched to modern minds, the relationship between the rhythm of the moon and the menstrual cycle is clear and unmistakable. Science has yet to confirm the ancient belief that the position of Mars in the sky affects aggression, the will, arterial blood flow and the male psyche, or that the position of Jupiter affects our liver biochemistry or intellectual ability, but we readily accept the fact that lunar cycles affect more than the tides. To summarize these effects would be a large task, but what is clear is that, in a way still partly shrouded in mystery, the rhythmical cycles of the moon influence the behavior or flow of fluids on the earth, including the watery realm of the human body.

The ebb and flow of the tides is a rhythm characterized by predictability, beauty and a profoundly healing quality. Throughout the earth, people walk the beaches for a sense of peace and renewed vigor. Yet tides can also be destructive, rising with relentless power. The source of both the healing and destructive nature of tides is the moon, molding the oceans of the earth, which are in turn the source from which all life has sprung. This is true both from the perspective of biology and evolution—our "objective" scientific viewpoint—and from the perspective of mythology and legend. Aphrodite, the archetypal female, emerges from the oceans to the Isle of Crete. Many cultures have similar legends about the origin of human life, or perhaps more specifically the human feminine soul, emerging from the oceans of the earth.

We have all felt a sense of beauty and awe at the sight of a brilliant full moon. No other visual phenomenon inspires us as much to explore the larger questions of our existence. Yet paradoxically, the beautiful moon that has haunted poets and lovers has no light of its own. What we see on those glorious moonlit evenings is really an illusion. The moon itself is a cold, dark, lifeless dusty rock circling our earth, held in an eternal grip by the power of gravity.

It should be no surprise that the system of medieval correspondences assigns to the moon the metal silver (*argentum* in Latin). Silver is the second most precious metal next to gold, much like the moon is the noble companion of the sun. If one condenses silver, taking it rapidly from the liquid to the solid state, it will pop and crackle until it forms a cratered surface that bears an eerie resemblance to the surface of the moon. Silver, like the moon, is characterized by clarity, brilliance, purity and, above all, perfection as a reflector of light. It is the perfect metal for mirrors, photographic paper and certain musical instruments, like flutes and bells. It is difficult to imagine a flute made from lead or a mirror of bronze. Silver is the most perfect vessel, receptacle or complement to the pure light of the golden sun, and yet this perfection is an illusion. It is not an accident, therefore, that even today we speak of the "light of the silvery moon."

The moon's relation to the feminine clearly manifests in the monthly cycle we call the menses. The normal female menstrual cycle lasts 28 days, exactly the same period as that of the moon. Many women report that they ovulate either at the new or full moon and menstruate on the opposite phase, although this kind of regularity seems to be less common today than in the past. Furthermore, the growth of the child in the womb is also governed by the moon, taking exactly 9 moon cycles of 28 days to complete under optimal circumstances. Animal gestation periods also occur as multiples or common fractions of the moon's cycle.

The menstrual cycle is divided into two relatively distinct phases of waxing and waning, each characterized by its dominant hormone. The first stage, from the end of bleeding to ovulation, is called the proliferative stage, during which the endometrium or inner lining of the uterus grows and thickens under the influence of the hormone estrogen. This phase prepares the uterus to receive the implantation of the ovum or fertilized egg. Of course many other events are happening simultaneously during this stage to prepare the uterus as a receptacle for a new human being, but the common theme is that estrogen stimulates new growth, more blood vessels and more nutritive supply to build up the uterus. Then ovulation occurs, and for a period of a few days, implantation can take place. The second phase follows, during which estrogen levels decrease while progesterone, the other female hormone, increases. Progesterone causes a decrease in the blood supply to the endometrium, and if no fertilization occurs, the endometrium is expelled ten to fourteen days later. The expulsion of the endometrium, or the menses, lasts three to five days.

It seems logical that when a woman is completely healthy and in tune with her surroundings, the first phase of her cycle would coincide with the lunar phase between new moon and full moon, when the moon is "growing;" and the second phase would coincide with the time between the full and new moon, when the moon "dies off." Furthermore, the uterus, governed so precisely by the phases of the moon, may be likened to a silver vessel. As the reflection of the moon is the light of the sun and the content of the silver flute is the tone and the "idea" of the composer, so the content of the uterus is the child. The silver vessel is sacred not in and of itself but for what it contains.

In recent decades, women have made great strides in the area of civil rights. But such progress on economic and political levels should not blind us to the true source of power for the feminine—the fact that only in the female menstrual cycle is the human being so closely and so obviously linked with external nature and the wider cosmos. This connection does not occur in the male. In a sense, men are freer from nature, but as a consequence, they feel more lost. What men perceive as feminine power is actually their awe-inspiring connection to the world outside themselves. As the moon governs the biochemistry of the womb, the most inward and secret place of the human body, so the connection of women to the cosmos reaches into the depths of their physical beings.

With this understanding of the healthy menstrual cycle and its relationship to the phases of the moon, we can find guidance on how to proceed when things go amiss.

As I have stressed throughout this book, health is a condition not of stasis but of balance. The basis of health for the female reproductive area must be a 28-day cycle in which ovulation occurs around the full moon and menses at the new moon. If you suffer from a gynecological problem—such as prolonged or shortened menses, endometriosis, dysmenorrhea (painful cramps), an abnormal pap smear or breast cancer—then the first step toward recovery should focus on bringing the menstrual cycle in sync with the moon.

1. PROLONGED MENSTRUAL CYCLE—ESTROGEN DOMINANCE

The most common disruption of the menstrual cycle involves abnormalities of the first phase. When a woman has too much estrogen in her blood and tissues—either because she makes too much or because she is exposed to estrogens in her food and environment—the first phase will be prolonged and the cycle will last more than 28 days. Prolonged menses are a common occurrence today because we are literally awash in a sea of environmental chemicals that mimic estrogen—pesticides, plastics, estrogens that find their way into meat and milk and phytoestrogens in plant foods, particularly in soy products that are used in so many of our processed foods. Due to modern farming methods, the very foods that provide us with cholesterol, the raw material out of which estrogen is made, also contain a "phony" copy of estrogen, which overstimulates our estrogen receptors. The result is that women's bodies are chronically exposed to foreign estrogen compounds, leading to reduced sensitivity to the body's own estrogen.

Prolonged menses and estrogen dominance can be associated with obesity—typically in a pattern of excessive weight in the upper body—because estrogen is stored in the fat cells. Overweight women are thus exposed to excessive levels in the blood.

On the soul level, disruption of menstrual cycles follows logically from the changes in life-style that accompanied industrialization. Modern women no longer plant seeds by the moon, gather herbs and harvest grain by the moon, make love by the moon or even look at the moon. We are not aware of where the moon is in its cycle, so the link between the lunar rhythm and the inner menstrual rhythm is lost.

The therapy for this type of imbalance follows from an understanding of the underlying cause and entails minimizing exposure to estrogens from all sources—from pesticides and plastics in the environment to soy foods and contaminated animal products in the diet. For overweight women with prolonged menses, the first step is losing weight (see Chapter 11).

Nutrition

 Animal products provide cholesterol, the raw material from which estrogen is made, while good-quality animal fats provide factors that nourish the entire endocrine system. The estrogen-dominant woman is often hooked on refined carbohydrates. While she can still continue to eat appropriate carbohydrate foods, she needs to put somewhat more emphasis on animal foods as they are very important for restoring regularity. This step will also help her lose weight if she is too heavy, or gain weight if she is too thin. However, all animal foods should be from organically raised, pasture-fed animals or wild, ocean-going fish. Milk products, including butter, cheese and yoghurt, should come strictly from grass-fed cows. The balance of the diet should be vegetables, fruits and properly prepared organic whole grains and nuts, but no legumes (beans and lentils), particularly no soy products.

It is important to prepare your own foods according to a regular schedule. Learn to use plenty of herbs, especially rosemary, thyme and basil.

Trans fatty acids in partially hydrogenated vegetables oils should be strictly avoided as these interfere with the conversion of cholesterol to estrogen and progesterone, and with many other biochemical processes that affect the reproductive system. Caffeine may also disrupt the endocrine system, affecting the menstrual cycles, and should be minimized.

As always, cod liver oil is essential. Women actually need more vitamin A than men as vitamin A is required for the production of female hormones. The dose should provide about 20,000 IU vitamin A per day.

Therapeutics

 Homeopathically potentiated silver is the medicine of choice for menstrual irregularities. I recommend Argentum D6 from Weleda, which provides the reproductive organs with a "picture" of healthy function. Giving silver as a medicine is like giving a small dose of the moon and can help the patient reconnect to the moon's 28-day rhythm. The dose is 1 pea-sized portion 3 times per day.

I also give Simplex F from Standard Process for virtually all problems associated with the female reproductive system. Simplex F is a protomorphogen designed especially for women. It contains bovine tissue of the pituitary, thyroid and adrenal glands as well as the ovaries. The compound helps relieve stress from the entire endocrine axis involved in the female reproductive system. The dose is 1-2 capsules 3 times per day.

Marjoram complex is a mixture of five herbs formulated for the restoration of harmony or rhythm to a disordered menstrual cycle. First suggested by Rudolf Steiner, it is currently produced by Weleda. The dose is 15 drops in water four times a day, omitting the days of the menses. Marjoram complex should be taken for at least one year as the menstrual cycle gradually takes on a more normal rhythm.

In addition, I frequently prescribe castor oil packs to improve the health of the uterus. They should be placed on the pelvic region 2-3 times per week. Castor oil packs increase circulation and stimulate detoxification by supplying warmth to the affected organs.

Movement

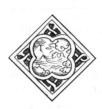 Our western society handles such themes as puberty, menstruation, and indeed the whole world of sexuality in a very clumsy manner. Even our discomfort in discussing the processes of digestion and excretion puts unnecessary chokeholds on these vital functions. We should not consider these functions as necessary evils, but as expressions of the very life processes themselves. The common phrase: "It hurts down there," indicates distance and separation—the abdomen, pelvic floor and sexual organs relegated to the nameless and unspeakable below. Although we have made considerable progress in recent years, taboos persist, for the genitals and organs of digestion and excretion are still often considered somehow dirty or less worthy. A further, often overlooked factor is chronic pelvic pain and discomfort in women who have suffered intimate or domestic violence, which lingers as an unwanted gesture long after the trauma has occurred.

We need to celebrate every part of the body as beautiful, as important and as virtuous as all the others. Failure to do so has resulted in physical, mental, developmental and emotional blockages that contribute to "dis-ease," to the disorders discussed here. When every part of the body is fully inhabited, fully cared for and enjoyed, there is greater energy, possibility and healing that comes from experiencing yourself as an integral whole.

The condition of estrogen dominance often manifests itself as a lack of clearness in the head. Tides can be helpful in stilling the brain and nervous system. It helps return the body to an "even keel." Likewise, the Lemniscate Dynamic can help clear the head and provide warmth to the abdomen. The Stomach Wave and Abdominal Massage can help bring the proper rhythm to the abdominal area. Downright-Upright, Grounding, the Body Space Imagination, the Water Level Gesture, the Spinal Stretch, Knee Mapping, Bestowing and the Dipole are also useful in rhythmically uniting the Nervous and Metabolic Systems.

A vigorous exercise program is important, particularly for a woman who is overweight. Participation in sport, dance or training activity can be especially helpful. These activities should should foster a reconnection of the head with the lower centers of balance. Fencing and dancing fall into this category.

Meditation

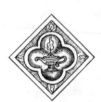

Women's liberation has brought great benefits, but women should beware of "liberation" from their connection with the moon, the source of their receptivity, sensitivity, mystique and power. As we all know, during the last forty years, women have had to act more and more like men, to compete in a man's world. But if they are to remain healthy, and retain their power and influence, at some point women need to draw the line. They can and should "compete" but not to the point of losing their femininity, their lunar connection.

I highly recommend that women take the simple step of noting the phase of the moon and correlating it with the stage of their cycle. In addition, women should take at least one minute every day to locate and look at the moon. When you engage in the *Rückschau* Meditation, be sure to focus your attention for a moment or two on the phase of your menstrual cycle, noting whether you are in the waxing or waning phase and how it corresponds with the phase of the moon.

If possible, take a long walk in the open air, preferably by the sea, when the moon is full. As the years pass your soul will deepen its connection to lunar rhythms and help restore your body to its proper health.

II.   SHORTENED MENSTRUAL CYCLE—ESTROGEN DEFICIENCY

The menstrual cycle can also be disrupted in the proliferative phase by estrogen deficiency, resulting in a cycle that is too short. In extreme cases, insufficient buildup of the endometrium results in complete failure of ovulation. This condition may be associated with scanty menses and painful cramps, not to mention anorexia, hypothyroidism or other chronic illnesses that disrupt hormonal activity. In the shortened cycle, the relative balance of estrogen to progesterone is shifted to excess progesterone, whereas estrogen excess characterizes the prolonged cycle.

Shortened menses involve excess breakdown as opposed to buildup. In other words, the sympathetic impulse to catabolism or breakdown overwhelms the parasympathetic anabolic urge to build up or repair. The processes that take place in the uterus involve competing tendencies to build up (which is watery or plantlike) and to break down (which is emotional or animal-like). Not surprisingly, when the forces for breakdown predominate, pain ooccurs, in this case, in the form of menstrual cramps.

With shortened menses, we could say that the consciousness or awareness of healthy female rhythms is lacking. (With prolonged menses, the opposite is true—there is often too much attention to this region of the body.) I often find a history of sexual trauma in women with painful menses or shortened periods. This experience seems to lock the soul into the area of the sexual organs where it becomes the seed of physical imbalance later in life. Or, scanty, absent or short menses often follows a stressful period in puberty, or a bout with anorexia or bulimia.

Metaphorically speaking, the overall challenge these women face is to become "earth-ripe." For one reason or another, they are struggling to find a happy relationship with their bodies and developing sexuality. If there are problems in these areas, the usual response is to blame fat intake. The progesterone dominant woman may also adopt a lowfat diet—yet another denial of "earth ripeness"—leading to weight loss and fatigue. The menses, already scanty, may stop altogether.

Nutrition

The goal in the treatment of shortened menses is increased estrogen production. Estrogen is made from cholesterol by our ovaries and adrenal glands. A diet high in fats, and the fat-soluble nutrients they contain, will nourish the endocrine system and provide the raw materials for estrogen production. The condition of shortened menses actually calls for more emphasis on animal foods than the condition of prolonged menses.

Many women with shortened menses suffer from anorexia, a condition in which the fat content of the diet and hence the body has become so low that the menses stop altogether. Women with this condition need to eat liberally of butter, cream and the healthy fat of all properly raised animals. Eggs—a symbol of fertility—are especially beneficial. Fish roe should be consumed frequently.

Once again, *trans* fatty acids from partially hydrogenated vegetable oils should be strictly avoided as these interfere with the enzyme system the body uses to produce estrogen. In addition, avoid all soy foods, which can act as potent endocrine disrupters.

Substances that put stress on the adrenal glands, including coffee, tea, chocolate and refined sugar, should be completely eliminated from the diet. For a hot drink, use warm broth or ginger tea.

For the first year or so, a diet of 40-50 percent high-fat animal foods is appropriate, complemented by a variety of vegetables, fruit, grains, legumes and nuts. When the menses become healthy again, the amount of animal foods can be reduced somewhat.

As always, cod liver oil is the supplement of choice for providing fat-soluble vitamins and supporting thyroid and endocrine function. The dose is one that supplies at least 20,000 IU vitamin A per day.

Therapeutics

For shortened menses, the best silver preparation to use is Bryophyllum Argento Culto 1%, 20 drops given in water, 4 times a day for six months. This is a Weleda preparation made from the bryophyllum plant grown in compost to which homeopathic silver has been added. The bryophyllum plant is a succulent, vital plant called the "Mother of Thousands" because at the end of each leaf grow numerous rootlets, each of which can be planted to form a new plant. Thus it makes sense to use this plant in a situation in which the powers of growth and regeneration are too weak to support a normal cycle. In a sense, the silver in the compost connects the vitality of the plant with moon rhythms and the female reproductive cycle.

In addition, I prescribe Symplex F from Standard Process, 1 tablet 3 times a day for 6 months.

Over and over in my years of medicine I have heard women with this condition tell me, "I don't want to be here." Often this is a result of a trauma they have experienced; or it may simply reflect their constitution. It is not difficult to grasp that to counteract this soul mood, the therapy must involve warmth—warmth that gently encourages a woman to make contact with her own body and involve herself in meaningful activity. This can be encouraged by the use of warm castor oil packs over the lower abdomen and nightly use of copper ointment, the Venus metal, over the uterus. I recommend Cuprum 0.4%, a formulation by Weleda. Hot baths and warming massage can also be helpful in restoring balance in these cases.

Movement

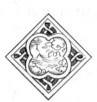

For problems of estrogen deficiency or progesterone dominance, the Horizontal Plane needs moving down. The Water Level exercise can help achieve this. With adolescence, part of the heart forces are—or should be—sequestered in the uterus, a phenomenon that can find its gesture in the exercise we call Bestowing. The Personal Space Gesture and Autumn Leaves are also helpful for this condition. The Stomach Wave brings rhythm and movement into the abdominal area. Latin dancing can be useful in transferring the sexual energy away from the upper body.

Highly athletic women with shortened menses may benefit from a less strenuous workout regime. Menstruation often ceases during hard athletic training. Gentle movement that has an artistic content should be encouraged.

Meditation

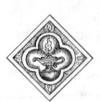

In addition to spending time each day locating and looking at the moon, women with shortened menstrual cycles should contemplate the quality of "earth ripeness." During your *Rückschau* Meditation, focus your attention on daily activities that have drawn you closer to the workings of nature.

Ultimately the medicine that works best for the condition of estrogen deficiency is love and acceptance, usually initially from one's family and then in the context of an intimate relationship. Often the acceptance of truly "being here" is not resolved until the woman falls in love and experiences firsthand the beauty and power that love enkindles. Fraught with pitfalls as it is, the acceptance of love and sexuality can often be the decisive step in becoming "earth-ripe" for many young women.

III.   DYSMENORRHOEA—PAINFUL CRAMPS

While this condition is usually associated with shortened menses, in fact it can happen with equal severity in prolonged menses, or even in menses of a normal cycle. Painful cramps often result from an imbalance of prostaglandins, localized tissue hormones that, among other things, control uterine contractions. The modern diet with its altered fats often results in the overproduction of prostaglandins that stimulate uterine contractions and the underproduction of prostaglandins that relax the uterus.

Nutrition

In addition to the appropriate diet for prolonged or shortened menses, I recommend one teaspoon daily of flax oil and six capsules daily of evening primrose oil to redress prostaglandin imbalance, along with cod liver oil. Saturated fats in butter and coconut oil also aid in prostaglandin production. Zinc is an important element in this process, available in red meat and oysters and other shellfish. Use Celtic sea salt, for vital sodium chloride and important trace minerals, and plenty of vegetables, both raw and cooked. Avoid all processed foods, especially vegetable oils, both liquid and hydrogenated.

Therapeutics

As with prolonged menses, the combination of castor oil packs, two to three times a week over the uterus, plus nightly applications of copper ointment from Weleda will often significantly relieve debilitating menstrual cramps.

Another medicine that has proved invaluable in the treatment of menstrual cramps is the herbal combination Cramplex from Mediherb. The primary ingredient in this preparation is *Corydalis ambigua* tuber, which traditional Chinese medicine values for its ability to relieve the cramps that occur in smooth muscle tissue. It can be used at the dose of 1-2 tablets every 2-4 hours when the cramps are occurring.

Movement

The most useful exercise for menstrual cramps is the Dipole. When women with menstrual cramps first do this exercise, the lower hand usually stops near the navel while the upper hand continues on with the exercise, often resulting in loss of balance and even a sideways fall. This inability to move the hand through the genital area reflects the fact that western culture does not honor the process of menstruation. We have no celebration, no rite of passage for girls when their menses begin. Instead, we often treat the transition into adulthood as an embarrassing, shameful and private event. In cases where this suppressive gesture was changed into one that accepted menstruation as part of the natural creative process, the cramping lessened and sometimes eventually disappeared. The Dipole exercise is a tremendous aid in this process.

Letting Go, Autumn Leaves and Bestowing can also be very helpful for release. Bestowing is a very graceful gesture, giving the menstrual fluids over to gravity and the earth.

The Breathing Exercise is also recommended. Allow the abdomen, not just the lungs, to increase in volume, thus supplying the lower organs with replenishment of oxygen and rhythmic movement.

In conjunction with these exercises, an imagination exercise, in which you create the spacial dynamic of gold melting down through the spine, has helped many women overcome painful cramps.

Meditation

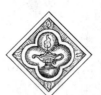

Use the appropriate meditation for prolonged or shortened menstrual cycles, noting the phases of the moon and cultivating "earth ripeness" as needed. If you have experienced a sexual trauma, gently consider its impact on your thoughts and actions as you engage in your *Rückschau* Meditation.

IV.   ENDOMETRIOSIS/ADENOMYOSIS

This condition usually goes hand-in-hand with a prolonged menstrual cycle and is accompanied by severe menstrual cramps, pain with defecation, painful intercourse and even pain with ovulation. In endometriosis, the endometrium, or lining of the uterus, actually begins to seed and grow in other sites, such as the intestines and the bladder. These islands of endometrium cause pain when they go through the cycle of menses and bleed as though they were normal uterine tissue. The usual therapy for this painful condition is surgical ablation or birth control pills to shut off excessive estrogen production.

Nutrition

Foods rich in vitamin A, including liver, fish and shellfish, eggs and butter from pasture-fed cows, are especially helpful for this condition. Cod liver oil should be taken at a dose that supplies *at least* 20,000 IU vitamin per day. In South Africa, this condition has been treated successfully with vitamin A dosages as high as 90,000 IU per day.

Therapeutics

The underlying pathology of endometriosis is severe estrogen dominance. To correct this imbalance, follow the instructions in the section on prolonged cycle with the addition of a natural progesterone cream. I recommend 1/8 to 3/4 teaspoon natural 100 mg/gram progesterone cream applied twice daily to the skin. Once the problem is under control, the progesterone can be gradually tapered off.

In addition, I recommend the herb chaste tree (*Vitex-agnus castus*) which helps increase progesterone production. Use tablets by Mediherb at a dose of 2 tablets every morning from ovultation until menses start, for 3-6 months.

Movement

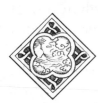

The condition of endometriosis has a gesture of withdrawal from the pelvic floor. As with the condition of painful cramps, the Stomach Wave, Dipole, Letting Go and Bestowing provide a way of changing this gesture to one of acceptance, balance and rhythm. Shoulder Muscle Mapping can also be helpful. Latin dancing can help transfer warmth into the abdominal region.

Meditation

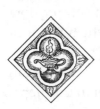

Follow the meditation for estrogen dominance, noting the phases of the moon and the phases of the menstrual cycle. As you engage in the *Rückschau* Meditation, note those activities of your day in which your thoughts and actions exhibited traits of estrogen dominance.

V.   VAGINITIS

Vaginitis is a common occurrence characterized by episodes of painful, itchy inflammation of the vagina, often with a thick vaginal discharge. Many microorganisms can cause vaginal infections. The specific type can be determined by laboratory tests and treated with specific drugs. However, we must remember that micro-organisms are scavengers, as we discussed in Chapter 1 on infectious disease. They live off of our waste products. Therefore, the most appropriate therapy involves determining the source of the "waste." In addition to the waste from processed foods, another source of "waste" in the vagina can be the male semen and sperm. Put another way, sex without love can deposit waste in the vagina, which can lead to infection. For many women, this crucial interaction must be addressed.

Nutrition

The most common cause of vaginitis, however, is chronic yeast infection, which usually responds to dietary changes without the use of drugs. First in the line of defense is the maintenance of a strong population of healthy bacteria in the bowels and vaginal orifices. Refined carbohydrates and sugars should be completely eliminated, along with improperly prepared whole grains, such as granola and extruded breakfast cereals. Total carbohydrate intake (grains and fruit) should make up no more than one-third of the diet. Butter and coconut oil should be eaten liberally as they supply short-chain saturated fatty acids that have strong antifungal effects. Include 2-4 tablespoons of each in the diet daily. (Coconut oil can be mixed with warm water or herb tea or added to smoothies.) Finally, the diet should include liberal amounts of lacto-fermented foods such as yoghurt, kefir, sauerkraut and beet kvass. These supply lactobacilli that keep yeasts at bay in the intestinal tract.

Therapeutics

Daily application of a small amount of plain, high-quality yoghurt rubbed inside the vagina can be very soothing and help establish the proper flora in the vaginal tract. Another useful remedy is tea tree oil, which has antifungal properties. It can be mixed with olive oil and applied to the vagina, or used in suppository form. Orally, the herbs pau d'arco, cats claw and echinacea can be used to dampen down the yeast population. They are mixed together in the preparation from Mediherb called Cats Claw Complex, and can be used at the dose of 1 tablet 4 times per day for 2-3 months.

Synthetic, non-breathable fibers can encourage yeast growth. Choose cotton underwear and clothes made of natural fibers such as cotton, wool and silk. Use loose-fitting cotton sleep wear and remove underwear for sleeping.

For very severe outbreaks, a three-day course of Monistat, an over-the-counter fungal drug, may be necessary. If the infection persists in spite of these measures, you should be checked for diabetes as vaginitis is often an early sign of a sugar imbalance.

Movement

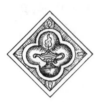

There should be a glow to the lower body, like embers. Infections in the vagina derive more from a coldness rather than a heat. The inflammation in vaginitis is like a prickly heat and is an attempt to create the heat or fire that is missing.

The Stomach Wave and the Dipole can help bring a glowing heat back into the lower body. When doing the Stomach Wave, imagine a glow as from embers to warm up this area from the center down and outward. Likewise, imagine embers in the lower body when doing the Dipole. Shoulder Muscle Mapping can also be helpful to increase the flow of blood downward, warming hands, buttocks and feet.

Meditation

As you engage in the *Rückschau* Meditation, pinpoint any emotions or actions that draw heat and light away from the vaginal area. Remember that fungus thrives in darkness. Also, if you are engaged in a relationship where love is absent, focus on those factors in your life that have contributed to this situation.

VI.   ABNORMAL PAP SMEARS

The purpose of the yearly pap smear is to detect cervical cancer when it is still at an early stage and when it can be treated with simple surgical procedures. In fact, by most accounts this has been a very successful approach to the illness as the number of deaths from cervical cancer has fallen over the past decades. When cancerous tissue is detected in an early stage and is still localized, I fully support the usual surgical approaches to this problem. This involves something called a cone biopsy, which is a minor procedure.

Nutrition

Follow the general dietary guidelines for prolonged or shortened menstrual cycles as appropriate. It is very important to avoid processed foods containing *trans* fatty acids. Most importantly, avoid exposure to estrogens in soy foods and in conventional fruits and vegetables. Eat organic or biodynamic foods as much as possible.

Therapeutics

 The diagnosis of cellular changes in a pap smear should serve as a warning signal that the cancer process is gaining a foothold. The dietary and life-style changes outlined in Chapter 2 on cancer should be strongly considered. I usually give women with abnormal pap smears one year of mistletoe therapy with Iscador Mali, described in Chapter 2.

Movement

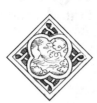 As in other problems with the female reproductive area, the Dipole, Letting Go and the Stomach Wave can all be helpful. As an abnormal pap smear is the first manifestation of cancer, the various movements outlined in Chapter 2 on cancer should be added to these exercises, including the Personal Space Gesture, the Wrestling Stance, Penguin Wrestling and the Sundial, which create buffer zones so that everything can be met outside of our organs.

Meditation

 I have found that women with abnormal pap smears are often undergoing problems with their relationships, or have unresolved underlying issues concerning their sexuality. Any resolution must begin with the observation that the sexual organs have two main functions. The first, of course, is reproduction. The second function—less recognized in the medical world, but equally important—is pleasure, fun and the exploration of passion. These functions are just as much a part of the physiology of the sexual organs as the reproductive functions—in fact, women have an organ, the clitoris, whose only function is to provide pleasure.

The goal is for every person to freely experience the pleasure and joy of their sexuality. Unfortunately this may be difficult for those with unhappy relationships, a history of sexual trauma or a difficult emotional relationship with their sexuality due to repressive childhood religious training.

The correlation that I find of abnormal pap smears with sexual difficulties leads me to believe that joy and pleasure are actually a primary source of nourishment for the sexual organs. An abnormal pap smear can be a great motivator for women to change not only their diets and their life-styles, but also their attitudes about sexual relationships. The most important question for a women with an abnormal pap smear, therefore, is this: "Is sex a source of pleasure and joy for me?" If the answer is not clearly yes, then this is the place for the soul work to start. As you engage in the daily *Rückschau* Meditation, try to determine which changes can be made to bring joy and pleasure back into your sexual relationships.

VII.   PROBLEMS OF MENOPAUSE

As a woman ages she gradually and naturally loses her connection with the moon. When her fertility wanes, her menses become irregular as she is liberated from the controlling rhythms of the lunar forces. In some women the transition is smooth and regular, with few symptoms other than the occasional hot flash. This was the usual situation with women in traditional cultures.

Today, menopause is a period of tremendous upheaval for many women. The first step in any therapy is to recognize an important law of nature, which is that whenever one connection is lost, another connection or influence takes its place. The question is, what is the new connection? What takes the place of the moon's influence when women go through menopause?

To answer this question, let us look at two of the most common symptoms of menopausal difficulties: vaginal dryness and hot flashes. These symptoms provide clues to the new connection women must forge during menopause.

Decline in estrogen production is said to be the cause of the diminution of vaginal secretions. For many women, this change is hardly noticeable, but for some the output of mucus declines to the point that intercourse becomes painful and difficult. Aging, in and of itself, can lead to dryness and loss of elasticity. With age, cellular water content decreases. The liver is said to control the watery or etheric realm of our bodies. This organ is associated with the planet Jupiter and represents not fertility, but wisdom. Before menopause, a woman's fluids, like the tides, are controlled by the moon. After menopause, they come under a new influence, that of Jupiter, god of wisdom, society and the political state. The change in women's bodies at menopause means that it is positive and natural for her to turn her attentions away from the family and the home and toward the world of politics, business and education. These changes also suggest that when there are problems of excessive dryness—either vaginal dryness of dryness of the skin—a treatment for the liver may be beneficial.

Hot flashes are often the first symptom the premenopausal woman experiences, sometimes occurring years before changes in the menstrual cycle. Most women experience this as a rush of warmth, often starting in the lower half of the body and moving upwards. In many cases, hot flashes are accompanied by sweating and flushing of the skin.

Taking the Fourfold Man as our model, it is clear that hot flashes represent activation of the mental or warmth body. The phenomenon involves the organ of the heart and the spirit of individuality. Seen in this light, hot flashes are not so much a symptom of disease needing treatment as a statement of the body's wisdom and a sign that the woman has reached a turning point in her biography. Even in modern societies, until menopause most women live their lives largely for others, first as a child and daughter, then as a mother and wife. It is only at menopause that most women can take control of their own lives and turn their full attention to the outside world. What is more natural, therefore, than hot flashes at menopause, a signal from the warmth body and a physical manifestation of human individuality, the call for a woman to take control of her own destiny.

When women take estrogen, in the form of hormone replacement therapy (HRT) drugs or even by consuming large amounts of soy foods, they maintain their strong moon connection well into their seventies. I am not going to state categorically that taking estrogen is always wrong, but only suggest that it may not be in a woman's best interest to prolong a phase of life past the time when nature intends for new links to be forged. She may end up with nothing more to do than over-mother her husband and children and mope about in an empty nest.

Nutrition

Although it is clearly stated in biochemistry textbooks, most practitioners are unaware of the fact that saturated fats like butter, coconut oil, beef fat and lamb fat are highly protective of the liver. These saturated fats also aid in the conversion of essential fatty acids into prostaglandins. Flax oil and evening primrose oil can be beneficial in small amounts, but only in a diet that also includes adequate saturated fats.

We know that alcohol consumption puts a strain on the liver, but fructose is equally harmful. All fruit juices, fructose-sweetened foods and drinks, and even a surfeit of honey and fruit should be avoided.

Bitter and sour foods such as greens, lemons and sauerkraut have a beneficial effect on the liver. One teaspoon of Swedish bitters mixed with a little warm water can be taken morning and evening and should also prove to be helpful.

As for supplements, cod liver oil will often produce immediate relief from both vaginal dryness and hot flashes. Start with a dose that provides 10,000 IU vitamin A per day, increasing to 20,000 IU if necessary.

Therapeutics

Treatment of the liver for dryness should include homeopathic Stannum, D8. Stannum is tin, the metal the ancients associated with the liver. The dose is 1 pea-sized portion, 3 times per day. Castor oil packs over the liver may also be helpful. If excessive dryness continues in spite of dietary changes, estrogen-stimulating herbs such as black cohosh may be used. I often prescribe Remifemin, an over-the-counter formulation that contains black cohosh. The dose is 1 tablet 3 times per day. In extreme cases, a small of amount of estriol, from Women's International Pharmacy, may be given, not orally but intervaginally, two times a week.

Genuine discomfort due to hot flashes can be treated with a Weleda homeopathic preparation of Aurum (gold) as gold is the metal most closely related to our warmth body. The dose is 10 drops 3 times per day in water of Aurum D10.

If symptoms persist, a last resort is Tri-Est by Women's International Pharmacy, composed of the three naturally occurring estrogens, given at a dosage of 1.25 mg 1-2 times a day. Continue with Tri-Est only as long as the symptoms are disruptive and do not respond to other medications.

Movement

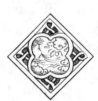

The reproductive organs have many purposes, including reproduction, pleasure and creation/communion. After menopause, they no longer function for reproduction, but should still serve as organs of pleasure, recreation and creation. Often with menopause, women handicap themselves because they cease using these organs completely. Those women who embrace menopause as a new lease on life and the "greatest thing that ever happened" will remain young throughout their remaining years—not only young but wise, as the womb can become the location of intuitive wisdom after menopause.

The sexual organs should be invigorated with every breath. When you do the Breathing Exercise, the pelvic floor should pulse with every breath. On the out-breath, the Kegel movement of the muscles of the pelvic floor should contract and release, as though they were a second diaphragm.

Menopause is a good time to enjoy horsebackriding again or to take dancing lessons!

Meditation

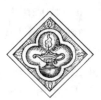

The word menopause contains the word "pause." Very often menopause represents the first time in a woman's life when she even has time to pause for meditation. Contemplation of the experiences that life has brought you should be a defining activity of your menopausal years—it is this contemplation that confers wisdom. As you engage in the *Rückschau* Meditation, consider well the meaning of everything that happens to you, the connections forged throughout your daily activities, and the opportunities presented for you to pass on your wisdom to others.

VIII. OSTEOPOROSIS

During the early 1980s, when I was working in my first job as an emergency room doctor, I encountered a patient whose condition made such a lasting impression on me that I have not forgotten her to this day. The patient was a frail, thin, almost emaciated white woman who came to our ER after having fallen at home. She told us that she had just stood up and then fell down. After that, she felt pain in both hips.

X-rays revealed that she had broken both of her hips at the neck of the femur. Her bones were so "thin," that is, devoid of calcium, that they were barely visible on the X-ray. But even more remarkable was the fact that on both sides, lying right next to the femur bone that had fractured due to insufficient calcification, there were "white pipes" running about one-fourth inch to the outside of each femur. The orthopedic surgeon came in to see about the woman, and I asked him about those white pipes next to her femur bones. He replied, "Those are her femoral arteries (blood vessels)."

I asked, "How come we see them on the X-ray."

He replied, "Well, they are completely calcified."

I scratched my head as I pondered this curious finding. Finally, it hit me, what this patient suffered from was bad aim! Her calcium missed by about one-fourth inch on either side, filling her arteries rather than her bones; if she had better aim, these fractures wouldn't have happened.

For many years after that, whenever a patient would say she wanted to take calcium to prevent bone loss, I would ask her, "How's your aim?" Clearly, taking extra calcium, and putting it in the soft tissues, like the arteries, does not do your bones any favor, and would only contribute to arteriosclerosis. It became imperative for me to discover how human beings "aim" their calcium. Endocrinologists, gynecologists and even specialists in osteoporosis provided no help in answering this fundamental question; what is the key factor in determining whether we put our calcium into our bones and therefore keep them strong and healthy, versus putting the calcium in our soft tissues, and thereby create arteriosclerosis, cataracts (calcification in the soft tissue of the lens of the eye), arthritis (calcification of the joints) and many other "diseases," the hallmark of which is excessive calcification?

As is often the case, examining the facts surrounding osteoporosis eventually led me to the answer. Here are the facts: osteoporosis is known to occur in three distinct groups. The first in thin, older white women, the second is astronauts during prolonged travel outside of the earth's gravity field, and the third is with people of any age and either sex suffering from anorexia (or any kind of severe weight loss). The common thread in these situations is that in each case the person experiences too little gravity. In other words, it is our weight that puts a variable amount of stress on our bones, and "tells" them how calcified they should be. If you carry too little weight, the bones must be thin so your body "aims" the calcium towards the soft tissue to lighten the bones. If there is sufficient weight then the bones must thicken to carry this weight and the "aim" is directed towards the bones. I am always amazed to discover how wisely and accurately our bodies are able to respond to our situation.

Over and over through the years I have seen women struggling to maintain the weight they had in high school and treat their developing bone loss at the same time. It never works! Without the stimulation of increased weight, all that calcium taken in will only exacerbate ongoing soft tissue calcification. The new drugs for osteoporosis, like phosamax, work by trying to move the calcium from the soft tissues to the bones. This may sound reasonable, but the result is an indiscriminate transfer of calcium from soft tissue to bone, inevitably resulting in problems with the soft tissues, which need calcium to function. This explains the esophageal and bowel disorders that inevitably result from the use of these medicines. There is simply no other way to stop the bone loss and rebuild bones than to increase body weight. Nothing else works, whether it be estrogen, increased calcium or vitamin D therapy, because none of these addresses the basic cause and each results in its own set of unwanted consequences.

In understanding this fundamental dynamic behind the progressive bone loss of postmenopausal women, a whole host of phenomena also became clear. First, why does "weight-bearing" exercise help (a little) for osteoporosis? The answer is that such exercise increases the weight or gravity the body experiences, at least temporarily. The problem is that in order to carry this much weight around for long enough to really help, you end up with sore arms. It is far better to do what nature intended for postmenopausal women and put the weight around the waist, hips and buttocks where it belongs. Second, as we all know, many peri- and postmenopausal women resist this inevitable process of gaining weight, usually by trying to starve them-selves, and sometimes through excessive exercise. Unfortunately, this is done in the name of "getting healthy," with the full blessings of society and the medical commu-nity. Many of these women then end up getting the most common "disease" of peri- and postmenopausal women, which is hypothyroidism, a condition in which your body, in its infinite wisdom, understands that drastic action must be undertaken in order to get you to gain weight. This drastic action takes the form of the mobilization of antibodies that partially destroy your thyroid gland, thereby decreasing the output of thyroid hormones, which has the effect of making you tired, which gets you to decrease the excessive exercise, and consequently makes you gain weight, thereby effectively addressing the gravity issue underlying the osteoporosis. Unfortunately, most doctors fail to understand this dynamic and prescribe some sort of thyroid supple-ment. The woman feels better, resumes her exercise, is grateful that she can maintain her slender figure, and her osteoporosis, better called the crumbling of her infrastruc-ture, continues apace. There is a better way!

The final phenomenon this dynamic explains is the prevalence of uncomfort-able hot flashes. As I mentioned in the previous section, mild hot flashes are a normal part of the change of life, not only normal but also pleasant. But severe hot flashes that prevent sleep and involve intense sweating represent a real problem for many women and indicate a precipitous drop in estrogen levels. (All humans need some level of estrogen in their blood, not only young women, but women in menopause and also men.) Increased fat stores not only protect against osteoporosis, they also help retain estrogen in the body. After all, estrogen is fat-soluble and the body uses the fat stores to keep enough estrogen available to protect the bones. Having enough stores of *healthy* fat also helps maintain enough estrogen in the body to prevent hot flashes. Very overweight women can also get hot flashes, of course, but this is due to the hyperinsulinemia and excessive sugar intake (see Chapter 5 on diabetes). The only true solution to the problem of osteoporosis, hypothyroidism, severe hot flashes and all the other associated peri- and postmenopausal symptoms is a life-style and an attitude about life that allows you to accept your body's fluctuating weight demands with the kind of reverence and respect it deserves. The diet you follow should not be one that keeps you eternally thin, but allows your body to find its ideal weight—which is at least two dress sizes greater than your weight as a young woman. Once that is accomplished, we can take steps to restore calcium to the bones as we can be confident that our aim will be right on target.

If I had to boil down into one sentence the essence of my "goal" when I see a patient I would say that it is to allow a situation to develop so that at some point during the visit he or she either laughs or cries. My experience has been that when either or both of these occurs, the patient has shifted to a new level of understanding about her situation, and as a result can make real changes in her life. With a few "diseases" I have noticed that at a certain point in the visit the same emotional reaction emerges. Many cancer patients cry as they tell their story, but curiously most of the people who tell me about their osteoporosis laugh. They laugh when I point out the connection between osteoporosis and lack of gravity or weight. After the laugh or chuckle they invariably say, "I could never gain weight, my husband would kill me" or "I hate being overweight" (usually in a woman who is 20-30 pounds underweight), or "Oh no, I feel awful when I can't fit into my high school prom dress." So, rather than give a single case history, I present all these women as a kind of a group, a group that desperately needs liberation, not liberation to go to work and join the rat race of the men, but liberation from the alienation—often, but not always, imposed by men— of an unrealistic image of their own bodies, liberation from the tyranny of trying to force their bodies into assuming a shape different from that which it naturally wants to assume.

The osteoporosis patient cries out for liberation from dieting, exercise regimens, advertisements and the male-dominated culture that alienates women from rejoicing in the sensuality of their own bodies. Have you ever seen a picture or statue of a Greek or Roman goddess that is thin? No, they are all rounded, even plump. This is a much more profound liberation than the ability to join the work force. This is the liberation of the feminine soul, which is the heart and soul of the world. The laughter of the unnaturally thin patient is the voice of this feminine soul wondering whether it is true that her days of enslavement can finally be over.

Nutrition

Having read this far in the book, you are all aware that excessive carbohydrate intake along with a lowfat diet will lead to a number of health problems, including, for many, obesity. The irony is that in some people, this type of diet contributes to excessive thinness rather than obesity. I find that women with osteoporosis often eat lots of carbohydrate foods such as pasta, dry breakfast cereals and sugar, often in the form of chocolate. Usually they consume lowfat milk and dairy products ("to provide calcium for their bones"), perhaps fish and skinless chicken meat, and low-calorie vegetables, usually salad without dressing. These women are literally starving, while using excessive exercise and "busyness" as appetite suppressants. As they chase the dream, or rather the illusion, of a slim, "healthy" body, totally unfit for their current physical needs, their very foundation of life crumbles away. The solution is a less "busy" life and more good fats in the diet. The diet for osteoporosis should contain 60-80 percent of calories as fat, mostly healthy animal fats. There is no need to restrict carbohydrates as they will stimulate weight gain, but the fat intake must be dramatically increased. There is no other way to bring about beneficial weight gain.

This new diet will have many physiological effects. First, the starvation will end and your body will find its ideal weight within six to twelve months. Second, the increased fats (good fats!) will provide adequate vitamin D, which will stimulate the absorption and deposition of calcium in the bones. Third, the increased fats will stimulate your circulatory pump (see Chapter 3 on heart disease), thereby making you warmer. Fourth, the increased fats will normalize estrogen production and help alleviate hot flashes. And finally, the increased weight will alleviate the need for your body to turn down the thyroid gland. This will result in the thyroid production returning to normal, also in about six to twelve months.

It is important during this period to insure adequate mineral intake. At least once a day, you should consume a good rich soup broth made by boiling bones a long time. Use only Celtic sea salt to ensure adequate trace mineral intake.

As usual for supplements I recommend cod liver oil to insure adequate vitamin D. Take a dose that provides at least 10,000 IU vitamin A per day, which will also supply at least 1000 IU vitamin D.

Therapeutics

The therapeutics for osteoporosis involve diet and exercise, not medicines. I do, however, also recommend Calcifood (a bone-broth supplement) from Standard Process at a dose of 1 scoop in water 1-2 times per day.

Movement

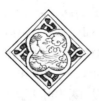
Traditional women, who suffer much less osteoporosis, spend a lot of their time walking slowly and carrying heavy objects, especially on their heads. Is it possible that this traditional practice of increasing the weight and equally distributing it over the whole body, which is what happens when we carry things on the head, is in fact an ingenious method of maintaining the crucial strength of their bones? It may well be that maintaining a healthy relationship to gravity and balance contributes strongly to the health of their skeletal systems.

The loss of bone might be seen metaphorically as a sacrifice of the material world to reach the spiritual. Preparing for the next life, however, does not mean ignoring this one! Continuing to enjoy your body's full potential is indeed spiritual activity right here on earth.

Rediscovering the ground is vital for the second stage of life. Enjoy the feeling of resistance when you climb stairs or walk up a hill—bone is built through resistance. The Grounding Exercise can be especially helpful and also Downright-Upright.

Exercises that increase our sense of balance should be part of daily movement repertoire, such as swinging in a swing, gardening, dancing and even rocking in a rocking chair. The Tides and the Crest can also be helpful. Such movements activate the inner ear and stimulate core muscles and the breath.

Meditation

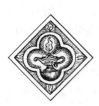

Above all, the desire or interest in being thin must stop. This is a task for individual women and for the society as a whole, which has conspired to create this epidemic disease through manipulation of women's attitudes. Individually and collectively we must allow our bodies to find the right weight and to recognize that the "ideal" weight is variable from person to person and within an individual person depending on activity level and stage of life.

When you engage in the *Rückschau* Meditation each day, note the times that you felt pressure to be thin—whether from articles, advertisements or casual remarks—and mentally place those influences in a trash can. At each instance, imagine yourself as robust and strong, able to carry heavy loads and important responsibilities. Above all, note the enjoyment you get from rich food and the vigorous metabolism it bestows.

IX.   BREAST CANCER

I have discussed the subject of cancer at length in Chapter 2, but the issue of breast cancer belongs with women's diseases. In 1920, breast cancer was rare. Today it afflicts one woman out of nine, many of whom are still in their childbearing years. Orthodox medicine offers few explanations for this alarming situation. Spokesmen for the medical establishment contend that the cause may be genetic, and that women should adhere to a lowfat diet. But how can so many women develop a genetic tendency to a disease that was virtually unknown just 70 years ago; and how can a lowfat diet be of help when Americans at the turn of the century ate much more butter and lard than we do today?

In October 1996, a lead article in *Scientific American* explored the role of xenoestrogens—estrogen-like compounds found in pesticides, industrial chemicals and plastics—in the etiology of breast cancer. In the same year, a group of Nobel-prize-winning scientists presented a statement to the US Congress, expressing their belief that the alarming incidence of cancer in the US is primarily a problem of environmental pollution, especially from excessive radiation and agricultural chemicals. These two events should have made the front-page news, but in fact neither was even mentioned in the popular press.

In the *Scientific American* article, the two authors concluded, after almost twenty years of research, that breast cancer is highly correlated with exposure to environmental estrogens. Xenoestrogens and estrogens manufactured by the human body are not the same, for whereas our natural estrogens link to estrogen receptors and are then removed, xenoestrogens are removed from the receptors in our cells with more difficulty and therefore have a more lasting effect. In the breast, these tightly bonded estrogen-mimicking chemicals overstimulate breast cell growth, eventually resulting in the development of cancer. The scientists based their conclusions on research from many sources, including laboratory and epidemiology studies. For example, almost 80 percent of the women exposed to chemicals in the Love Canal incident developed breast cancer. The Nobel laureates expressed a similar opinion in their statement to Congress.

It should be no surprise that the female breast, which is the veritable foundation of nourishment for the infant, is also so sensitive to mankind's environmental poisons, from the chemicals sprayed onto our crops to the altered fats added to our processed foods. The real question is why there has been no call to action as a result of the findings implicating environmental chemicals and processed vegetable oils. Meanwhile, we spend billions of dollars per year testing and using antiestrogen drugs such as Tamoxifen to blunt the effects of excess estrogenic chemicals in the environment.

The breast cancer epidemic merits a national campaign, a grass roots expression of outrage against the use of toxic chemicals in the environment and poisons in our food. Yet few have spoken out on these issues. In the absence of leadership on the part of our politicians, it is left to the consumer to make a statement by simply refusing to buy foods treated with toxic chemicals, refusing to purchase the fabricated concoctions that line the grocers' shelves and by opting out of the fast food culture.

Nutrition

Besides the use of environmental chemicals, the other factor involved in the huge increase in breast cancer is a fundamental change in the American diet—the switch from animal fats to vegetable oils. Orthodox nutritionists have demonized animal fats, but in fact they contain many factors that protect us against cancer. One nutrient that scientists have studied extensively is CLA, a compound found only in the butterfat and adipose tissue of pasture-fed animals. (The richest source of CLA is the fat of pasture-fed lamb.) Animal studies indicate that CLA is highly protective against breast cancer. Unfortunately, today most dairy animals are raised in confinement and never eat green grass. As a result, there is no CLA in their butterfat or adipose tissue.

Commercial polyunsaturated oils, such as soy oil, safflower oil, corn oil, cottonseed oil and canola oil, create serious imbalances on the cellular level. They are invariably rancid and a source of cancer-causing free radicals. Furthermore, they are loaded with hormone-like chemicals. The scientific literature indicates that overconsumption of polyunsaturated oils is especially damaging to the reproductive organs like the breasts. Even worse, most of the vegetables oils in our food come in the form of partially hydrogenated vegetable oils. When these altered fats are built into the cell membranes, they inhibit thousands of chemical reactions on the cellular level. Several major studies have definitely correlated consumption of partially hydrogenated vegetable oils with increased breast cancer but this fact is rarely mentioned, even in books that espouse alternative treatments to breast cancer.

As with all types of cancer, a supplement of cod liver oil to provide at least 10,000 IU vitamin A is essential.

Therapeutics

For breast cancer therapies, follow the protocols outlined in Chapter 2 on cancer.

Movement

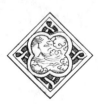

As we have said in Chapter 2, cancer patients need to reclaim their Body and Personal Spaces. This is especially true for women with breast cancer. Breast cancer patients may take things too much "to heart," they may indulge in over-mothering and often tend to have a contracted space in front of the chest. This gesture of withdrawal leads to crystallization, and hence lumps in the breast and difficulty in healing. The Personal Space Gesture, Wrestling Stance and Penguin Wrestling can help open up this space and expand the chest area, as can the Water Level walk and the Sundial. These movements can help the breast cancer patient meet the world at the borders of her personal space. The impluse to over-mother and draw her family members towards her subsides as she is able to create a space next to her in which they can stand now as friends.

Meditation

 The solution to the breast cancer epidemic is a return to food preparation in the home, performed with wisdom and love. Cooking is a form of meditation, and one of highest importance for the woman suffering from breast cancer—it allows her to express her creativity and desire for service without at the same time interfering in the lives of others. In the daily ritual of food preparation we can reunite with the natural rhythms of the cosmos—marked by the cycles of planting and harvest, and nourishment and growth in the animal world; the delight of fresh foods and the alchemy of fermentation for storage; the seasons of the year marked by feasts and festivals; and a reverence for the mysterious lunar forces that govern the female form. As you perform the *Rückschau* Meditation, note the meals you have prepared, the passage of seasons and the cycles that govern our lives.

SUGGESTED READING
> *Garden of Fertility* by Katie Singer
> *The Goddess of the Gospels* by Margaret Starbird

Summary

1. PROLONGED MENSTRUAL CYCLE—ESTROGEN DOMINANCE

Nutrition

* Avoid

Refined carbohydrates

Trans fatty acids

Legumes, particularly soy products

* Emphasize

Foods you have prepared yourself,
    according to a regular schedule

High-quality animal products and their fats

Wild, ocean-going fish

Milk products from grass-fed cows

Whole grains and nuts, properly prepared

Rosemary, thyme and basil

* Supplements

Cod liver oil to supply 20,000 IU
    vitamin A per day

Therapeutics

* Argentum D6 from Weleda, 1 pea-sized capsule 3 times per day.
* Symplex F from Standard Process, 1-2 capsules 3 times per day.
* Marjoram complex by Weleda, 15 drops in water 4 times per day, omitting the days of the menses.
* Castor oil packs on the abdomen 2-3 times per week.

Movement

* Vigorous exercise, fencing and/or dancing.
* Symmetry Walk and Lemniscate Dynamic.
* Stomach Wave and Abdominal Massage.
* Downright-Upright, Grounding, the Body Space Imagination, the Water Level Gesture, the Spinal Stretch, Knee Mapping, Bestowing and the Dipole.

Meditation

* Correlating the phase of the moon with the stage of your cycle.
* Locate and look at the moon at least one minute every day.

Summary
II. SHORTENED MENSTRUAL CYCLE

Nutrition

* Avoid   *Trans* fatty acids
  Soy foods
  Coffee, tea and chocolate
  Refined sugar

* Emphasize   High levels of animal foods, especially animal fats
  Eggs
  Fish roe
  Ginger tea
  Bone broth

* Supplements   Cod liver oil to supply at least 20,000 IU
  vitamin A daily

Therapeutics

* Bryophyllum Argento Culto 1% by Weleda, 10 drops in water 4 times per day for 6 months.
* Symplex F from Standard Process, 1 tablet 3 times per day for 6 months.
* Copper ointment by Weleda over the uterus.
* Hot baths and warming massage.

Movement

* Water Level Gesture, Bestowing, Personal Space Gesture, Autumn Leaves and Stomach Wave.
* Latin dancing.
* Avoid rigorous exercise regimes.

Meditation

* Contemplate the quality of "earth ripeness."

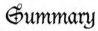

Summary

III. DYSMENORRHOEA—PAINFUL CRAMPS

Nutrition

In addition to the appropriate diet for prolonged or shortened menses

* Emphasize   Butter and coconut oil
                Red meat
                Shellfish, especially oysters
                Celtic sea salt
                Flax oil, 1 teaspoon daily

* Supplements   Evening primrose oil, 500 mg capsules, 4 per day
                 Cod liver oil to supply 10,000-20,000 IU
                         vitamin A daily

Therapeutics

* Castor oil packs, 2-3 times per week over the uterus.
* Copper ointment from Weleda over the uterus.
* Cramplex from Mediherb, 1-2 tablets every 2-4 hours when the cramps are occurring.

Movement

* Dipole, Letting Go, Bestowing and Autumn Leaves.
* Breathing Exercise.

Meditation

* Appropriate meditation for prolonged or shortened menses.
* Gently consider the impact of any sexual traumas.

Summary
IV. ENDOMETRIOSIS/ADENOMYOSIS

Nutrition

* Avoid   Same foods as prolonged menstrual cycle

* Emphasize   Liver
                         Fish and shellfish
                         Eggs from pasture-fed chickens
                         Butter from pasture-fed cows

* Supplements   Cod liver oil to provide at least 20,000 IU
                         vitamin A per day

Therapeutics

* Remedies for prolonged cycle.
* Natural progesterone cream, 1/8 to 3/4 teaspoon natural 100 mg/gram applied twice daily to the skin until condition clears.
* Chaste tree tablets from Mediherb, 2 tablets in the morning from ovulation to menses for 3-6 months.

Movement

* Stomach Wave, Dipole, Letting Go, Bestowing and Shoulder Muscle Mapping.
* Latin dancing.

Meditation

* Meditation for estrogen dominance.

Summary
V. VAGINITIS

Nutrition

* Avoid — Refined carbohydrates and sugars
Improperly prepared whole grains, especially
   granola and extruded breakfast cereals.

* Emphasize — Restricted carbohydrate intake
Butter and coconut oil
Lacto-fermented foods such as yoghurt,
   kefir, sauerkraut and beet kvass

Therapeutics

* Yoghurt or tea tree oil mixed with olive oil rubbed
inside the vagina.
* Cats claw complex from Mediherb, 1 tablet 4 times per day
for 2 -3 months.
* Loose fitting clothing of natural fabrics.
* For very severe outbreaks, a 3-day course of Monistat.

Movement

* Stomach Wave and Dipole.
* Shoulder Muscle Mapping.

Meditation

* Consider emotions or actions that draw heat away from
the vaginal area.
* Focus on any factor that contributes to a relationship in
which love is absent.

Summary
VI. ABNORMAL PAP SMEARS

Nutrition

In addition to the appropriate diet for prolonged or shortened menses

* Avoid   *Trans* fatty acids from partially hydrogenated
                    vegetable oils
                Soy foods
                Conventional fruits and vegetables

* Emphasize   Organic and biodynamic foods

Therapeutics

* Iscador Mali (see Part 2, Chapter 2).

Movement

* Dipole, Letting Go and Stomach Wave.
* Space Finding Gesture, Wrestling Stance, Penguin Wrestling
  and Sundial.

Meditation

* Explore the question "Is sex a source of pleasure and joy for me?"

Summary
VII. PROBLEMS OF MENOPAUSE

Nutrition

* Avoid   Alcohol

Fruit, fruit juices and honey

* Emphasize   Butter, coconut oil, beef fat and lamb fat

Flax oil, 1 teaspoon daily

Bitter and sour foods such as greens, lemons
and sauerkraut

* Supplements   Swedish bitters

Evening Primrose oil, 4 capsules per day

Cod liver oil to provide 10,000-20,000 IU
vitamin A daily

Therapeutics

FOR VAGINAL DRYNESS

* Homeopathic Stannum, D8, 1 pea-sized portion 3 times per day.
* Castor oil packs over the liver.
* Remifemin, 1 tablet 3 times per day.
* Estriol, from Women's International Pharmacy, intervaginally.

FOR HOT FLASHES

* Aurum (gold) D10 by Weleda,10 drops 3 times per day in water.
* As a last resort Tri-Est by Women's International Pharmacy,
1.25 mg, 1-2 times per day until symptoms disappear.

Movement

* Breathing Exercise using the Kegel movement.
* Horseback riding and/or dancing.

Meditation

* Contemplate the meaning of your daily experiences and the opportunities to pass on your wisdom to others.

Summary
VIII. OSTEOPOROSIS

Nutrition

* Avoid   Lowfat foods
                   Refined and processed grains

* Emphasize   Plenty of good animal fats
                   Bone broth
                   Celtic sea salt

* Supplements   Cod liver oil to supply at least 10,000 IU
                     vitamin A daily

Therapeutics

* Calcifood from Standard Process, 1 scoop in water 1-2 times per day.

Movement

* Working and walking while carrying heavy objects.
* Exercises that increase your sense of balance (swing, dancing and rocking chair).
* The Grounding Exercise and Downright-Upright.
* Symmetry Walk.

Meditation

* Practice conscious resistance to all influences to be too thin.

Summary
IX. BREAST CANCER

Nutrition

*	Avoid	All commercial vegetable oils
		Trans fatty acids from partially hydrogenated vegetable oils

*	Emphasize	Butter from grass-fed cows
		Fat of grass-fed beef and lamb

*	Supplements	Cod liver oil to provide at least 10,000 IU vitamin A daily

Therapeutics

* Follow the protocols for cancer in Part 2, Chapter 2.

Movement

* Personal Space Gesture, the Wrestling Stance, Penguin Wrestling, Water Level Gesture and the Sundial.

Meditation

* Home food preparation.
* Reverence for cycles of the season and the year.

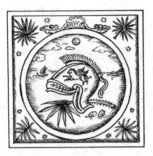

Chapter 10
Men's Diseases

M. d'Artagnan will conduct the prisoner to the ile Ste. Marguerite. He will cover his face with an iron visor, which the prisoner cannot raise without peril of his life.
Alexandre Dumas
The Man in the Iron Mask

As we have seen in previous chapters, we can achieve an understanding of human illness by studying a corresponding process in nature. Insights into the treatment of women's diseases come to us from the mythology of the moon and the metal silver. So too, we can look to nature for enlightenment on the subject of men's diseases. Not surprisingly, the challenges to the health of the male anatomy are bound up in the metal iron, the characteristic metal of Mars or Ares.

The correspondence of iron to the biochemistry of the male organism shows up at puberty, which usually occurs around the age of 13 or 14. Puberty marks the entrance into the third phase of a boy's life and the beginning of a third major physical transformation. The first physical transformation in any life is, of course, the birth of the physical body. After an average of seven years, most individuals begin the next major physical transformation, marked by the loss of baby teeth and the development of adult or permanent teeth.

The eruption of permanent teeth heralds an important step in the development of the child. The whole face undergoes a dramatic restructuring. The child begins school and embarks on a more independent life, often preferring the company of friends of his own choosing to that of parents and siblings. According to Steiner, the age of seven marks the birth of the etheric body, in which the force of pure growth becomes at least partially freed from the demands of physical growth and available for the development of other faculties. For example, academic learning is possible for the first time during this second seven-year period.

257

We then come to the start of the third seven-year stage, the stage that affects the underlying dynamics of men's health. Many traditional cultures mark the transformation called puberty with a ceremony, such as the Jewish Bar Mitzvah, the Christian confirmation and the traditional African rites of passage. All these traditions mark the boy's passage into manhood, both in his physical body and in that portion we call the soul. We must therefore look at what actually happens both physically and in the soul of the boy at this time.

Physically, we see a number of changes. Pubic hair begins to develop under the arms, followed by the gradual growth of hair all over the body. The musculature of the boy's body starts to develop, growing heavier, thicker and stronger. The voice deepens, the penis enlarges and the production of sperm and semen begins.

Another change that takes place, one that is not visible, is a slight rise in the iron content of the blood. This change is especially striking because it contrasts with the blood changes of adolescent girls, who experience a slight lowering of their blood iron levels at this time. This phenomenon has perplexed the medical profession for many years. No one knows just why this happens, but the fact that it occurs is unmistakable. Researchers have devised many experiments to help them understand how or why these changes come about and in the process have discarded many theories. One explanation was that the decline in blood iron levels in girls was due to loss of blood in the menses. However, studies of girls who never menstruate have shown that this drop still occurs. Other explanations, such as lower activity levels and differences in the diet, also fail to provide a conclusive answer.

The answer can be found in the relationship between the human being and iron, and to the soul changes we undergo during puberty. For it is during this period that the characteristics of the inner life manifest in the physical world. During this phase, boys generally become more inward, more withdrawn and less communicative. Those who have been parents of teenage boys count themselves lucky to get one sentence a week. Girls, on the other hand, often turn outward. They can become very social, very chatty and, in more extreme cases, even coquettish. The manifestation of these inner changes—highly "feminine" for girls and "masculine" or "macho" for boys—usually lasts throughout this seven-year phase, after which a more balanced personality emerges.

How, then, does this essential male process shed light on the illnesses men experience later in their lives? One conclusion is that the challenge of the male lies in balancing the heaviness or inwardness to which he is first subjected at puberty with more buoyant and outward tendencies. According to Steiner, it is during puberty that the emotional body or soul force is born. Consequently, for the first time, the developing man can work with the world of emotions. However, this newborn emotional life finds itself trapped in a world characterized by the qualities of iron—martial, somber and heavy.

Iron is an interesting substance. It is the only metal found in significant quantities in the human body, and therefore the only metal not called a trace metal. Instead, it is a substantial metal, substantial not only in quantity but also in its effect. It is the component of red blood cells that carries oxygen throughout the body. Iron is also a component of certain enzyme systems where its ability to change easily from a $2+$ to a $3+$ valence allows for the transference of oxygen in the cellular respiratory cycle.

Thus, the metal associated with clanking armor and impassible barriers (the iron mask, the iron curtain) is the very metal that allows oxygen to be transported in the body and used by the cells. And because iron can exist as a $2+$ or $3+$ valence with equal ease, this weighty metal can transform itself according to the amount of oxygen available. We are all familiar with the phenomenon of iron oxidation because when iron becomes saturated or filled with oxygen, rust forms. The more oxygen it takes on, the heavier and more weighed down it gets.

Metaphorically speaking, iron is the perfect substance to modulate the process of puberty, and even to physically distinguish man from woman. Increased iron brings more robust life to the youthful frame while its heaviness presages the weightier matters of adult life.

As we have seen, illness often results from a normal process taken too far. For example, mineralization is the normal way we form our bones. However, mineralization in the gall bladder can lead to gall stones and excessive mineralization in the joints can lead to osteoarthritis. Likewise, the process of oxidation as mediated by the iron in our blood is normal, but oxidation is akin to burning and brings about tissue destruction when it becomes excessive. Heaviness is also not an illness in and of itself, for heaviness also confers strength and power to our muscles. However, when we are too subject to the forces of gravity, we can become stiff, even leaden.

Heaviness in the soul is not a pathology either, for emotional heaviness leads to depth of ideas and feelings. However, when taken too far, the result can be the uncommunicative, somber, middle-aged man so common in our culture. It is a sign of the biochemical dominance of the traits conferred by iron.

Thus, the intriguing phenomenon of elevated serum iron levels in men tells us that being male is intimately connected to the properties of iron. Just as iron assumes its unique place in our physiology because of its ability to change valences and become heavier, so, too, is the male physiology largely dependent upon the mediation of this tendency to become heavy. If the attribute becomes extreme and stiffness and inflexibility prevail, the stage is set for the appearance of the illnesses to which men are subject later in life.

Many traditional forms of medicine associate the metal iron with the planet Mars. Mars was the patron and protector of Rome, a culture that epitomized the masculine or macho tendencies of the human spirit. The Martian properties thought to rule the male character include aggression, passion, dominance and fire, in contrast to the more feminine or Venusian attributes of passivity, receptivity and openness.

An interesting confirmation of the thesis that excess iron causes disease, especially in men, comes in the form of reports that men who donate blood regularly live longer, healthier lives than those who don't. Besides the positive feedback from the altruism involved, regularly losing some blood helps keep the iron stores low and prevents the kinds of oxidative and inflammatory diseases to which men are prone. The ancient practice of bloodletting may indeed have some basis in fact.

In the chapters on heart disease and hypertension, we saw that diseases of the blood vessels and circulation are connected with the interaction of the forces represented by iron and copper, and that these metals work via the arterial and venous blood vessels respectively. Our discussion of iron helps explain why coronary artery disease is predominantly, although by no means exclusively, a male disease. As we discussed, the tendency toward oxidation is intimately related to the development of coronary artery disease. The standard explanation of the sex difference in the incidence of heart disease is that estrogen is somehow protective against its development, a theory that recent studies have negated.

It is clear, however, that iron serves as one of the body's primary modulators of the oxidative processes. We know that excessive iron in the blood has a toxic effect on the heart and liver and can be a primary cause of early coronary artery disease. We can also say that, in general, the higher level of iron in men predisposes them to a greater tendency for oxidative damage. Chronic inflammation follows, with scarring and sclerosis (hardening). This conclusion is supported by epidemiological data which suggests that coronary artery disease is highest in the same geographical areas where other diseases of oxidative stress are high—diseases like cancer, diabetes and macular degeneration. All of these diseases are thought to be caused by oxidative damage to the tissue.

In addition, oxidative damage in the blood vessels leads to other developments characteristic of male tendencies, causing the arteries to become stiffer, harder, heavier and constricted. It is as though the blood vessels themselves show the physical corollary to the physiological and soul tendencies of men. The situation is aggravated when a man demonstrates all the typical or exaggerated male characteristics. Repeatedly, studies have shown that dominant, aggressive, uncommunicative men—men with the "Type A" personality—have a greater tendency to coronary artery disease.

We might say that the working of iron is too strong in their physiology. As a result, they become subject to the oxidative damage characterized by iron excess.

Unbeknownst to many patients and even some physicians, the understanding of the underlying dynamics of coronary artery disease has undergone a major change in the past decade or so. The old theory was that plaque in one of the coronary blood vessels blocks the blood flow through that vessel downstream to the heart muscle. According to the old theory, when sufficient blockage occurs, ischemia or lack of blood supply in the heart muscle causes that part of the heart muscle to die. However, a recent study, reported in a major cardiology journal, found that only 10 percent of heart attack victims have greater than 70 percent occlusion or blockage in one of the major coronary blood vessels. (An occlusion level of 70 percent is considered necessary for a heart attack to occur.) The authors commented that heart attacks seemed to occur not so much because of the amount of occlusion but because of what goes on within the arteries. They found that arteries that had friable plaque, that is plaque that is easily broken apart, were much more likely to lead to heart attacks than arteries with stable plaque. It only remains to find the source of friability of this plaque. Although excess iron has not yet been studied as a cause, it is tempting to compare friable plaque to rusted iron, which easily flakes off. Interestingly, new data indicates that adequate levels of copper protect against the breaking off of plaque. When copper, the feminine element, is adequate, the plaque in the blood vessels is stable, and heart attacks do not occur.

The diet, therapies and movement exercises for coronary heart disease are explained in Chapters 3 and 4. These guidelines also have relevance in the treatment of the male reproductive system—impotence and prostate problems, including cancer of the prostate gland, all of which have been linked to excess oxidative stress.

Another substance that plays an important role in reproductive and prostate health is the trace mineral zinc. While the connection between zinc and iron is not immediately obvious, a deeper examination of the characteristics of zinc reveals important similarities to iron, as well as interesting distinctions. In nature zinc is mostly found in carbonate deposits, always in conjunction with iron. Zinc has the same relation to the process of oxidation as does iron, in that it forms different oxidative states known respectively as carbonates, hydrates and oxides. Like iron, zinc is necessary for mammalian life, and also like iron, it is needed in substantial, not minute, amounts. The mammalian organs richest in zinc, besides the prostate gland, are the muscles and bones, exactly the organs that outwardly differentiate the male from the female physiognomy. As shown by the sites in which it localizes, zinc participates with iron in the process of heaviness or earthiness of the male muscle and bone structure. Brittle bones and weak muscles are a defining sign of zinc deficiency.

Zinc's opposition to iron most clearly reveals itself in the fact that while iron may be called the central element of the red blood cells, zinc has an analogous role in the white blood cells, the cells that mediate our immune function. Zinc functions as a kind of inner armor, protecting us from invasion and occupation by invaders of many sorts. Like the physical outer armor made of iron, we also have an inner armor in the form of white blood cells, which contain large amounts of zinc.

Semen, the secretion product of the prostate gland, contains large amounts of zinc and the prostate gland concentrates this nutrient. In animal studies, zinc deficiency results in complete sterility. In addition, zinc is a cofactor in many reactions involving our immune system. Zinc deficiency is often associated with immune dysfunction, resulting in a number of disease conditions, from chronic viral infections to cancer. Zinc deficiency is also related to prostate enlargement. Many researchers believe that chronic zinc deficiency results in gradual enlargement of the prostate in much the same way that chronic iodine deficiency results in enlargement of the thyroid gland.

As recently as 20 years ago, when I was in medical school, doctors avoided discussion of male reproductive disorders. Male impotence, now called "erectile dysfunction," was relegated to the domain of sex clinics. Doctors considered benign prostatic hypertrophy a normal part of aging, and prostate cancer occurred much less often than it does today.

Other issues affecting the health of the American male have yet to receive the same national attention. For example, the average sperm count of today's adult male is about 50 percent lower than it was 50 years ago. Infertility rates among American couples now approach 25 percent, a heartbreaking situation that can be partially explained by lower sperm counts and decreased viability of the sperm. These changes parallel the findings seen in other mammalian species, including lowered fertility rates, decreased sperm counts and anatomical changes in the male reproductive organs.

Clearly, environmental changes that have accelerated during the past 40 to 50 years affect the reproductive health of males of different species. In Chapter 9 on women's health, we discussed the problem of exogenous estrogens in our environment and their effects on the modern female. These pervasive environmental hormones undoubtedly contribute to the feminization of males in many mammalian species, as well as the lowered sperm counts of the American male.

Another cause, one far less recognized or discussed in scientific circles, involves the huge change in the American diet during the past 80 years. The decline in soil fertility translates into lower mineral content in our food, and the substitution of vegetables oils for animal fats has robbed the developing male of the fat-soluble vitamins (vitamins A and D) that he needs to make testosterone out of cholesterol. In addition, the vegetable oils are invariably rancid, causing irritations and inflammation in the arteries. The *trans* fats in margarines and shortenings used in processed foods also interfere with the production of testosterone.

Another nutrient that has declined in the modern diet is vitamin E, normally found in whole grains, cold pressed vegetable oils, egg yolks, butterfat and dark green vegetables. Modern processing destroys vitamin E in grains and oils, and consumption of vegetable oils actually increases the body's need for vitamin E. The scientific name for vitamin E is "tocopherol," which in Greek means "to beget or carry offspring." Numerous experiments with animals have shown that vitamin E, originally used in the form of wheat germ oil, is absolutely necessary for an animal to achieve and maintain fertility. Studies have also shown that the purified products, such as alpha-tocopherol, are not nearly as effective in maintaining fertility as feeding whole wheat germ oil or an ample supply of whole grains. In addition, vitamin E is a powerful antioxidant and can protect us from overly exuberant oxidation of substances like iron.

Nutrition

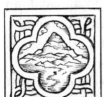
The best dietary sources of zinc are red meat and seafood, especially oysters. Any man suffering from problems with the reproductive tract should eat oysters once or twice a week. Other animal foods include wild, ocean-going fish, butter from pastured cows and eggs (particularly the yolks) from pastured chickens.

An important source of zinc is unrefined sea salt, another commodity that has disappeared from the American diet during the past 50 years. When salt is refined, most of its minerals, including zinc, are removed. Today, the typical American male will never eat any salt in his whole life that contains even a trace of this valuable mineral. Nutritionists have been relatively successful in spreading the word about the dangers of refined sugar, but few voices warn us about an equally severe problem of mineral deficiencies caused by the consumption of refined salt. This is why I strongly encourage all my patients to use Celtic sea salt exclusively for all their cooking, as this is one of the few commercially available salts that still has its full complement of minerals, including valuable zinc.

Another dietary component vital for men's health is sufficient fatty acids of the omega-3 type, including the forms with two double bonds found in flax oil, organic whole grains and leafy green vegetables. The longer and more unsaturated forms occur in cod liver oil, seafood (especially wild salmon, fish eggs and shell fish), organ meats and eggs from pastured chickens. These foods also provide many of the nutrients mentioned earlier—vitamins A, D, E, iron and zinc. Fish eggs, in particular, provide a complete packet of minerals, fat-soluble vitamins and elongated omega-3 fatty acids—many traditional cultures value fish eggs as an aphrodisiac.

In addition to incorporating certain nutrient-dense foods in the diet, men should also avoid consumption of foods fortified with iron. Most men have no need for any more iron than that which occurs naturally in food. Consumption of iron-fortified foods, or of supplements containing iron, can cause a toxic overload and contribute to heart disease, liver disease and perhaps even cancer—numerous studies have shown a relationship between high iron levels and increased cancer incidence. Plentiful fat-soluble vitamins in the diet help the body absorb the iron it needs without accumulating an excess.

My caveat against iron-fortified foods does not include liver. Although liver is rich in iron, it is also our best dietary source of copper, so vital for healthy arteries. I recommend including liver in the diet at least once a week.

Any therapy for reproductive disorders and prostate problems must incorporate the dietary elements discussed in Chapter 1, Section I. All processed foods, vegetables oils, white flour products ("fortified" with inorganic iron) and extruded grain products must be avoided. Cold whole-grain breakfast cereals made by the extrusion process not only contain rancid vegetables oils, they are also high in phytic acid, an organic acid that blocks zinc. All grain products must be properly soaked to neutralize phytic acid. Soy foods not only block zinc, but they contain plant-based estrogens that can have feminizing effects.

Caffeine, found in coffee, tea, soft drinks and chocolate, is best avoided as it stresses the adrenal glands, ultimately affecting male potency.

Supplements include cod liver oil for vitamins A and D (providing at least 10,000 IU vitamin A per day) and wheat germ oil for vitamin E. I recomment Standard Process wheat germ oil, 4 capsules per day. For those who don't like oysters, I recommend zinc-liver chelate from Standard Process, 1-2 tablets 3 times per day. Avoid supplements of vitamin C as the synthetic form increases iron absorption and blocks copper.

Therapeutics

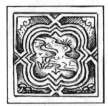

I. ACUTE PROSTATITIS

The prostate gland is a walnut-sized muscular organ responsible for making and secreting semen. As with any muscular structure, it is susceptible to contractions, spasms and overuse. Many cases of acute prostatitis result from overworking the gland, as in a burst of abnormally high sexual activity (when previously there was no sexual activity). The prostate becomes enlarged, painful and swollen, often felt as an uncomfortable lump in the rectal area, occasionally accompanied by difficulty or pain in urination. Often the patient has a fever and occasionally a pus-like discharge from the penis. On examination of the prostate through the rectum, the gland will be very painful to touch. It often feels swollen and even warm or hot.

One of the controversies surrounding the etiology and treatment of prostatitis is whether or not this condition is an infection or an inflammation of the gland. As a result, it is unclear whether the conventional treatment with oral antibiotics really addresses the problem. In my experience, only the most extreme cases require antibiotics.

Taking our cue from the fact that the prostate is a muscular gland, one can treat acute prostatitis in the same way one treats other strained and inflamed muscles, with rest and Epsom salts. Ejaculation should be avoided for at least two weeks. I recommend regular soaking in a warm or hot bath, to which is added 1 cup of Epsom salts. If possible, soak in the bath 20 minutes, 2 times per day for 10 days. This bath treatment will relax the muscle as the Epsom salts help cleanse the gland by promoting secretion of its contents. Many patients experience immediate relief with this intensive bath therapy.

I also suggest oral medicines that work in an anti-inflammatory way on the prostate including Echinacea Premium (Mediherb), 2 tablets every 2-3 hours until better, saw palmetto extract (Mediherb), 1 teaspoon 2 times per day, Prostate PMG (the Standard Process protomorphogen extract) 1-2 tablets 3 times per day, and Erysidoron 1, an anthroposophical anti-inflammatory medicine, at a dose of 10-15 drops 4 times per day. This regimen should resolve the problem in less than one week. If not, antibiotics may be prescribed.

II. BENIGN PROSTATIC HYPERTROPHY (BPH)

BPH is relatively easy to control with the proper intervention and the cooperation of the patient. The major symptom is difficulty in urination, which happens as the gland swells and puts pressure on the urethra, directly adjacent to the prostate gland. As a result of this pressure, the caliber of the urethra gets smaller and the urine has a more difficult time passing through. The patient experiences this as a weakening of the urine stream, a need to urinate more often while passing only small amounts at any one time, and finally, nocturia, or the need to make frequent trips to the bathroom during the night. This is the symptom that usually brings the male patient to the doctor, as the disturbed sleep begins to interfere with his ability to function optimally during the day.

I should stress that as far as we know there is no relationship between BPH and prostate cancer. The current understanding is that large, swollen glands are no more likely to be prone to cancer than glands of normal size.

As BPH is a chronic rather than an acute condition, its treatment must be based first and foremost on the dietary protocols given above. The medicine that many practitioners, including myself, have found effective is a lipid extract of the saw palmetto plant. Saw palmetto is a small woody shrub that produces berries with high concentrations of a medicinal oil rich in a cholesterol-like substance that has a direct influence on testosterone metabolism. It may seem surprising that a kind of plant cholesterol would be the therapy for BPH, but a closer examination makes sense of this phenomenon. Research shows that chronic overstimulation of certain types of the hormone testosterone is one of the reasons for enlargement of the prostate gland. As mentioned earlier, testosterone, like the other sex hormones, is a derivative of cholesterol. Men who take medicines that block the action of testosterone, or men who have been castrated, do not suffer from prostate disease. This is why doctors consider prolonged exposure to excessive testosterone as one of the causes of BPH. The active ingredient in saw palmetto seems to act as a kind of testosterone mimic that binds to the testosterone receptors in the prostate and thereby prevents the testosterone from having its influence. As we have seen, a common way for plants to exert their effect is to mimic the normal action of an endogenous hormone or neurotransmitter. Thus it is with saw palmetto, which mimics the body's own testosterone, thereby blocking its exuberant and injurious effects on the prostate gland. I use the saw palmetto extract from Mediherb, 1-2 teaspoons per day, sometimes along with nettle root extract by Mediherb, another plant with a therapeutic effect on BPH, also at the dose of 1-2 teaspoons per day.

III. PROSTATE CANCER

Just a few decades ago, prostate cancer was uncommon and considered nonvirulent. Today it is the second most common form of cancer leading to death in men. In addition, a study of autopsies suggests that more than 70 percent of men older than 70 who die from other causes have some prostate cancer which may not have been detected. Thus, prostate cancer truly qualifies as an epidemic in our time.

In many ways the epidemiology of this disease is like that of breast cancer; it has had the same recent dramatic rise in incidence, it has the same pattern of growth, and even shares in the medical controversies on the best type of treatment. As we discussed in Chapter 2 on cancer, this controversy centers on a fundamental issue with cancer in general and these two cancers in particular, which is whether cancer is a localized phenomenon or a general, systemic illness. In conventional medicine, cancer is believed to start in one location, then spread to many sites in the body. This view holds that while the cancer is still encapsulated, one can effectively remove all traces of it by removing the tumor. Both breast and prostate cancer, with their often confounding histories, frequently contradict this rule. In both these cancers, removal of the encapsulated tumor does not necessarily render the patient cancer-free, although in some cases the cancer will not return until almost 20 years later. This phenomenon has led some prominent breast and prostate cancer doctors to claim that the only true way to say that someone has been cured of these cancers is for them die of some unrelated disease after a long period during which they were cancer-free. What this means is that removal of the gland or the breast does not eliminate the disease, for it doesn't change the underlying dynamics that led to its emergence.

The practical consequence of this conclusion is that the physician has difficulty in counseling the many men who have newly diagnosed prostate cancer. Usually their cancer is discovered by a prostate specific antigen (PSA) screening test and then confirmed by biopsy. At this point the patient often goes through an agonizing decision process. On the one hand, removal of the prostate results in the best chances for five-year survival, according to current statistics; on the other hand, we all know that removal cannot be considered a cure. In addition, a high percentage of men have symptoms of incontinence or impotency following prostate removal. We also know that because removing the prostate cannot be considered a complete solution, the patient still has many other issues to address.

My advice at this point is to go ahead with the prostatectomy only if there is a very high chance that the disease is still totally confined to the prostate gland. This is usually the case when the PSA is relatively low, the biopsy shows encapsulation, and all the other tests (liver enzymes, CT scan of pelvis, and bone scan) are normal. I then encourage the patient to follow the advice given about diet and mistletoe therapy in the cancer chapter. Even in those patients who choose prostatectomy, I still urge them to follow the cancer diet, and to do mistletoe therapy for at least three years.

Like breast cancer, prostate cancer has a profound effect on the body and soul of the patient. It provides a kind of life-training in living with uncertainty in that the patient can never be sure the disease has truly been eliminated. As a result, many prostate cancer patients find they have to reorient how they think and feel about their life. There can be no more waiting another five years to reconcile with an estranged loved one, no more putting off beginning the type of work one has always longed to do. One of the clarion calls of this disease is that the time to act—the time to change, the time to make of one's life what one wants, the time to fulfill one's goals—can only be in the present. For many, life becomes clearer, as though the camera lens of perception is brought into a sharper focus through the very uncertainty that this illness presents.

The epidemic of prostate cancer is a message to all of us that it is time to clean up our environment, improve our diet, enjoy relationships and apply ourselves to meaningful work in the present, before we are forced to do so under the threat of cancer. Cancer is the modern voice that reminds us of the uncertainty and transitory nature of all of our lives and urges us to live as though we really knew this truth.

IV. IMPOTENCE

Surprisingly, the treatment of impotency has a long history. Over two thousand years ago, traditional Chinese physicians theorized about the causes and treatments of this common dilemma. In fact, almost without exception, all traditional medical schemes have included the treatment of male impotency as one of their central concerns. Curiously, when one looks behind the disparate terminology, one finds a general uniformity of opinion as to the cause and treatment of this situation. In many ways, the traditional views on impotency and its treatment are in agreement with current scientific information about this condition.

Impotency is not an isolated event, but is closely related to aging and loss of vitality. The Chinese held that this vitality was closely aligned with overall physical vigor and was also organ-specific. They associated male potency with Kidney Yang energy, which refers to the ability of the kidney area, particularly the adrenal glands, to generate warmth or fire. Many other traditional medical schemes relate loss of "fire" to the problem of impotency and conclude that the kidney/adrenal system is the generative organ for this fire. According to the principles of anthroposophical medicine, the kidney/adrenal system is the house of the Emotional or Soul body. It is not a huge stretch to conclude that the Emotional body has some role to play in our ability to engage in healthy sex, one of the most important manifestations of our emotional life.

The interconnection between the kidney/adrenal system and male sexuality contains further mysteries. If asked which organ is most related to impotence, most modern physiologists would choose the testicles or, if they were more emotionally inclined, the brain. Why the adrenal gland? As we have learned in the Chapter 6 on diseases of adrenal insufficiency, the adrenal gland is the master organ of the endocrine system. Through their adaptation to stress mechanisms, the adrenal glands direct the synthesis and flow of virtually all the other hormones. The adrenals also have the ability to produce hormones that are normally made by other glands. A particularly striking example of this is the hormone estrogen. After menopause, when the ovaries reduce the production of estrogen and progesterone, healthy adrenal glands can make up the difference and set the basis for a long healthy life with little or no repercussions from the loss of ovarian function.

In a similar way, while science has clearly demonstrated that sexual drive and performance in both men and women relates to testosterone levels, the traditional medicines for treating impotency have had their main field of action on the production of adrenal hormones. Herein lies the mystery and brings together some of the main points of this book. That is, there is no sense in speaking of a therapy for impotence that does not address the patient's overall health. You cannot separate sexual function and treat it as though it were unrelated to the whole.

Moreover, the level of potency is intimately related to the emotional, or soul health, of the man, as well as his overall physical vigor. When a boy or man suffers undue pressures on his emotional life, either through childhood traumas, repressed feelings, or the everyday strains of life in modern America, his emotional balance and sexual ability may suffer.

Impotency is not primarily a problem of testicular dysfunction or testosterone deficiency. Rather, it involves an imbalance of the entire hormonal axis—pituitary gland, adrenal glands, testicles and even the thyroid gland. All of these glands are governed by the same feedback loops between the brain and the body. They function as a group and have much to do with determining our overall health. Impotency is not simply due to deficiency of testosterone—or Viagra; the treatment of impotency must involve the restoration of health. Science actually corroborates the practices of ancient physicians, who treated impotency by restoring male vigor. This is best accomplished by relieving emotional blocks, often old lingering impediments that still stand in our way, and by taking steps to restore the health of the adrenal gland, described in Chapter 6.

In addition to the diet and the work on soul connections and our relationships, I recommend several interventions that have proven useful in treating impotency. The first is the herbal extract of *Tribulus terrestris*, from Mediherb. Tribulus is adaptogenic, meaning that it helps our bodies adapt to stress by improving adrenal hormonal production. A number of studies involving both animals and people indicate that the herb improves erectile function, decreases the latency period (that is the time between ejaculations), and increases the length of time that an erection can be sustained. It does not provide any testosterone, nor is it clear that it improves the ability of the testicles to produce testosterone. Rather, the herb seems to directly stimulate the adrenal glands to produce their hormonal products and therefore adapt to stress, even the stress of aging. Studies also indicate that tribulus improves cardiovascular endurance and slightly dilates the coronary arteries, thereby allowing improved oxygenation of the heart. The recommended dose is 1 tablet 3 times per day, for at least 6 months. Many men report an improvement in their potency during the third to fourth month of treatment.

In more severe cases, or with men who have lost overall vitality in addition to sexual potency, I recommend Bacopa complex, a Mediherb preparation that combines schisandra (a liver herb) and Siberian ginseng (a well-known adaptogenic herb) with bacopa (an adaptogenic herb that has a specific effect on improving memory). Together these herbs help strengthen the nervous system, liver and adrenal glands. The dose is 1 tablet 3-4 times per day for at least 6 months.

Finally, to help restore the glandular health of the entire pituitary-adrenal-testicular-thyroid axis, I use the Standard Process preparation Symplex M, which contains the protomorphogen extracts from each of these glands. In fact, it was the genius of Royal Lee who recognized, well before it was appreciated by normal science, that effective treatment of any of these glands requires treatment of the whole group or axis, rather than treatment of each in its own fiefdom. The dose is 1-2 tablets 3 times per day for 6 months.

Movement

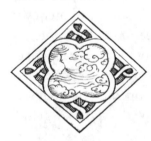

I. PROSTATITIS

Unlike women, men do not experience a monthly rhythm in their reproductive organs. The Breathing Exercise can bring a sense of rhythm to the pelvic area. The whole abdomen should be involved in the exercise, so as to gently massage the intestines and the prostate. Be sure to involve the Kegel muscles in the pelvic floor during exhalation as these are the muscles that control urination and give power to ejaculation. This also tones the rectal muscles to avoid hemorrhoids. Then do the Stomach Wave and the Abdominal Massage to further bring warmth to this area.

All men, but especially those prone to prostatitis, need to give attention to the position and way in which they urinate. As a preventative measure against prostate problems, it is important to urinate in a sitting position. Always urinating standing up often encourages constipation—it is often when we first sit down that we feel the need to evacuate. Urinating sitting down results in more frequent elimination and provides better conditions for the prostate. In the beginning of urinating, hold, release, hold, release, hold and then fully release. This brings a rhythmical contraction to the prostate area and is good for both impotence and prostatitis.

"Tough" men with hard bodies tend to identify their strength with being hard. But the swollen hardness of the prostate in prostatitis needs to be balanced. This can be accomplished by the element of water. Swimming is an excellent antidote. Having learned to move rhythmically in water, apply this flow in dancing, your work, your play and your sex life. When you participate in a sport, spend less time on the competitive part (a hard game) and emphasize enjoyment of the rhythmical activities and social interactions (a soft game) within the sport.

II. BENIGN PROSTATIC HYPERTROPHY

As with acute prostatitis, the Breathing Exercise, Stomach Wave and Abdominal Massage can bring warmth to the area of the prostate. Other helpful exercises include Carriage Down/Carriage Up, the Body Space Imagination, the Spinal Stretch, Shoulder Muscle Mapping, Bestowing and the Dipole to help you let go.

III. PROSTATE CANCER

As we have said, the cancer patient needs to enlarge his personal space. The Personal Space Gesture, the Wrestling Stance and Penguin Wrestling can help the cancer patient meet the world at the edge of his personal space, along with Autumn Leaves, the Crest, the Sundial and the Dipole. To these should be added the Abdominal Massage and the Stomach Wave to bring warmth and rhythm and release to the abdominal area.

IV. IMPOTENCE

Many men are overly trained and specialized in highly intellectual and abstract thinking. These activities are gestures of condensing information, of extracting and bringing information to a point. If the rhythmical/metabolic/sexual system begins to do these same gestures, the rhythmical forces and the forces of reproduction can strongly reduce and wither. The phrase "down there" indicates a feeling of separation from the lower abdomen and sexual organs; but the phrase "get down" indicates not only the process of getting into music, but also of sinking one's attentiveness spacially to the area of the hips and sexual organs. The inability to "get down" describes someone whose life is taken up with intellectual activity and whose sexual functions have suffered.

Those who engage mostly in intellectual activity live from the chest up. They tend to have their "water level" at the chin and are often considered "uptight." The lower part of the body is often neglected and becomes "frigid," engaging in the constrictive movement gesture of the head, where the blood is actually about one degree cooler. The Water Level Gesture can help bring the focus of attention down to the heart level. The Coat Hanger and Lowering the Sails can help release the upper body from a sense of constriction. These should be followed by the Abdominal Massage and the Stomach Wave. The Dipole helps integrate the energies of the upper and lower body.

Meditation

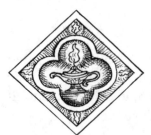

Rudolf Steiner made an interesting remark when speaking about the nature of the genders. He stated that the soul of the human being has the opposite gender to that of the physical body. Thus, those living in male bodies have feminine souls. Many other religious traditions have hinted at the dual nature of the human being. In Hinduism, for example, the road to salvation is depicted as the merging of opposite genders in one person. In contemporary thought, Carl Jung's psychological philosophy includes the notion that each of us harbors the opposite gender within our souls. According to Jung, one of the main tasks of self-actualization involves the reconciliation of these opposites. For men this means blending one's feminine side into the overall personality—a notion that has taken on a certain triteness these days with frequent repetition. Nevertheless, it is a profound insight, one that has reemerged after centuries of darkness. In fact, it is the most important challenge any man faces in working with his soul life.

The soul that dwells in a masculine body can automatically express the typical masculine attributes of aggression, action and decisiveness. However, to achieve optimal health, these need to be balanced with the more feminine, intuitive nature that most males struggle so mightily to comprehend. As predicted from our earlier discussion, iron and the male attributes may lead to action but they also lead to disease, particularly to the sclerotic diseases that afflict so many in our culture. The feminine, on the other hand, is the healer. Most traditional cultures clearly recognized this fact and consigned the healing arts to the hands of women. In our time we need both, and each person needs to make space within to accommodate both genders. Living in a culture that struggles to value the feminine side of life only makes this reconciliation harder for today's males as they find themselves caught between the outer demands of their culture and their own, often weak inner voice.

There is no magic formula for finding one's inner feminine aspects. But the most important step is simply to understand that this is necessary and then to try to open oneself to what life brings, paying particular attention to the feelings and intuitions that arise. As you engage in the daily *Rückschau* Meditation, focus on those actions that integrated feeling and intuition with action. Those who carry out this process in earnest will find themselves on the path that transforms the sword of iron and destruction into the plowshare of peace and good health.

Summary

Nutrition

* Avoid

    All vegetable oils

    Trans fatty acids from partially hydrogenated
        vegetable oils

    Iron-fortified grains; extruded grains

    Soy foods

    Caffeine

    Synthetic vitamin C

* Emphasize

    Oysters, at least once per week

    Red meat

    Fish eggs

    Liver, about once per week

    Butter from pastured cows

    Eggs from pastured chickens

    Wild, ocean-going fish

    Unrefined sea salt

    Flax oil, 1 teaspoon per day

    Organic whole grains, properly prepared

    Leafy green vegetables

* Supplements

    Cod liver oil to supply 10,000 IU vitamin A
        per day

    Wheat germ oil from Standard Process,
        4 capsules per day

    Zinc-liver chelate from Standard Process,
        1-2 tablets 3 times per day

Therapeutics

I. ACUTE PROSTATITIS

* Hot sitz baths with 1 cup of Epsom salts, 20 minutes, 2 times per day for 10 days.
* Echinacea Premium by Mediherb, 2 tablets every 2-3 hours.
* Saw palmetto extract by Mediherb, 1 teaspoon 2 times per day.
* Prostate PMG by Standard Process, 1-2 tablets 3 times per day.
* Erysidoron 1, 10-15 drops 4 times per day.
* In cases unresolved by the above, antibiotics are usually needed.

II. BENIGN PROSTATIC HYPERTROPHY (BPH)

* Saw palmetto extract by Mediherb, 1-2 teaspoons per day.
* Nettle root extract by Mediherb, 1-2 teaspoons per day.

III. PROSTATE CANCER

* Use the cancer therapeutics described in Chapter 2 of Part II.

IV. IMPOTENCE

* Tribulus herbal extract by Mediherb, 1 tablet 3 times per day, for at least 6 months.
* Bacopa complex, 1 tablet 3-4 times per day for at least 6 months.
* Simplex M by Standard Process, 1-2 tablets 3 times per day for 6 months.

Movement

I. ACUTE PROSTATITIS

* Breathing Exercise.
* Stomach Wave and Abdominal Massage.
* Swimming and Dancing.
* Emphasis on the rhythmical activites and personal interaction in a sport, rather than on winning.

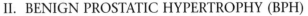

II. BENIGN PROSTATIC HYPERTROPHY (BPH)
* Breathing Exercise, Stomach Wave and Abdominal Massage.
* Carriage Down/Carriage Up, the Body Space Imagination, the Spinal Stretch, Shoulder Muscle Mapping, Bestowing and the Dipole to rhythmically inhabit the pelvic area.

III. PROSTATE CANCER
* Personal Space Gesture, Wrestling Stance and Penguin Wrestling.
* Autumn Leaves, the Crest, the Sundial and the Dipole.
* Abdominal Massage and Stomach Wave all release the iron grip of concerted effort and compressed drive.

IV. IMPOTENCE
* Water Level Gesture.
* Coat Hanger and Lowering the Sail.
* Abdominal Massage and Stomach Wave.
* Dipole, all exercises contribute to "getting down."

Meditation

* Accept the necessity of developing the feminine qualities of your nature, then try to open yourself to what life brings, paying particular attention to the feelings and intuitions that arise.

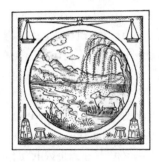

Chapter 11:
Weight Loss

Three is a number of great strength because it represents the threefold nature of the one God. In scripture it stands for a completed period of time. . . . Three represents the third spiritual center, the adrenal glands, the use of power on earth, self-preservation. Earth is a three-dimensional experience. Some strengths associated with this center are that the person participates, takes responsibility, strives to improve, has patience.

Jo Jean Boushahla and Virginia Reidel-Geubtner
"The Dream Dictionary"

And I will send grass in thy fields for thy cattle, that thou mayest eat and be satisfied.
Deuteronomy 11:15

Obesity is one of the most pervasive problems of western culture. Not only does obesity predispose us to a number of medical risks—diabetes, heart disease, arthritis, digestive problems, breathing difficulties and even sleep problems, but it also constricts our daily activities and creates emotional distress

Overweight is one of the most difficult medical conditions to treat. Successful long-lasting weight loss poses a tremendous challenge that involves permanent lifestyle changes. In general, simple solutions, pills, magic bullets and miracle diets only add to the dieter's frustrations and, in the long run, make matters worse. Yet long-lasting weight loss can also be a most rewarding accomplishment. When a person loses 50 pounds, he feels as though he has gotten his life back, and when a dieter is able to maintain her weight loss for more than a year, she feels that she has literally been transformed. A new person emerges from a successful diet—happier, more involved and more productive.

A comfortable weight cannot be achieved without a clear understanding of the problem, without a clear plan for addressing the problem and without the support necessary to carry this plan through to a successful conclusion. I say "comfortable" weight because the goal of any weight-loss program should not be extreme thinness, but rather a weight that is optimal for your age, body type and genetics. Most of us know what this weight is by how our bodies feel and by what we are able to do. We should feel unencumbered but strong. Our ideal weight may fluctuate over the years—it is normal, for example, for women to gain 10-30 pounds at menopause—but if we start to feel heavy or sluggish, and if the scale keeps climbing, it's time to address the situation with a weight-loss program.

The key to weight normalization is to relearn the difference in feeling between hunger and satiety. Through years of improper eating, most overweight people have lost this sense. Their eating habits are chaotic, and the food they eat is so devoid of nutrients that neither the appetite nor the body's nutrient requirement is satisfied.

The first step in restoring the body's ability to sense hunger and to feel satisfied is to take advantage of our universal healer, which is rhythm. This means eating three meals a day with no food whatsoever in between. (Water between meals is, of course, permitted, as are dilute lacto-fermented beverages.) I recognize that this is an "antisocial" act insofar as social eating often takes place as between-meal or late-night snacks. But remember, we are trying to restore health in a situation that begs to be understood as a serious medical condition. The rhythm of three meals a day not only teaches the body to experience hunger followed by fullness, it also creates a healthy rhythm for the digestive organs. In fact, the rhythm of three meals a day, especially one in which the food is eaten slowly, carefully and with a sense of thankfulness, will often resolve the digestive problems common to overweight conditions. The number three stands for completion, self-preservation and power in the material realm; the adoption of a three-meal-a-day rhythm can literally be a lifesaving step that allows us to function at full capacity in the physical world.

To institute the three-meal-a-day rhythm, there must be an absolute prohibition against eating anything between meals. Otherwise, the body never feels hungry. At the same time, it is strictly forbidden to skip meals. With regular meals, the body becomes accustomed to experiencing first hunger and then satiety on a regular basis, without suffering any long periods of deprivation. It is especially important to eat breakfast every morning. In one study comparing people who were overweight with those whose weight was normal, researchers actually found no difference in the number of calories consumed; the only difference found between the two groups was that those of normal weight always ate breakfast, while those who were overweight tended to skip breakfast. When a person skips breakfast, either she begins snacking around mid-morning, or is so famished by lunch time that she over-eats in reaction to a prolonged fast.

The second principle for weight loss is to eat only foods that supply an abundance of nutrients. The feeling of satiety is designed to tell us when we have taken in enough to nourish the body. Weston Price was the first to note that primitive diets were relatively low in calories but high in nutrients. The food was highly nourishing and therefore completely satisfying, whereas most modern food is high in calories and low in nutrients. Modern processed food satisfies only momentarily because the body continues to signal the brain that it needs more nourishment. Ironically, overweight is actually a symptom of malnutrition, a sign that the "appestat" never receives the signal to turn off.

Refined foods—sugar, fructose, white flour and commercial vegetable oils—are high in calories and almost completely lacking in nutrients. In any weight-loss program, these must be completely eliminated. *Trans* fatty acids from partially hydrogenated vegetable oils must also be avoided. In a comparison of individuals eating the same amount of calories, those who consumed *trans* fats weighed more.

Processed foods containing MSG must also go—and virtually all processed foods contain MSG. MSG, used to add flavor to tasteless processed foods, is an unrecognized cause of weight gain. In the laboratory, researchers induce weight gain in mice by feeding them MSG!

Even our animal foods lack nutrients today because of the way we farm. Milk, cheese, butter, eggs, meat and organ meats from animals kept in confinement—and fish raised in pens—lack minerals, important amino acids and adequate levels of vitamins, particularly the vitamins found in the fats. In fact, one fat-soluble nutrient called CLA is found chiefly in the fat of grass-fed ruminant animals—in butterfat and the fat attached to beef and lamb. In studies involving both animals and humans, CLA has been shown to encourage the buildup of muscle and the reduction of adipose fat. When animals are raised in confinement and given dry feed, the CLA content of their fat disappears.

The two trends that have paralleled the rise in obesity in America—the trend toward empty, processed food and the trend toward animal confinement—must be counteracted by the individual initiative of the dieter. A successful weight-loss program requires a return to whole, unprocessed foods grown in mineral-rich soil and from animals that feed on grass grown in mineral-rich soil.

One of the most important food components the body needs to feel satisfied is animal fat. That is why I never recommend lowfat diets for weight loss, even though the vast majority of books on weight loss promote a lowfat regimen. Our brain is specifically designed to sense the fat content of our food and to tell us to stop eating when the proper amount of fat has been ingested. When the need for fats and the nutrients they contain is satisfied, we stop eating. Lowfat diets may give temporary results, but they almost never work in the long run. The body's requirements for fats is so great, and the appetite that spurs the body to obtain those fats is so strong, that

Diet Plan A

BREAKFAST
Two eggs scrambled or fried in butter or coconut oil with no-nitrate bacon
    with one cup whole milk or yogurt or
Raw Milk Tonic (see Appendix A) or
Yoghurt Smoothie (see Appendix A)

LUNCH
Chicken broth with coconut milk, wild salmon with butter
    with salad and olive oil dressing or
2-3 ounces raw cheese and 1/3 cup crispy nuts (see Appendix A) or
Several thin whole grain crackers spread with butter and chicken liver paté

DINNER
Chicken, lamb, beef or fish; cooked vegetables with lots of butter;
    and sauerkraut or
Calves liver and bacon with sautéed onions and sauerkraut

Diet Plan B

BREAKFAST
4 ounces (1/2 cup) animal protein and fat, 1/2 cup (measured uncooked)
    cooked oatmeal or other whole grain (soaked first overnight), 1 cup fruit

LUNCH
4 ounces (1/2 cup) animal protein and fat, 1 cup cooked vegetables with
    1 tablespoon butter, 1 cup raw vegetables with dressing containing
    1 tablespoon oil, clear soup broth

DINNER
Same as lunch with addition of sauerkraut and 1 cup fruit.

binge eating is likely to occur if fats are omitted from regular meals. Those who have the will power to avoid fats often exhibit lack of control in other areas, engaging in bouts of anger, criticism or overspending.

Along with animal fats, another fat that greatly supports a weight-loss program is coconut oil. Studies have shown that the medium-chain fatty acids in coconut oil raise body temperature and increase metabolism. The body uses these types of fats for quick energy and never stores them in the adipose tissue. Use of coconut oil prevents the depression of thyroid function that so frequently occurs in dieters, which results in renewed weight gain even when calorie levels remain restricted. Coconut oil supports thyroid function, resulting in steady, even weight loss over a long period of time, until the optimum weight is achieved.

Of course, there is a psychological component to obesity. A typical patient who comes to me for weight loss is a woman in her early forties who is about 40 to 50 pounds overweight and who has suffered difficult emotional episodes and even abuse at some point in her life. While counseling can help resolve these issues, it does not, in my experience, lead to weight loss. The problem of overweight must be addressed directly, with practical actions that restore the body's rhythm of hunger and satiety, and with foods that provide for the body's nutritional requirements. Followed carefully, these guidelines can result in weight loss of about 40 pounds over three months and kept off, with consistent effort, for years.

Nutrition

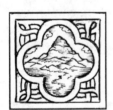
I have devised two slightly different programs to help my patients achieve weight loss. Both are preceded by a period when the patient eliminates refined grains, refined fats and oils and all sweeteners except for about 1 tablespoon of raw honey per day. Otherwise the patient eats normally of nutrient-dense foods three times a day for eight weeks. This is a period of normalization, during which, in general, little or no weight loss occurs. Then, for a two-week period the patient follows Plan A, a diet containing about 80 percent animal food from pasture-raised animals (meat, fish, chicken, eggs, whole raw milk, raw cheese and butter) and the other 20 percent mostly as vegetables—raw, cooked and fermented. Water or fermented drinks can be drunk liberally throughout the day, but no grains or fruit are allowed. There are no caloric restrictions in Plan A as we let your natural fat "sensors" regulate your intake. In fact, people discover that if they eat too much at any one meal, they feel nauseated and may even vomit.

This diet is a variation on the ketogenic diet although not as stringent. It takes advantage of the fact that the low-carbohydrate intake causes a shift in the metabolism and mobilizes the stored fats in our cells. With people who tolerate the diet, the weight loss is dramatic, often 20 pounds in two weeks. The dieter generally feels well although sometimes slightly nauseated.

A typical day during this two-week weight loss period for Plan A is shown on page 280.

After the two weeks of the stringent diet, the usual diet is followed for six weeks and then by another two weeks of the weight-loss approach. Usually 7 to 10 pounds will be lost during each subsequent two-week period until the comfortable weight is attained. To maintain weight, the patient follows the normal diet, eating three times a day and avoiding all refined carbohydrates, vegetables oils and sweeteners.

Those who do not do well with the high-fat intake of Plan A can follow a different approach. The diet for Plan B contains more carbohydrates but fewer calories. Once again, the patient eats three meals a day, but there is less restriction on carbohydrate consumption and lower levels of fat in the diet. However, refined carbohydrates and vegetable oils are completely eliminated. A typical day during this two-week weight loss period for Plan B is shown on page 280.

Typically this approach results in a 20-pound weight loss every 2 to 3 months until the comfortable weight is reached. At this point the patient should resume the normal diet suggestions with the same caveats as for Plan A.

It is important for dieters to eliminate all synthetic vitamins, minerals and other pills except those that are absolutely necessary. Supplements of cod liver oil and other super foods are fine. In both plans, the dieter should take 2 tablespoons melted coconut oil mixed with warm herb tea or warm water about 20 minutes before each meal.

Therapeutics

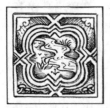 Successful treatment of obesity requires acceptance of the paradoxical fact that overweight is a condition of malnutrition and not excessive nutrition as is commonly assumed. Overweight individuals are literally starving for nutrients, while at the same time awash in "junk food," in particular refined carbohydrates. One can help this renourishment process along simply by supplying extra nutrients. The best way to do this is by using the organic whole food concentrate from Standard Process called Catalyn. This supplement, which has essentially remained unchanged since the early 1930s, contains the dehydrated organic juices of a number of different plant and animal tissues. It has been shown to contain all the known vitamins and minerals important to human nutrition. Catalyn should be the supplement of choice

for any patient or doctor interested in whole foods nutrition. For patients trying to lose weight, I advise 3 tablets 3 times per day with each meal.

The other medication I frequently use in overweight patients is Paraplex, the Standard Process protomorphogen extract from the adrenal gland, thyroid, pancreas, and pituitary. I recommend Paraplex because the condition of obesity is both caused by and contributes to adrenal stress, digestive stress and stress on the thyroid gland. Supporting these glands with the appropriate protomorphogens helps strengthen these already overburdened organs. The dose is Paraplex, 2 tablets 3 times per day, not taken with meals (mid-morning, mid-afternoon and before bedtime).

Movement

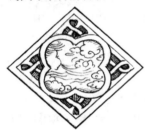

One of the most important rhythms to establish in a weight-loss program is that of regular exercise. In fact, in order to lose weight, it is absolutely essential to engage in some sort of continuous movement for 20 minutes every day. The simplest way to accomplish this is to take a vigorous walk. Swimming is also excellent, as is exercise on a small trampoline or rebounder. Rebounding can be done indoors, even in inclement weather. Best of all would be a program that combines 10 to 20 minutes on the rebounder daily with 20 minutes of brisk walking or swimming.

During exercise on the rebounder, the body alternates between heaviness and lightness as it goes up and down. On the rebounder, even a very overweight person can experience rhythmical alternations of exaggerated heaviness and lightness. These alterations are stimulating to the lymph and circulatory systems.

The best way to use the rebounder is simply to walk in place, pushing down with the heels but keeping the feet on the rebounder at all times. The action of pushing down the heels stimulates the adrenal glands and can help relieve the sense of fatigue that is so common in conditions of overweight. Ten minutes of pushing through the heel may be followed by more vigorous jogging in place or jumping, but this is optional.

In my experience, many people embarking on my weight-loss programs omit regular exercise from the therapy, and the results are undermined. They claim that it is inconvenient, that they have no time, or that there is too much pain involved. My answer is that regular exercise is an absolute requirement for success. Even if you start with just a few minutes a day, you will soon build up endurance and stamina for longer periods. Remember that calories are not meant to be counted, but enthusiastically burned.

It is ironic but true that the person who is overweight often has a very constricted personal space. When we learn to create an enlivened personal space, then the need to create a buffer of excessive fat between ourselves and the world becomes less. To enlarge the personal space, start with the Personal Space Gesture. Make the biggest gesture you can, starting with your arms parallel in front of you, then slowly rounding your arms so that you are indicating a sphere encompassing the body from behind. Follow with the Body Space Imagination and the Silhouette, and then move on to the Wrestling Stance and Penguin Wrestling. Downright-Upright, the Crest and Foot Streaming are also recommended. Foot Streaming is excellent for providing relief to sore feet, so common in those who are overweight.

There is no one ideal body type. Learn to love and enliven yours. We need to distinguish between cold and warm fat. Abhorring the fat is an actual withdrawal from it, which leaves the area cold and foreign. Fat cells are some of the most vibrant of the whole body. Like the stem cells, they are very versatile. Fat cells may have more important roles in health than we know to date. While you may want to reduce them in size, it is important to honor and respect the fat that you carry. People who are considered "heavy" carry around weight that is not enlivened. Yet there are many full-bodied people who can move and dance with an uncanny, unexpected lightness. Their shape may not fit the "modern ideal," but it expresses levity because the body space is completely inhabited and enlivened.

Meditation

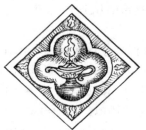

The Plan B diet that I have outlined was developed by Overeater's Anonymous. This group has had excellent results with weight loss because it combines a sensible diet plan with a spiritual component—participants are advised to actively integrate a spiritual component into their daily lives.

Overweight people tend to be reluctant to seek help and guidance from others. According to one popular book on the psychology of various diseases, overweight is an expression of oversensitivity, fear and anger, all of which result in a lack of ability to call on others for help. The fat that covers the overweight person's body might be likened to a shield to protect him or her from the insensitivity of others. When difficulties arise, participants in the Overeaters Anonymous program are specifically advised to actively seek the help and guidance of friends, spouses and fellow participants in the weight-loss program and, most important, their higher powers. On this program, many experience for the first time in their lives an active cultivation of an individual relationship with some being or "power" outside of themselves. The impact of this action is often profound, leading to a dramatic transformation in the overall health and psychological outlook of the patient.

In his daily *Rückschau* Meditation, the patient suffering from obesity should specifically ponder any incidents in which he refrained from seeking outside help or neglected to acknowledge the guidance of a higher power. This is the first step to overcoming these tendencies through self-determination and conscious thought. Gradually the barrier of excess fat will fade away as the patient realizes that he no longer needs that sort of protection from the outside world. The higher power that created this world has provided all that is required to satisfy every need—from grass in the fields to nourish the animals who provide us with food, to the loving support of family and friends.

SUGGESTED READING
    Eat Fat, Lose Fat by Mary G. Enig, PhD and Sally Fallon

Summary

Nutrition

Meals should be taken 3 times a day, with no snacking in between

*	Avoid	Refined carbohydrates
		Commercial vegetable oils
		Grains
		Fruit
		All processed foods containing MSG

*	Emphasize	Pasture-fed animal foods
		Traditional fats, especially butter from grass-fed cows
		Vegetables
		Lacto-fermented beverages

*	Supplements	Cod liver oil to provide 10,000 IU vitamin A daily
		2 tablespoons melted coconut oil with warm water or herb tea 20 minutes before each meal

Therapeutics

* Catalyn, 3 tablets 3 times per day with meals.
* Paraplex, 2 tablets 3 times per day, not with meals.

Movement

* Twenty minutes of daily continuous exercise, such as walking, swimming or rebounding.
* The Personal Space Gesture, Body Space Imagination and the Silhouette.
* Wrestling Stance and Penguin Wrestling.
* Downright-Upright, the Crest and Foot Streaming.

Meditation

* Recognize a power higher than yourself.
* Strive to reach out for help from family and friends.

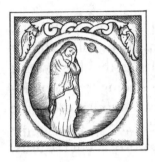

Chapter 12:
Depression

Deep in the shady sadness of a vale
Far sunken from the healthy breath of morn,
Far from the fiery noon, and eve's one star,
Sat grey-haired Saturn, quiet as a stone. . .

Knowledge enormous makes a god of me.
> *Hyperion, Books I and II*
> *John Keats*

Insight into the treatment of depression comes from a story told by a Waldorf school teacher. In the Waldorf system, teachers usually begin with a group of about 25 children in the first grade and continue with them through grade eight. Obviously, the children and the teacher get to know each other quite well during their eight years together, and when things work well they become a kind of extended family.

The teacher's story was about his class of boys and girls who had been together for seven years and were then entering the eighth grade. Up to that time, there had been no romantic relationships in the class as the children thought of themselves more as brothers, sisters and friends. Then in the eighth grade a new girl joined the class. She had recently moved to the area and, for whatever reason, was interested in having a boyfriend. As the year went by she had a series of three or four boyfriends. Each time she would pursue one of the boys, and he would get involved for a short time. Then she would break up with the boy and start again. Naturally, this caused a lot of turmoil and hurt feelings in the class, and some of the parents of the boys called up the teacher asking him whether he could help the new girl "cool it a bit." The teacher talked to the girl's mother, but she seemed relatively unconcerned and told the teacher that this behavior was normal for her daughter's age. "After all," she said, "it's just hormones."

Toward the end of the year, the new girl "fell in love" with another of the boys. They went out briefly, but the boy did not want to alienate himself from his friends of eight years, so he dumped the new girl. She now had no boys left in the class to serve as her boyfriend, and she was heartbroken. She could not face going to school. Instead she stayed in her room crying for days on end. Finally, the mother called the teacher, urging him to do something about her daughter's grief and tears. After patiently hearing the story, he calmly said to the mother, "Don't worry about the tears, it's only her tear ducts."

Depression is a huge and serious issue in our country today. Recently a patient of mine asked the guests at her wedding party how many were taking antidepressant medication. Out of about one hundred guests, more than 40 percent replied that they were taking or had taken antidepressant medication in the previous year. In my own practice, I find that at least one-fifth of my new patients ask questions about the appropriateness of taking either an antidepressant medication or some alternative such as St. John's wort.

So depression is a huge national problem, but I believe that the rationale for its treatment is completely wrong. Let me explain with a scenario that occurs in my practice at least one hundred times a year. A new patient—usually someone I have never met before—tells me that after many months or years of feeling poorly, and often after a long period of psychotherapy, he went to his family doctor, or a psychiatrist, who told him that he had "chemical depression"—or, sometimes, "clinical depression." The patient is then told that the best approach to the treatment of his "genetically determined, chemical imbalance" is to take certain medications, usually a serotonin reuptake inhibitor such as Prozac, Paxil or Zoloft.

Usually the patient is not sure that she wants to take this kind of medication. Unfortunately, she does not ask me to help her look carefully at her life or understand the meaning of her depression; rather, she wants to know whether I have a different medicine for treating her condition. I don't like the terms of this debate.

Here's the problem. First, when the family doctor or psychiatrist says the patient has chemical depression, we are entitled to ask about the basis of his diagnosis. Has he pinpointed this chemical imbalance through some laboratory tests that showed abnormal blood or brain chemistries? After all, we don't tell a patient that he has hypothyroidism or anemia without first checking his blood for the levels of thyroid hormones or red blood cells. But in the case of depression, no tests are performed because no blood or spinal fluid tests have ever shown any value in making the diagnosis of depression.

Perhaps the doctor bases his diagnosis of chemical depression on careful research indicating that people with depressive emotional symptoms tend to have altered brain or blood chemistry? Yet I know of no blood or spinal fluid test that indicates any consistent blood level abnormalities of any substance we know about in persons who exhibit depressive symptoms. PET scans, which measure levels of activity in various regions of the body, may indicate that patients with depression have low levels of activity in certain areas of the brain thought to relate to emotional expression. Otherwise, the evidence for a biochemical or physical basis of depression is scanty at best.

Physicians and psychiatrists argue that the medications are justified because they elevate the mood of the depressed patient, at least for a short period of time. Thus, according to the current medical logic, the problem has a biochemical origin or cause. But this explanation only leads to more questions. For instance, why assume that when a chemical or medicine alters a symptom, it does so because the patient had a deficiency or an imbalance of that chemical? Cocaine also elevates mood but no one is suggesting that a deficiency or imbalance of cocaine is the cause of the depression.

And how do we distinguish cause and effect? How do we know, for instance, that having a depressed mood results in suppressed serotonin output in the central nervous system, and not vice versa? Why should we assume that chemical imbalances cause depression when we know that changes in our emotional state can cause changes in our body chemistry—fear results in adrenaline secretion, for example, and stress often leads to excessive acid production in the stomach. The Waldorf school child cried tears because she was sad, not because she suffered from some defect in her tear ducts!

The reason patients are told they have chemical depression is because that is the current theory of depression. When the psychiatrist believes that depression is largely a biochemical event, then every patient who is depressed must have a chemical imbalance. As Plato said; "Let me choose the assumption and I can prove anything."

Patients who are depressed find themselves in the midst of uncertainty and despair. They often ask questions about issues of love, family, God, meaning and their own purpose. The mindset of the depressed person is most certainly linked to biochemical effects, but it is a huge leap to say that one's mood is merely a biochemical event. Moreover, the theory that depression can be solved with pharmaceuticals points the patient in the wrong direction, pushes him down the black-and-white path, paved with the extreme scientific viewpoint, where uncertainty finds no haven. Instead, the most important step for any person who feels trapped in an unpleasant or destructive mood is to learn about the rules that govern the world of mood, the world of emotion, the world of the soul.

The realm of soul is the astral or airy realm. The very word "emotion" suggests that this realm is in constant motion, like the wind rustling the leaves or the gale of the hurricane. The airy realm, the world of soul, needs to be in motion or it becomes frozen and stiff, eventually hardening into illness. This is the point I try to get across to all my "depressed" patients. The important thing is to stop identifying oneself with only one of the emotions, to stop labeling oneself with only one emotion, and to stop expressing only that one emotion. Sadness is not a pathology. Everyone I meet carries some sadness. Life can be hard, life can be unfair, some parts of the world are in an awful state, and truly none of us knows what this business of being is all about. We live through hurts, we experience pain in ourselves and in those we love. Of course, we should not be numb to loss or heartache, but the laws of the emotional realm teach us that on the heels of sorrow come laughter and joy. The world of emotion is like the constellations of heavenly bodies, each with a different mood or influence. The ancients understood this and assigned to every planet a mood or state of mind.

The ancients described a depressive person as someone living with the mood of Saturn—dark, foreboding, heavy, carrying the weight of the world. Each planet symbolizes one of the major moods experienced by the human being, and each mood has a negative and positive aspect. The negative side of Saturn occurs when one becomes fixed in this heavy, dark mood, as fixity in Saturn leads to illness. The positive side of Saturn, however, is insight and wisdom.

The treatment of depression, therefore, should not so much help the patient suppress his bleak mood, but rather help him avoid becoming stuck in that mood, unable to experience—or even acknowledge—that other moods exist. How can this person experience the intelligence of Mercury, the beauty and romance of Venus, the expansiveness and joviality of Jupiter, the reflectiveness of the moon, or even the forceful activity of Mars? The answer to this question is and must be a paradox because in the realm of soul and emotion, logic and the intellect do not hold the answers. Nor, in my opinion, do the compounds of organic chemistry. No, in this realm, magic prevails. Only the ridiculous, the absurd, the surprising hold any weight. So what is the answer? What is a depressed person to do?

My answer to this question is that when we are depressed, we must begin to pay attention to the realm of soul, to the world of emotion. We must resist the temptation to condense the understanding of our inner life into a biochemical explanation. This is a very difficult task for many of us because so-called mental illness carries the weight of shame and guilt. Patients often believe that it is their own fault that they are depressed or not making the best of their lives. The feeling of guilt and shame often drives people into taking antidepressive drugs to "fix" their faulty biochemistry. The reality, however, is that depression is not solely a biochemical phenomenon, nor is it the "fault" of the patient. It is more a matter of attention and focus.

I wish to emphasize this matter of focus because my personal and professional experience has taught me that when you begin to focus on your inner life, on your soul, a crescendo effect occurs in which your understanding and your experience of your inner life build and grow simply as a result of giving it attention. Your dreams, for example, will become richer and easier to remember, your encounters with people will become deeper, you may notice more things in the world around you, you will feel more emotions and feel them more deeply. But you must pay attention so that this realm can speak to you.

Other specific activities that might help to encourage more flow in your emotions include taking walks, writing down your dreams in a notebook kept by your bed, listening to music that calls forth all the various emotions, eating food that you particularly enjoy or cooking a special dish. Above all, pay attention to the world of your soul, and learn to experience your depression as just one emotion among many and an important avenue to wisdom and self-knowledge.

Nutrition

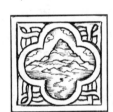 The scientific world does indicate a relationship between diet and mood, although this information is sketchy at best. Traditions about food and behavior include the belief that potatoes make people dull-witted, excessive meat-eating leads to aggressive behavior and dairy products make people docile. Modern research has focused more on the connection between specific single nutrients and various moods. We have learned, for example, that tryptophan, an animo acid, has a calming effect and makes people sleepy. We have also learned that cholesterol levels are related to depression.

One of the most interesting findings to emerge from the hundreds of studies on cholesterol and heart disease is the fact that whenever cholesterol levels are successfully lowered through diet or drug therapy, there is a corresponding significant increase in depression and aggressive behavior in those whose cholesterol has been lowered the most. Researchers at first dismissed this finding as an unimportant and artificial relationship. Later, however, scientists in the field of neurology discovered that the serotonin receptors in the brain cannot work when cholesterol levels are too low. These are the same receptors that are affected by Prozac and other antidepressant drugs. Serotonin is the body's "feel good" chemical, and when the receptors for serotonin are compromised, the brain gets less of it and depression follows.

I do not mean to argue that depression is caused by low cholesterol levels—to do so would be tantamount to the assertion that depression is a biochemical event and would contradict what I have said earlier. Unless an individual is pathologically upbeat at all times, he or she is going to experience Saturn's dark moods on occasion. A good diet cannot, and should not, enable us to avoid periods of sadness; but the right foods can make these somber emotions easier to bear.

When we are under stress, cholesterol levels rise. This is a natural and protective reaction because the hormones that the body uses to deal with stress are made from cholesterol. When we try to lower our cholesterol levels during periods of stress, the body no longer has the building blocks it needs to make these protective compounds.

During the past thirty or forty years, Americans have abandoned traditional animal fats for vegetable oils. During this same period, we have seen a steep rise in the levels of chronic depression. I believe there is a connection. Vegetable oils will lower cholesterol levels, and the partially hydrogenated vegetable oils interfere with the enzymes the body uses to make stress hormones out of cholesterol.

In shunning animal fats, Americans have also cheated themselves of other important nutrients that the body needs to maintain optimistic moods. One is vitamin A, which is rapidly depleted during periods of stress. Vitamin A is stored in the liver, which the ancients believed was the seat of Jupiter. Jupiter symbolizes the expansive, jovial mood—the antidote to Saturn. When the liver is depleted of vitamin A, it cannot well serve as the seat of optimism nor provide the balance to our periods of sadness. Depletion of vitamin A from the liver occurs even more rapidly when a diet low in vitamin A is also high in protein. Consumption of low-fat milk, lean meat, egg whites or protein powders found in meal-replacement drinks rapidly depletes the body's stores of vitamin A.

Another vitamin provided by animal fats is vitamin D, the sunshine vitamin. Depression is more frequent during the winter months, particularly in northern latitudes. When depression is linked to lack of sunlight, it is called Seasonal Affective Disorder or SAD. In the Arctic and in Scandinavia, foods rich in vitamin D, such as oily fish and blubber, were consumed in the winter months. Vitamin D is found in cod liver oil, butter, egg yolks, organ meats, seafood and lard.

Animal fats also contain certain long-chain fatty acids, which are essential for the function of the brain and nervous system. These are called DHA and EPA and are found chiefly in organ meats, eggs and seafood. Cod liver oil is an excellent source of DHA and EPA and, in fact, has been used successfully to treat depression.

Another important contribution of dietary fats is the role they play in maintaining stable blood sugar levels. When fats are removed from the diet, the fat calories are usually replaced by carbohydrate calories. During digestion, carbohydrate foods flood the bloodstream with glucose. The body reacts to this rapid rise with hormones that send blood sugar levels lower, often too low. Low blood sugar levels are frequently associated with depression.

When fats are lacking in our food, we do not feel satisfied. Satisfaction from food is an important first step for the depressed individual who feels that life does not satisfy his basic desires. I also suggest that the depressed person follow the recommendations of three meals a day in the chapter on weight loss. This will instill a regular rhythm of hunger and satiety.

For all of these reasons, I recommend that individuals suffering from depression include plenty of good-quality fat at every meal, along with a supplement of cod liver oil to supply at least 10,000 IU vitamin A daily and additional vitamin D derived from cod liver oil, at a dose to be determined by the 25(OH)D blood test. (See Appendix B on Vitamin D Therapy.) Beet kvass, with its liver-cleansing properties, may also be helpful.

One final note: Those suffering from depression will find it helpful to eat nothing at all after 7 pm. This technique alone can help turn one's attention to the inner world, which is more active at night. Dreams may be more frequent and easier to remember if sleep begins after digestion has finished.

Therapeutics

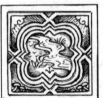

Several medicines can be of great help in the treatment of depression, particularly in cases in which the patient has difficulty adopting the optimum diet. Furthermore, in examining the rationale for these treatments, much can be learned about the proper merging of the scientific and poetic views of life.

In the treatment of depression the best single natural medicine I have seen is St. John's wort, also known as *Hypericum perforatum*. While the mechanism of action of St. John's wort is unknown, scientists have presented some interesting information about its mechanism of action. First of all, numerous studies have failed to show that St. John's wort has the same mechanism of action as any of the current classes of conventional antidepressants. It is neither an MAO inhibitor nor a serotonin reuptake inhibitor. The most consistent findings about St. John's wort is the fact that it up-regulates, or makes more efficient, certain enzymes in the liver. This is perfectly consistent with the theory espoused by the ancient physicians that the real cause of depression is excessive Saturn (or heaviness), which can be countered by the joviality of Jupiter, associated with the liver. Hypericin, the so-called active ingredient in St. John's wort, also has antiviral properties and has been used to treat various chronic viral infections. In Europe, herbalists have used St. John's wort to treat depression for at least 70 years.

My first experience with St. John's wort occurred a number of years ago when a young male artist came to me so that I could administer daily injections of hypericum. He had come to New Hampshire to do a six-month residency in music. As he prepared his musical compositions, he had a recurrence of the severe depression he had experienced years before. His physician in Germany had given him 100 ampules of hypericum to use intravenously. At first, he took the injections daily and then tapered off to two or three times a week. As the weeks and months went by, his mood became lighter, his compositions became more varied, and he found that he could see the light shining through the darkness. He left New Hampshire feeling very different about his life.

We know the science of St. John's wort. What about its poetry? St. John's wort gets its name because it flowers on St. John's Day, which is very near the day of the summer solstice, June 21. It is a common and inauspicious plant with an unusual shape. Most plants have a conical shape: they are largest on the bottom and taper or "lose their substance" at the top. Then the "normal" plant forms a flower. We say that this transformation of leaf into flower is the first transformation. The second is the transformation of flower into scent, which then expands into the air and metaphorically reaches out to others. Hypericum, however, does not follow these normal conventions. Rather, it shapes itself as a pyramid facing downward rather than upward. It flowers low down in the body of the plant rather than at the top, and it gives no scent. Its direction is clearly not outward into the world with beauty and scent like a rose, but rather downward or inward.

What are the qualities that St. John's wort directs inward? The five-petaled flowers dispersed throughout the body of the plant have a bright yellow color, like the sun. It is the qualities of the sun that are directed inward, and these qualities appear at the time of the summer solstice, a time of madness, magic and passion, a time for breaking out of the confining walls of the ego. These qualities are celebrated in Shakespeare's play *A Midsummer Night's Dream* and, in traditional cultures, by a huge bonfire and wild dancing on St. John's eve. The bonfire was lit even though the ritual occurred during the warmest part of the year in order to symbolize the qualities of warmth, light and passion. St. John's wort is the plant version of this yearly event. It brings passion, magic and even a bit of madness into the body to help dissolve the confining bonds of depression.

The qualities that help us break out of depression are also symbolized in the life of John the Baptist. His message was one of passion, one of breaking down the confines of the old ways. He carried this message even to the point of utter madness, a madness about the love of God similar to the madness about human love in *A Midsummer Night's Dream*. The life of St. John symbolizes a break from the past, an unfreezing of depression's chains, and his plant, St. John's wort, helps bring this passion, this fire, and even some madness, into our frozen souls.

Hypericum has another aspect that also deserves mention. The second part of the Latin name is *perforatum*, which means perforated. When we hold the leaves up to the light and view them from the underside, we can see that they are perforated with a shimmering red oil. It is highly unusual for a plant to have oil droplets perforating the leaves. In fact, it is in this extracted red oil that the highest concentration of hypericin is found. Remember that oils or fats are related to our warmth body. These oils are the part of the plant that can be burned for warmth and light. The substance of the oil that perforates the leaves of St. John's wort also perforates the cold walls of depression.

Other therapies for depression help stimulate and nourish the liver, the seat of Jupiter. One is a preparation from Weleda called Hepar-Magnesium D4, which is given 20 drops in water four times per day for six months. Magnesium is the light-producing mineral found in the chlorophyll molecule; like vitamin D, it is a kind of trapped sunlight. Hepar-Magnesium is a special preparation in which the magnesium is bound to a liver substance. In a sense, this therapy brings sunlight into the liver, the seat of optimism and expansion. Castor oil packs over the liver area, one hour each day, three to five times per week, are also recommended.

The Standard Process liver protomorphogen, Hepatrophin, 1-2 tablets 3 times per day, can be helpful, as can Livaplex (Standard Process) which contains many liver nutrients. This is used at a dose of 1-2 capsules 3 times per day.

Movement

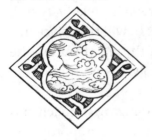

For no other medical condition is exercise so important as it is for depression. This statement is supported not just by common sense, but also by scientific studies, many of which document the biochemical benefits that come from regular, consistent and vigorous exercise. Exercise raises the levels of mood-enhancing chemicals called endorphins in the brain. Depressed individuals often have the feeling that they are going nowhere. A most important therapy for patients suffering from depression is 20 minutes of outdoor walking, six times a week, preferably in a setting that provides a rich and varied scenery. I suggest walking as vigorously as possible. An occasional long walk on the beach or hike up a gentle mountain will help gauge improvements in endurance. When it is not possible to walk outdoors, use a rebounder indoors.

Depression in its most extreme expression is a kind of paralysis in which the patient wishes to withdraw most of the time, a state in which he loses all interest in the activities of the world, a state in which his whole being feels frozen in a single mood. The patient tends to meet positive suggestions with a downcast look and a flat statement that "it is all too hard" or "too impossible" to do. The depressed state of mind is one devoid of creativity. We can gather information through books, television and computers, but wisdom comes from moving these ideas in three-dimensional space where ideas prove themselves through the feedback of the world. Self-focused motivation promotes increased loneliness but motivation stimulated and led by the world "out there" makes us part of the world community. Consider Hamlet in Shakespeare's famous play. Highly intellectual and self-absorbed, Hamlet's behavior, soliloquies and inability to act are a classic demonstration of a depressed state. The depressed patient is not literally paralyzed, of course, but suffers from a paralysis of the will. He is trapped within his body. This is a situation that cries out for movement therapy.

In Steiner's model of the threefold man, the metabolic system is connected with the limbs, and this region correlates with the soul force of the will. The best way to extend out of the body is through one's hands, the head remaining sovereign and still. The quieter you can make your head, the more open you can be to objective ideas. There are certainly ideas that come from the body, such as the need for food, water, warmth and so forth. But we must also be receptive to ideas that come from outside the body. Steiner called for the need to develop "body-free" thinking as well. Movement and stretching of the limbs and hands away from the body can actually change your spacial orientation and help replace self-centeredness with an awareness of ideas "out there."

An excellent activity for the depressed patient is fencing, an activity that involves the arm reaching out with a long sword while the head remains relatively still. It is no accident that Hamlet's release from depression and lack of will take place in a fencing match. In taking up the sword and extending himself through his limbs he connects again and can act. Any rhythmical activity that involves extention of the limbs can help with depression—dancing, tennis and badminton.

Classic gestures of depression include sagging shoulders, hanging stomach and inwardly turned feet and knees. These gestures can be retrained with the appropriate movement exercises: Personal Space Gesture, Wrestling Stance and Penguin Wrestling to enlarge the personal space; Carriage Down/Carriage Up to train the body to assume a posture that expresses interest; Downright-Upright to experience levity and gravity; Shoulder Muscle Mapping and the Cowl to correct the slouched shoulders;

and Foot Streaming, which moves the toes figuratively forwards (depressed people often have crunched back toes) while the retreating motion carves out a free space under the arch of the foot that is necessary to experience levity in the arch area. Often depressed people have a severe loss of the longitudinal arch (the main arch) resulting in feet that turn inward and down. Any foot exercise can be helpful and so can insoles that raise the arch. Knee Mapping, continues this process of "rising from the depths" in that it connects the lower limbs to the hips and brings the knees outward into a more assertive position.

Autumn Leaves and the Water Level Gesture can help bring the Frontal and Horizontal Planes to the place of the heart. Then follow with the Sundial.

Finally, creating the following spacial dynamic has helped to bring levity to depressed persons: stand and imagine that you are on a sphere that swells like the promise of a sunrise, buoying up both the arch areas as it expands.

Meditation

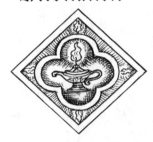

More than any other emotion, the dark mood of depression challenges us to self-analysis, challenges us to stand back and take account of how we live our life. Depression often occurs because changes are needed—changes in life-style, diet, work, relationships and outlook. This is why antidepressant drugs, whatever may be their short-term relief, can only be counter-productive in the long run, for if we suppress our depression, we remove our incentive to change. One goal of our treatment is to strengthen the will so that the patient can begin to make the changes his spirit requires.

When you engage in your *Rückschau* Meditation, analyze each event of the day with a view to determining which facets of your life need change. Start by choosing one or two small items that can be changed most easily. The various movement exercises will help strengthen the will so that you can initiate these changes.

Depression is also the soul's way of telling us to live more fully in the emotional realm, a world that defies logical thought. Remember that depression is not solely a biochemical event. It is also a clarion call from your soul. Your soul demands—is craving—attention. Give it attention. Begin to explore the riches to be mined in the inner life of soul. Numerous books and guides have been proposed to help people in their quest to explore their inner life. Perhaps none is as helpful or relevant as Tom Moore's original book *Care of the Soul*. Its point is simple and straightforward: each of us has a soul; it works in specific ways; ignore it at your peril, or embrace it and unlock its riches.

RECOMMENDED READING
Care of the Soul by Thomas Moore

Summary

Nutrition

* Avoid   All vegetable oils and *trans* fatty acids

* Emphasize   Traditional fats, including butter and lard
Eat three meals a day and nothing after 7 p.m.
Beet kvass for the liver

* Supplements   Cod liver oil to supply 10,000 IU vitamin A daily
Carlson's vitamin D from cod liver oil, dosage
determined by the 25(OH)D blood test

Therapeutics

* St. John's wort by Mediherb, 1 tablet 4 times per day
for at least 2 months.
* Hepatrophin, 1-2 tablets 3 times per day.
* Livaplex, 1-2 tablets 3 times per day.
* Hepar-Magnesium D4 by Weleda, 20 drops in water 4 times per
day for 6 months.
* Castor oil packs over the liver 3-5 times a week.

Movement

* 20 minutes of exercise daily outdoors or on a rebounder.
* The Personal Space Gesture, Wrestling Stance and
Penguin Wrestling.
* CarriageDown/Carriage Up and Downright-Upright.
* Shoulder Muscle Mapping and the Cowl.
* Foot Streaming and Knee Mapping.
* Autumn Leaves, Water Level Gesture and the Sundial.

Meditation

* Give your soul attention.

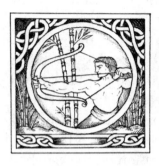

Chapter 13:
Back Pain

In Asia, the bamboo is employed in the construction of all kinds of agricultural and domestic implements and in the materials and implements required in fishery. Bows are made of it by the union of two pieces with many bands. . . it is employed in transmitting water to reservoirs or gardens. . . . The outer cuticle of Oriental species is so hard that it forms a sharp and durable cutting edge, and it is so siliceous that it can be used as a whetstone. This outer cuticle, cut into thin strips, is one of the most durable and beautiful materials for basket-making, and both in China and Japan it is largely so employed. Strips are also woven into cages, chairs, beds and other articles of furniture, Oriental wickerwork in bamboo being unequalled for beauty and neatness of workmanship. In China, the interior portions of the stem are beaten into a pulp and used for the manufacture of the finer varieties of paper. . . Small diameter poles are flexible and can be used as slings for pails. Large poles are lashed together to make scaffolding many stories high. The young shoots are prized as a vegetable and considered a salutary combination with meat. In short, the purposes to which the bamboo is applicable are almost endless, and well justify that "it is one of the most wonderful and most beautiful productions of the tropics and one of Nature's most valuable gifts to uncivilized man."

Adapted from
The Encyclopedia Britannica

*L*ike the bamboo plant, a healthy back is both flexible and strong, capable of numerous tasks. But when back pain strikes, even the simplest of tasks can be unbearable. The costs of missed work and lost time, added to the costs of treatment, make back pain an expensive problem indeed for the estimated 40 million adults who suffer from back pain at some point in their lives.

The most common causes of back pain, especially lower back pain, are degenerative arthritis, disc disease, lumbar strain, sciatica, trauma and arthritis, resulting in any combination of back pain, back spasms, weakness in the back, pains and weakness traveling down the legs, or just stiffness and an achy feeling in the neck or back. Sadly, back pain due to muscle wasting is often a side effect of cholesterol-lowering drugs, which, although unnecessary, are prescribed to millions of people.

As the bamboo is the wonder of the plant world, so the spinal column is the wonder of the human anatomy. It consists of 33 vertebral bodies or spinal bones which are stacked one on top of the other. In between are the soft, intervertebral discs, gelatinous, fluid-filled sacs that form a cushion between the bony vertebrae parts. The nerves emerge from the protective covering of the spine at regular intervals and travel to all the muscles of the torso and limbs. Muscle surrounds the spine, encasing and protecting it. These muscles also control the tension on the vertebral bodies to keep the spinal bones in alignment in both the vertical and horizontal planes. Finally, ligaments attach the muscles to the spinal bones and also play a role in maintaining balance.

Back pain occurs when some part of this system breaks down or goes out of alignment. Misalignment results in pressure on the nerves as they emerge from the spinal column, causing pain. Spikes or bony growth of the vertebral bodies can also irritate the spinal nerves at the point of emergence from the vertebrae. Another cause of pain is arthritis or osteoporosis, which can cause the vertebral bodies to collapse, squeezing the intervertebral discs out of the column and putting pressure on the nerves. Another source of trouble is weak muscles that are unable to maintain an equal tension on both sides of the spine. Uneven tension pulls the vertebral bodies out of alignment, once again putting pressure on the nerves.

Mr. G.H., a 40-year-old male came into my office some years ago having spent the previous weekend lying on the floor, unable to even get up due to severe back pain and spasm. As is often the case, NSAIDs like aspirin, Advil or Aleve provided only minimal relief. In taking the history I discovered that my patient, who works as a car salesman was under a lot of continous stress. As a result, he ate irregularly, exercised hardly at all, and used coffee and soft drinks to maintain his energy levels at work. This is a typical scenario of patients I have seen with serious back pain. This gentleman had suffered a similar episode previously, once having a diagnosis of ruptured disc based on an MRI exam. He was told that the next episode would necessitate back surgery and it was to avoid this questionable intervention that he sought out my care.

My experience with treating back pain is that unless there are clear neurological deficits, the results of MRIs or CT scans can be ignored. If neurological findings (such as weakness of the legs, or absence of reflexes) are present, referral to an orthopedic doctor is warranted; otherwise most people with back pain respond successfully to treatment regardless of their X-ray findings. Mr. H. was put on the program I will outline below, which included a "remineralization" diet; total exclusion of caffeine, soft drinks, and sugar; Injection of Disci Complex three times per week; Salegesic, 1 tablet 4 times per day for two months; and California poppy extract 1 teaspoon 4 times per day for three days, 3 times per day for 1 week, then twice per day until the pain subsides. With this medication protocol usually the severe pain is quickly reduced, and the patient is able to return to work within the week. At this point the all-important back exercises and movement therapy assume a crucial role. I recently met Mr. H. again, now about 3 years since I first saw him as a patient. He has religiously maintained his diet and exercise program and reports no back pain of any sort.

Nutrition

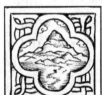

The two most important elements for bone health are silica for structure and calcium for strength. The diet should therefore emphasize foods rich in silica and calcium, with raw milk products and bone broth for calcium, and whole grains, seeds and leafy greens for silica. Celtic sea salt should be used liberally.

Remember that calcium absorption is dependent on vitamin A and D from animal fats, particularly butter from grass-fed cows and cod liver oil. The dose should provide 20,000 IU vitamin A daily.

Evening primrose oil, borage oil or black currant oil along with high-vitamin butter oil are useful for combating stiffness.

Strict avoidance of soft drinks is a must, as the phosphoric acid in sodas leaches calcium from the bones. Coffee and tea should also be limited. Fluoride in drinking water can cause calcium spurs. Water used for drinking and cooking should be filtered or processed to remove fluoride.

Therapeutics

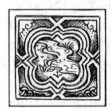

For about 40 years, anthroposophical doctors have been treating back pain with a therapy based on an extract made from the bamboo plant called Disci Complex by Uriel Pharmacy. The bamboo extract is mixed with various homeopathic medicines and given by intradermal (into the skin) or subcutaneous injection over the spine either daily or three times per week, depending on the severity of the symptoms.

As I have explained, when searching for a medicine or therapy for a particular illness, one looks in nature for a substance, plant or animal extract that, through its form or life habits, exhibits a pattern or characteristic similar to the disease. Such is the case with the relationship between bamboo and diseases of the spine.

Bamboo is a member of the grass family. It grows best in warm, moist climates and thrives in swampy soil. Surprisingly, it can attain a height of more than 40 feet in a single season, with stalks so large that a grown man can barely fit his arms around them. Bamboo is not woody and stiff but flexible. Nevertheless, it can be very hard.

The structure of bamboo is virtually identical to that of the spinal column. It is arranged as a series or stack, each unit separated by protruding areas like the protruding spongy discs between the vertebrae.

Bamboo also has a remarkably high silica content. Silica is the element used in nature to provide a scaffold onto which harder, more structural components can be laid. It is a misconception to think that a highly calcified bony structure is the key to good spinal health. A highly calcified spinal column would be too rigid and inflexible to allow any freedom of movement. Conversely, a mineral like sulfur with its inherent volatility, would be too soft to provide the strength the spine needs. As always, nature finds a perfect balance by using silica as the basis, both of bamboo and of the spinal structure; and by using the internodal form to provide the perfect blend of strength and flexibility.

As a medicine, bamboo extract not only provides extra silica and stimulates our body's ability to absorb and utilize silica, but it also gives us an image or a blueprint from nature for the dynamics of a healthy spine. Given as a medicine over a period of weeks or months, it will help form and give health to our spine regardless of the etiology of the disease.

Many other components are used in the various disci preparations, but two deserve special mention. The first is formic acid, a substance secreted by red ants to digest wood, leaves and other organic wastes on the forest floor. The second is *Arnica montana*, the best known and most valuable of homeopathic medicines, extracted from a member of the daisy family that grows in alpine meadows.

Problems with the musculoskeletal system can occur when the process of mineralization, particularly the laying down of calcium, becomes too strong. As a result, calcium deposits often develop in places where they don't belong, including the softer areas of the spine. These deposits can cause back pain, leading to such conditions as ankylosing spondylitis, degenerative disc disease and sciatica. Pain also occurs when the ligaments and muscles supporting the spine become calcified and inflexible.

Nature must have a mechanism for dissolving all the dead trees, animal bodies, bones and fallen leaves that would otherwise clutter up and suffocate our earth. Such a mechanism is provided by red ants producing formic acid to break down organic matter, which creates humus. Courtesy of red ants, we have food, vitality and new life instead of death and suffocation. Formic acid can also rejuvenate the spine by breaking down excess mineral deposits in our bones.

No book concerned with natural healing would be complete without a description of *Arnica montana*. This remedy, which comes in oral and ointment form, deserves a place in every cupboard. *Arnica montana*, with its sunny yellow flowers, is distinguished by its preference for high altitude and its utter dislike of the element calcium. According to folk tradition, if one throws even one handful of lime onto a field, arnica will not grow there for the next seven years. Like bamboo, arnica is a silica-rich plant that is antagonistic to calcium assimilation. Its effect in our bodies is to dilate the capillaries and bring more blood into an area that needs healing. Increased blood supply helps flush out and reabsorb debris and heal injuries. One can see how arnica acts therapeutically in cases of trauma, spasm or pain, where inflammatory substances settle in the tissue.

I use the preparation Disci Complex from Uriel Pharmacy, containing bamboo extract, formic acid and *Arnica montana*, injected subcutaneously three times per week to daily, depending on the severity of the pain.

The other medicines I use are Saligesic and California poppy, both Mediherb extracts. Saligesic is a preparation derived from willow bark which functions like its chemical "cousin" aspirin to relieve pain and inflammation. Unlike aspirin, which is a simple chemical medicine, Saligesic is a plant complex with many other beneficial effects. Furthermore, no side effects on any system have been reported with the use of willow bark extract.

California poppy extract is an opiate-like herbal drug, although it contains too little actual narcotic to explain its pain-relieving effect. Again, the effectiveness of this medicine for acute pain speaks to its complex and as-yet-unexplained mechanism, one which is far safer and in many instances more useful than conventional narcotics with their well-known side effects.

Three other therapies work well for the treatment of back pain. The first is castor oil packs, especially in situations involving muscle spasms, pain and inflammation. Castor oil acts much like arnica, and its warmth and anti-inflammatory effects do much to relieve acute lower back pain. Castor oil packs should always be used immediately after an injury that involves the back or neck.

The second therapy involves hydration. The intervertebral discs act as a hydraulic cushion, keeping the disc spaces intact and allowing the nerves to exit freely from the spinal column, without impingement. If one becomes even slightly dehydrated, the discs can shrink, thereby losing their effectiveness as cushions. Unfortunately, many liquids are actually counterproductive in that they cause dehydration, especially coffee, tea and alcohol. Lacto-fermented drinks such as kombucha and beet kvass, on the other hand, hydrate very well, as do any slightly salty beverages. Water, by the way, is not a particularly good hydrator. Back injuries often occur during physical activity in the hot sun when water and many mineral salts are lost. Traditional groups realized that fermented and mineral-rich drinks, such as haymakers' oat water (see Appendix A), were actually better than plain water for quenching thirst and combating dehydration.

The third intervention I have used successfully many times, especially in an acute situation and when nothing else has worked, is a three-day fast on pineapple juice and water in conjunction with frequent hot Epsom salts baths. Pineapple contains an enzyme called bromelain that has strong anti-inflammatory effects and that encourages the dissolution of mineral deposits and other debris. Inflammation can be relieved and pain reduced by flooding the bloodstream with bromelain for three days. After that, the patient returns to the other therapies with the addition of two to three glasses of fresh pineapple juice per day. I also suggest taking an enzyme preparation called Wobenzym, available through Emerson Ecologics and other sources, which contains bromelain plus many enzymes helpful to the detoxification process. The dose is 2-10 tablets 2-3 times per day between meals until the condition resolves.

These methods will usually relieve back pain without resort to conventional anti-inflammatory or strong pain medicines. I have found that long-term relief occurs in a high percentage of cases of back pain using these methods unless clear neurological findings are present.

Movement

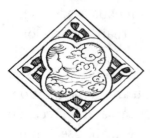

The essence of back health is proper alignment, a complex process that involves strength, flexibility and balance. Ironically, many exercises promoted in fitness classes contribute to misalignment of the spine and subsequent back pain. Chiropractors and osteopaths make adjustments to the alignment of the spinal bones, but relief is often temporary. Massage can be helpful for those whose back pain is caused by muscles that are too tense, but ongoing back health requires an ongoing dynamic of alignment.

Note that we speak of alignment as a "process" or a "dynamic." Most books on the subject of back pain say that it is caused by "poor posture" and can be alleviated by "correct posture." But posture implies stillness, a "position" or a "pose" rather than gesture, and conjures images of soldiers at attention or ramrod-stiff schoolboys, arms straight by their sides and shoulders hiked up to their ears.

The word "carriage" is better, as carriage is a process, not a position. Posture implies holding muscles to keep the body straight. But no bone or muscle in the body is straight. Good carriage or bearing results from a wonderful blend of curves working in harmony. The beautiful carriages of the horse-drawn age were not straight-edged juggernauts, but light and flexible works of art.

Exercises to improve carriage should be aimed at achieving balance within the three dimensions of space. We can orient the three planes of space so that they carry the chest, the area of rhythmical exchange between the head and the limbs. It is also the most economical area of intersection for the conservation of energy. When the three planes meet in the chest, our carriage is such that it spares energy and relieves muscles. Male dancers pick up their partners from this area because it is the place of maximum mechanical advantage. For centering the three planes, start with the Tides and then continue with the Crest and the Water Level Gesture.

The Pulley exercise will help achieve a graceful carriage as well as restore flexibility to the spine. Let the head and torso hang forward and the arms flop down. Then reverse the process by imagining a series of pulleys connected by a cord on the spine. As we pull down on the cord, the vertebrae straighten one by one and the head comes up. Thus we straighten up not by putting the head forward, but by pulling down on the spine. When we pull down on the spine, the head comes up.

The Coat Hanger will help put the fulcrum of balance for the Horizontal Plane at the level of the heart, between the fifth and seventh vertebrae. Shoulder Muscle Mapping will help with this as well. Knee Mapping can be helpful.

After these initial exercises, practice the gesture of good carriage with the Carriage Down/Carriage Up movements. When we try to stand up straight by protruding the torso and head and throwing the shoulders back, we get a rigid "straight up" posture that imitates uprightness. This stance is achieved by straining the muscles. In its most extreme expression, it is a gesture of self-righteousness that lacks mercy. These two gestures combined confer good carriage through motions that are both lifting and grounded.

The Spinal Stretch and the Victory Stretch can help relieve constriction in the spine. A final exercise for back pain is the Dipole, which gives an elongation of the spine as well as expansion and integration of the right and left sides of the body.

Meditation

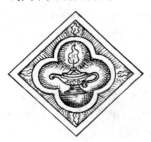

Just as the deliberate and graceful movements described above help us to maintain the dynamic of balance, so our meditation should focus on maintaining the dynamic of balance in the life of the soul. Remember that the spine maintains its shape and performs its work through a combination of strength and flexibility. So, too, our meditations must help us achieve a balance between justice and mercy, discernment and innocence, confidence and humility. Think about the qualities of the marvelous bamboo plant, capable of a thousand uses, from the flexible bow to sturdy scaffolding. So too the healthy spinal column makes possible the upright, graceful carriage with which we move forward to meet our destiny. As you engage in your *Rückschau* Meditation, analyze the various events of the day in terms of their qualities of justice and mercy, strength and flexibility, noting any items where a tendency to inflexibility has prevailed over the qualities of humility and balance.

Summary

Nutrition

* Avoid   Soft drinks
Coffee and tea
Fluoridated water

* Emphasize   High-vitamin butter from grass-fed animals
Whole milk and dairy products
Bone broths
Whole grains (properly prepared)
Green leafy vegetables
Celtic sea salt
Lacto-fermented beverages

* Supplements   Cod liver oil to supply 20,000 IU vitamin A daily
Evening primrose, black currant or borage oils,
    500 mg capsules, 4 per day

Therapeutics

* Subcutaneous Disci complex from Uriel Pharmacy, applied 3 times per week to daily.
* For acute conditions, Saligesic from Mediherb, 1 tablet 4 times per day in the short term and 2-3 tablets per day long term or until the back is much stronger; and
* California poppy extract 1 teaspoon 4-6 times per day, then tapering off over 1-2 weeks.
* Castor oil packs.
* Hydration through lacto-fermented beverages.
* Pineapple fast with Epsom salts baths.
* Wobenzym from Emerson Ecologics, 2-10 tablets 2-3 times per day between meals.

Movement

* The Tides, the Crest and the Water Level Gesture.
* Coat Hanger, Shoulder Muscle Mapping and Knee Mapping.
* The Pulley.
* Carriage Down/Carriage Up.
* Spinal Stretch and Victory Stretch.
* Dipole.

Meditation

* Strive for balance in all activities of life.

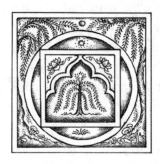

Chapter 14:
Arthritis

Madame Balionte must have neglected to fasten the window. A gust of wind blew it open, and the chill night air filled the room. The deep murmur of the blasted and tormented pines filled Argelouse, but, despite this sound, as of a fretting sea, the silence of the place was there. . . in summer at dusk, when the sun had come so near its setting that only the very lowest sections of the pine trunks were reddened with its light, and a belated cicada was still scraping away for dear life. . .

Therese Desqueyroux
Francois Mauriac

The poor soul sat singing by a sycamore tree,
Sing all a green willow;
Her hand on her bosom, her head on her knee,
Sing willow, willow, willow.
Her salt tears fell from her, and soft'ned the stones—
Sing willow, willow, willow—
"I called my love false love; but what said he then?"
Sing willow, willow, willow:
"If I court more women, you'll couch with more men."
Sing willow, willow, willow.

Othello
William Shakespeare

W hat is arthritis? Picture first of all a forest of pine trees that creak and grate against each other in the wind. The scene is one of stiffness and desiccation and describes metaphorically a young woman who has no outlet for her passions, whose relationships are blasted and tormented.

Such is the metaphoric image that describes osteoarthritis, the "wear and tear" kind of arthritis. The typical sufferer is an elderly man who seems worn out by life, bent over and thin, with a limp. He relates some of the trials he has lived through and describes the shooting pain and swelling in his hands and the pain in his left hip.

The inflammation of his joints is the result of progressive wearing away of cartilage and other structures that cushion bones where they meet. Weight-bearing joints such as the hips and knees are the most affected, but any joint can be involved. The typical osteoarthritis patient has actually worn away his "cushion" in the course of his life, which finally brings about a state of painful, debilitating arthritis. The osteoarthritis sufferer watches his ability to stay flexible erode; he can no longer move smoothly and easily; he is cold and stiff, even into his bones.

In osteoarthritis, the primary imbalance is one of excessive mineralization. In other words, in this illness, the forces of mineralization outweigh the ability of the body to keep its minerals in solution in the living, watery sphere.

Our description may seem metaphorical and impractical, but in fact it leads directly to some very powerful therapeutic options for osteoarthritis sufferers. For it is clear that what is needed to bring resolution or balance to this situation is warmth, flexibility and an increase in the body's power to dissolve the mineral element. Metaphorically speaking, this warmth with its physiologically correlated inflammation, can wash away the stiffness and pain, bringing with it new possibilities for flexibility and healing. If we can increase the body's "dissolving" forces, we can loosen the grip of excessive mineralization, thereby dissolving the painful deposits affecting the joints.

Inflammatory arthritis can be considered the opposite of osteoarthritis. This condition includes such specific illnesses as rheumatoid arthritis, lupus, psoriatic arthritis and Reiter's syndrome. These inflammatory conditions are also closely aligned etiologically with many other so-called autoimmune inflammatory conditions, each with its own particular characteristics, such as sarcoidosis, iritis and rheumatic fever. How can we describe these diseases in a metaphorical way?

Let me present this metaphor in the form of a story that actually happened to me and my family. We moved to a lovely house near a forest and beaver ponds on a lonely road in New Hampshire. For several years, we wondered whether there were some way of bringing more light into the house. Finally, with some reluctance, we chose the only solution available and cut down the large, old willow tree that guarded the property. Next spring the basement filled with cold, stagnant water that seeped in through the foundation. Clearly, the old willow tree performed a valuable function for our house. It kept the fluids in the earth circulating and flowing so they did not become stagnant and destructive.

Before the modern era of medicine, physicians looked to the willow tree for relief from any condition involving stagnant, unhealthy fluid collection in the body, particularly in the joints. Willow bark tea was given for all rheumatic conditions. They did not know, of course, that willow bark is nature's richest source of salicylates, from which we derive our modern-day aspirin and other nonsteroidal anti-inflammatory drugs (NSAIDs), such as Advil and Aleve. However, they understood very well the gesture of the willow tree, how it functions in nature and how the essence of its nature could be used for the treatment of rheumatism or inflammatory arthritis.

Inflammatory arthritis is the condition in which our tissues, in particular the tissues of our muscle-skeletal system, become waterlogged and have unhealthy, stagnant pockets of fluid. The patient feels sluggish, tired, stiff and achy. There is pain, often severe pain, not the piercing pain of osteoarthritis but rather a heavy, dull ache, akin to the continual battle of moving oneself through heavy water.

Our model provides two views of rheumatoid arthritis. First, it is the polar opposite of osteoarthritis, as the joint effusions (swellings) come from too much inflammation, not too little. This inflammation is directed, in particular, against the cartilage and cushioning structures of our joints causing effusions and pain, which, if left untreated, will eventually destroy the affected joint. Second, our model points to the fact that in rheumatoid arthritis, our water or life-force body is sluggish and stagnant. As we all know from observing nature's stagnant fluids, ponds or streams that are not continually refreshed soon become breeding grounds for all manner of pathogenic microorganisms that cause fever and illness.

Let us compare two patients I had, one with osteoarthritis and one with rheumatoid arthritis. Mr. R.B. was an 88-year-old gentleman who came to me with pain and swelling, primarily in his right knee. This situation was very tragic for him because otherwise he was in good health. His wife of many years was still alive and he enjoyed life. However, for five years he had been confined to a wheelchair with constant pain in his right knee. He had found that aspirin and other NSAIDS gave him no relief, and his surgeon said he was too old for a knee replacement. His whole family came with him for his first appointment, looking to me as his last hope. Examination of the knee revealed the virtual absence of any joint-cushioning structures and severe pain with any movement or weight-bearing.

By contrast, Ms. L.A. was a 46-year-old airline stewardess who, of course, spent a lot of time on her feet, often in stressful situations. About two years earlier she developed the classic symptoms of rheumatoid arthritis—fatigue, weight-loss, pain in numerous joints and multiple joint effusions. Aspirin and other NSAIDs gave only temporary relief, and she was unable to tolerate prednisone or methotrexate, the next level of pain-killers used to treat rheumatoid arthritis. Ms. L.A. was about to leave her job, as her symptoms would not allow her to continue—a difficult decision for her as she had no other financial support. The laboratory tests I ordered confirmed the presence of rheumatoid factor.

While there are some common factors in treating both types of arthritis, the remedies and certain dietary factors are specific to the type. I will come back to these two cases and describe the results of treatment after further discussion.

Nutrition

Both types of arthritis respond to a good, wholesome diet based on the principles outlined in *Nourishing Traditions*. All empty and devitalized foods should be avoided, particularly devitalized oils, fruit juices and sweets made from white sugar. Broth made from animal bones, which will be rich in factors that nourish cartilage, should be included daily as an ingredient in soups, stews and sauces.

Depending on the type of arthritis one has, I suggest an emphasis either on animal fats or certain types of oils. As a treatment for osteoarthritis, we can look to folk wisdom, which valued butter, cream and other animal fats for their ability to keep the elderly from getting stiff. People in nonindustrialized societies recognized that the animal fats needed to be very fresh and not overcooked, and that the butter or cream should not be heated at all. This intuitive wisdom suggests that these pure, unheated fats, the carriers of warmth in the world of food, can protect us against the cold, dry stiffness of osteoarthritis. In 1943, a scientist named Rosalind Wulzen discovered what came to be known as the *anti-stiffness factor*, a fat-soluble, heat-sensitive fraction found primarily in butterfat, certain animal fats and—surprisingly—sugar cane juice. Experiments performed at the time conclusively demonstrated that virtually any animal can be made arthritic by feeding it a lowfat diet, especially one that emphasizes skim or lowfat milk products. Wulzen further demonstrated that this arthritic syndrome can be reversed by feeding the animals fresh, raw (unheated) cream or butter. This comes as no surprise when we consider that in osteoarthritis one loses one's warmth and cushion, which can be countered by the warmth-giving, insulating qualities of fat.

Thus the emphasis in treating osteoarthritis is on the use of *raw* butter. Lacto-fermented vegetables are also important, as they supply enzymes that help the body process this anti-stiffness factor.

Betachol, made by Standard Process Labs, is the only supplement form of this anti-stiffness factor. Using a low-heat extraction method, the anti-stiffness factor is isolated from sugar cane juice and mixed with certain bile factors that help in fat digestion. I recommend one to two capsules, three times daily with meals, for my osteoarthritis patients, particularly those who cannot obtain raw butter and cream.

Natural, traditional fats are also important for the treatment of inflammatory arthritis, but with more of an emphasis on certain oils. On the cellular level, the chemicals that initiate and control inflammation are called prostaglandins, which are a kind of tissue hormone. Researchers have found that it is the balance of tissue prostaglandins that determine the amount and quality of inflammation. The absence of certain oils, out of which the anti-inflammatory prostaglandins are made, can lead to the kind of excessive inflammation found in rheumatoid arthritis. These anti-inflammatory oils include oils of the omega-3 family, like cod liver oil and flax seed oil. Most commercial vegetable oils and hydrogenated oils interfere with these anti-inflammatory prostaglandins and should be strictly avoided.

A special oil of the omega-6 family is gamma-linoleic acid (GLA), found in evening primrose oil, black currant oil and borage oil. It seems to help both types of arthritis, as both inflammatory and anti-inflammatory prostaglandins derive from GLA. Likewise, liver, and other organ meats, egg yolks, butter and other animal fats can be made into either type of prostaglandin and are important foods for anyone suffering from arthritis. However, for the sufferer of rheumatoid arthritis, it is not so important that the butter be raw.

Finally, beet kvass and kombucha, while good beverages for everyone, are especially helpful in cases of inflammatory arthritis, because they have detoxifying effects on the liver. As we have seen, the liver is intimately involved with the watery, life-force body, and requires detoxification when the fluids in the body become stagnant.

Therapeutics

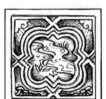 The remedy of first choice for the pain and stiffness of both types of arthritis is castor oil packs. Castor oil supplies stimulating warmth to the cold, over-mineralized joints of the osteoarthritis sufferer, but also has an anti-inflammatory and detoxifying effect for the swollen joints of the rheumatoid arthritis sufferer.

I prescribed castor oil packs for Mrs. H.B., a 44-year-old woman who slipped and fell on ice while skating. She suffered a mild concussion and a sprained neck. She was taken to a local Emergency Room and given a CT scan of the head and X-rays of the neck. Even though the scan indicated that the neck was normal, she began to experience headaches and neck spasm. Castor oil packs were applied, warm to the back of the neck, cool on the forehead. (We used cool compresses on the forehead because the head is the one area of our bodies that must remain cool.) These were kept on all night. We were all relieved to learn that the next morning she had minimal pain in her neck and only a mild headache. She had no repercussion from her concussion.

Castor oil packs should be considered the treatment of choice, the first line of defense, for all local pain and inflammation.

A specific therapy for osteoarthritis, and one that is more controversial, is bee venom therapy. Although use of bee stings to treat osteoarthritis may raise eyebrows, it is in fact a therapy that was widely used in folk medicine. Peasants throughout the world have used the practice of placing honey bees on their sore joints and muscles to treat their arthritis and pain.

We do not know the exact reasons why bee venom therapy works, or which specific components of bee venom have a healing effect. Consider, however, the fact that conditions like osteoarthritis, bursitis and tendinitis are due to a gradual process of sclerosis or mineralization. The body attempts to bring balance in these situations by creating an inflammation, but in many cases the body's attempt to heal through inflammation is too weak. Stinging the sore joint with a honey bee dramatically increases inflammation and brings more blood to the area. In addition, bee venom has a component that relieves pain. This inflammation becomes the agent for bringing warmth to the affected area. The warmth and inflammation from the bee sting also increases the body's ability to dissolve excessive mineralizations. As a potent local stimulator of inflammation, bee venom thus fulfills exactly the healing requirements for osteoarthritis. It increases the heat or warmth in the joint, and it increases the ability of the body to dissolve the excessive mineral deposits that are the hallmark of arthritis.

Let's return to Mr. R.B., the elderly man with the swollen knee. I prescribed raw butter and cream along with fermented vegetables; Betachol supplements; castor oil packs on the knee; and bee venom therapy three times a week. At the end of six weeks he had no further pain in his knee, was able to walk with a crutch and his whole mood and sense of life were uplifted. His family was thrilled. One year later, he was still without pain and able to walk using only a crutch.

Bee venom therapy also worked for Mrs. L.L., a 76-year-old woman with painful arthritis in both knees. She was overweight and suffered from high blood pressure, atrial fibrillation and congestive heart failure. Aspirin and other NSAIDs bothered her stomach and were not compatible with her coumadin, a blood-thinning medicine she was taking. She was also judged to be a poor candidate for joint replacement. Mrs. L.L. made it clear to me that she wanted a therapy that worked and that did not interfere with her lifestyle. I agreed to try and suggested bee venom therapy. On her initial visit she limped in, using a cane. After eight weeks of four injections to each knee, two to three times a week, she was free from pain and walking normally. Each year since then she comes back for two- to three-week booster sessions when she feels some twinges in her knees.

The use of bee venom and, indeed, the story of the honey bees themselves, is truly fascinating. Bee venom therapy for arthritis, tendinitis or bursitis is effective, simple, inexpensive and can be used by anyone. (For instructions, See Appendix C.)

What kind of treatment do I recommend for rheumatoid arthritis? Remembering our metaphor of the stagnant pond that breeds pathogenic bacteria and all sorts of pests, the following story makes sense. In the 1950s, a famous rheumatologist, Dr. Tom Brown, was able to show that a key component in the development of inflammatory arthritis was infection of the joints with a microorganism called mycoplasma. Orthodox medicine would claim that mycoplasma is the cause of the disease, whereas the holistic view sees the mycoplasma merely as a symptom of a more basic cause. Nevertheless, the treatment that Dr. Brown used, namely very small doses of tetracycline, an antibiotic that kills mycoplasma, can be very helpful in the treatment of rheumatoid arthritis.

I used tetracycline to treat our airline hostess, Ms. L. A. Along with an elevated erythrocyte sedimentation rate, a clear indication of active, excessive inflammation, she also tested positively for antibodies to mycoplasma. I also suggested dietary changes, including the addition of omega-3 oils and evening primrose oil. She took only one 250 mg. tablet of tetracycline, 3 times a week, but within two months she was off all her NSAIDs, her sed rate was down and she was working virtually pain-free.

The other therapy I use for rheumatoid arthritis takes direct advantage of the metaphor of the willow tree. For just as the willow tree relieves stagnation in the fluid body, a process analogous to swelling in the human being, so too does willow extract have a positive effect on the course of inflammatory arthritis. The Bayer drug company used willow bark extract, which is rich is natural salicylates, as the model for the original synthesis of aspirin, the prototypical anti-inflammatory. In its native or unprocessed form, willow bark extract is still a very valuable treatment for chronic pain and inflammation. And, while it doesn't have the same immediate effect as its chemical brother aspirin, neither does it have the side effects or cause the disruption of platelet function. Furthermore, unlike aspirin, the longer you use willow bark extract the more it seems to work, which is the direct opposite of what occurs with aspirin therapy. I use Mediherb Saligesic, 1 tablet 3-4 times per day, for inflammatory arthritis, and this therapy can be continued for as long as necessary.

Another excellent therapy for inflammatory arthritis is the Mediherb combination called Boswellia Complex. The ingredients in this preparation are boswellia (also known as frankincense), ginger, turmeric and celery seed extract. Boswellia, one of the gifts of the Magi to the Christ child, is also an old Ayurvedic medicine used for purification and to bring warmth. The boswellia plant contains an oil or resinous gum which when burned generates a pleasing aroma and warmth. We have described inflammatory arthritis as a chronic process of excessive warmth which, unlike an acute febrile illness where the fever "guides" the inflammation to its proper conclusion, lacks any guiding process. As a result, the inflammation wanders around endlessly as though lost. With the introduction of boswellia gum, we introduce a "guiding" warmth into the human organism, thereby slowly releasing the inflammatory process from the body. The other ingredients, ginger and turmeric, also provide warmth and have been shown to have anti-inflammatory effects. The celery seed extract acts as a diuretic, helping the body excrete toxic waste products. The dose of Boswellia Complex is 1-2 tablets 3 times per day, again usually long term.

Next we must address the liver, which always needs strenthening in the case of chronic inflammatory diseases. As we said, the primary cause of inflammatory arthritis is the stagnation of fluids, or a weakness in the life-force body. The ancients associated this etheric or watery realm to the liver. In fact, the derivation of the name of the liver comes from the word "to live." In former times, when mankind still understood the world in pictures, he had a sense of the intimate connection between the fluid realm and the liver. We know today that if the liver is sick, as in cirrhosis, stagnant fluid begins to build up in the abdomen, a condition called ascites.

The main medicines I use to treat the liver are Livaplex by Standard Process (1-2 capsules 3 times per day), which contains the liver protomorphogen Hepatrophin PMG, or Livco by Mediherb, which is a combination of herbal extracts of schisandra, rosemary and milk thistle, 1 tablet taken twice daily.

Another remedy that can be used in patients with virtually any autoimmune disorder, that is, disorders like rheumatoid arthritis in which the body attacks itself, is oral tolerance therapy. Discovered by Dr. Royal Lee, the theory of oral tolerance therapy is simple. When the body has an excessive immune or antibody reaction against a particular tissue, such as cartilage, we can "trick" the body by giving it large oral doses of the same tissue from an animal. For rheumatoid arthritis, Dr. Lee formulated oral Ostrophin or cartilage tissue from a bull. According to Dr. Lee, Ostrophin stimulates destructive antibodies, many of which are located in the intestines, to direct their attack against the medicine instead of the body's own tissue. This theory may explain why chicken soup, containing an abundance of dissolved cartilage, is such a time-honored method for treating rheumatism. The use of cartilage-rich broths, along with Ostrophin from Standard Process, often provides enough relief from inflammation to permit the patient to address the more fundamental causes of his disorder.

Finally, rhythmical massage, as practiced by an anthroposophical massage therapist, includes very specific techniques for encouraging the healthy circulation of fluids and is a remedy I often suggest for inflammatory arthritis.

Movement

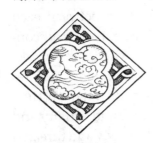

Arthritis manifests when the emotions, and hence our motions, get caught inside the body. The emotions should flow in and out; when they don't, either excessive mineralization or excessive inflammation occurs. The gesture of arthritis involves improper use of the limbs to meet the world and our daily activities. In osteoarthritis, the energy that should flow out is dammed up in one particular spot. In rheumatoid or "roaming" arthritis, areas of inflammation and pain move from one place to another in the body. The motions that lead to osteoarthritis are repetitive and constricting, while those of rheumatoid arthritis mimic flailing ineffectiveness.

For arthritis of the fingers and hands, the Magnet exercise is recommended. When you carry out the exercise with conscious thought, you can transfer the place of perceived pressure to a point outside the hand, and not by restraining the movement, thus straining the muscles and tendons in the hand.

Shoulder Muscle Mapping and Knee Mapping can help alleviate pain in these areas by relaxing tension and shifting muscles into more advantageous groupings. In these exercises, gentle moving pressure is applied to the affected area to retrain it to the proper gesture and space. Correct movement mapping of the knee begins on the inside of the knee and moves over the thigh to the outside of the hips. This helps correct a tendency to be knock-kneed, a gesture that creates strain and fatigue. Similarly, the Coat Hanger and Lowering the Sails can help move the shoulders and arms down to the point where they have greatest ease of movement.

I. OSTEOARTHRITIS

Beyond these basic exercises, the contrasting images of osteoarthritis and rheumatoid arthritis suggest very different types of exercise for each condition. In osteoarthritis, there is a coldness in the joints, the minerals start to deposit and the cushions wear out. Patients with osteoarthritis are crying out for more warmth, more flexibility. For this reason, anything that warms up the osteoarthritis patient is beneficial. This includes virtually any movement, particularly movement accompanied by enthusiasm. In other words, find a kind of movement you enjoy. The more enthusiasm and vigor, the better, as this will produce more heat. Begin each exercise period by loosening up and stretching, and then by rubbing arnica massage oil, which is a warming oil, into your tender joints. After exercising, stay warm and reapply the arnica oil. Remember that osteoarthritis is a cold illness that must be countered with warmth, movement and enthusiasm.

In osteoarthritis there is excessive wear and tear on the joints. The free space has been compromised by over-use, mis-use and even dis-use. To avoid and alleviate the degenerative symptoms, move as if there were lungs in each joint, between each bone. For example, let the spaces between each of your vertebrae expand and contract with every breath, and expand the space between your joints whenever you take on any pressure, force, or weight. Think of the grace of women from older cultures who walk with elongated and elastic spines while carrying jugs of water on their heads. This pulsing space between the joints encourages synovial fluid activity and brings warmth. Emotional weight can also weigh heavily upon the body and threaten the health of the joints. When you feel heavy, create the spacial dynamic of expanding sponges where you have felt squeezed and compromised. Breathe with all your joints while doing the Spinal Stretch and the Victory Stretch.

II. RHEUMATOID ARTHRITIS

In contrast to the focalized, fixation of osteoarthritis, in rheumatoid arthritis the joint space slowly disintegrates and diffuses from the periphery. The body's own defense mechanism begins to attack the joint, dispersing it from the outside. The joint is immobilized by self-destruction and by seeping fluids which have come to a standstill and dissolve the joint. Heat follows. In rheumatoid ("roaming") arthritis, these processes of inflammation are not set, but move about. The gestures appear in the Emotional Body as well and show themselves in the tendency towards "letting yourself go" such that you are literally "giving yourself away." While in osteoarthritis an exaggeration of point-centered tendencies can lead to physical and emotional antipathy, rheumatoid arthritis exhibits the danger of peripheral tendencies leading to unchecked sympathy. Indiscriminate dispersing gestures can lead to dissolution of both inner (joints) and outer (interpersonal and social) meeting spaces.

In rheumatoid arthritis, overly vigorous activity can actually damage the joints. Instead, begin with Carriage Down/Carriage Up and then move into rhythmical motions, such as the Tides, the Water Level Gesture and the Sundial. Light dancing such as the waltz, balance board and juggling to music are all appropriate.

Emphasizing the fluid moments of transition in all the Spacial Dynamics exercises is particularly helpful. Remembering that the image for rheumatoid arthritis is stagnation in a pond, we can see the logic of water exercise for this disease. Moreover, in water, the strain on the joints in counteracted by the buoyancy of water. Water aerobics or swimming in local lakes and ponds can be uniformly helpful to patients

suffering from rheumatoid arthritis. Playing in the ocean can be particularly beneficial as it combines movement in water with the detoxifying effect of a salt bath.
Producing warmth is not the goal, but rather redistributing warmth by stimulating
the movement of fluids.

Meditation

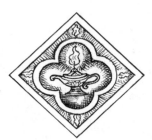

Our poetic images of the two types of arthritis suggest two
different attitudes needed for true healing to take place. The
metaphorical description of osteoarthritis is the dry, creaking
sounds of pine trees and the grating of cicadas, describing an
existence that lacks warmth and enthusiasm. The true healer
for osteoarthritis is passion, passion that activates our capacity for warmth, our dissolving powers, our juices. I have seen
many cases in which the joint pains and destruction of cartilage worsen when the
patient loses a loved one. We all need to put the pursuit of our passion, that activity
for which we feel the most enthusiasm, at the top of our "to do" list. Often this takes
the form of a warm, loving, passionate relationship, which certainly warms us and
literally gets our juices flowing. But it can also take the form of a passion for music,
for writing or even studying a variety of butterflies. No person can truly live a full life
when it is devoid of passion and true enthusiasm, and the osteoarthritis sufferer manifests the lack of passion in his very bones.

In rheumatoid arthritis, the patient suffers not so much from lack of warmth,
but warmth in the wrong place. Consider the image of the sorrowful, weeping willow
and the unhappy Desdemona, who "loved not wisely but too well." There may be
passion, love and warmth, but the patient lacks discrimination, leading to overindul-
gent, over-mothering behavior. Whereas the osteoarthritis patient may be overly critical, the sufferer of rheumatoid arthritis tends to be too obliging. The patient has
warmth, love and enthusiasm, but it is misapplied, perhaps as a love of sugar or
alcohol instead of healthy food, or overly protective behavior toward one's children
as they grow into adulthood. In more extreme cases, this can manifest as the inability
for incest survivors to separate themselves from abusive parents, or extreme hyper-
sensitivity to constructive criticism.

Those who suffer from conditions of stagnated warmth must take an honest
look at their lives, their relationships and their emotions. While engaging in the
Rückschau Meditation, they would profit from visualizing an antidote to the image of
suffocating warmth by comparing their emotional life to a flowing stream, nourishing the life-forms along its shore with clear, sustaining waters that never linger, but

always move on; or replacing the thought form of the weeping willow tree with its downward branches to that of a towering oak whose internal waters move with the seasons, rising up as sap in the spring and falling in showers of autumn leaves.

The goal in both types of arthritis is a state of emotional balance in which nurture and sympathy for others are balanced by passion and enthusiasm for one's own work, love and play.

RECOMMENDED READING

The Arthritis Breakthrough by Henry Scammell

Summary
OSTEOARTHRITIS

Nutrition

*	Avoid	All processed vegetable oils and hydrogenated fats
		Processed foods, especially those containing white sugar
		Fruit juices
*	Emphasize	Raw butter and unheated animal fats
		Liver and other organ meats
		Organic eggs
		Bone broths
*	Supplements	Evening primrose, black currant or borage oils, 500 mg capsules, 4 per day
		Betachol, 1-2 capsules 3 times a day with meals

Therapeutics

* Castor oil compresses over the affected joints or painful tissues.
* For more serious cases, bee venom therapy for 6-12 weeks.

Movement

* Any exercise that produces warmth and is done with enthusiasm.
* Magnet, Shoulder Muscle Mapping and Knee Mapping.
* Coat Hanger and Lowering the Sail.
* Spinal Stretch and Victory Stretch.

Meditation

* Determine that for which you have passion and enthusiasm.
* Avoid negativity and criticism.

Summary

RHEUMATOID ARTHRITIS

Nutrition

* Avoid   All processed vegetable oils and hydrogenated fats
Processed foods, especially those containing
white sugar
Fruit juices

* Emphasize   Flax oil, one to two teaspoons daily
Good quality cultured butter
Liver and other organ meats
Eggs from pastured chickens
Bone broths
Beet kvass and kombucha

* Supplements   Cod liver oil, to supply 10,000 IU vitamin A daily
Evening primrose, black currant or borage oils,
500 mg capsules, 4 per day

Therapeutics

* Livaplex 1capsule 3 times per day or Livco,
1 tablet 2-3 times per day.
* Saligesic,1 tablet 3-4 times per day.
* Boswellia complex, 1-2 tablets 3-4 times per day.
* Ostrophin, 1 tablet 3 times per day.
* In severe cases, use Tetracycline, 250 mg 1 tablet
3 times per week.
* Massage once a week for 2-3 months.

Movement

- * Magnet, Shoulder Muscle Mapping and Knee Mapping.
- * Coat Hanger and Lowering the Sail.
- * Carriage Down/Carriage Up.
- * The Tides, the Water Level Gesture and the Sundial.
- * Light dancing, balance board and juggling to music.
- * Swimming and any movement in water, especially salt water.

Meditation

- * Temper your nurturing tendencies with clear vision.
- * Release yourself and your loved ones to movement and freedom.

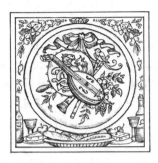

Chapter 15:
Neurological Diseases

In you come with your cold music till I creep through every nerve.
Robert Browning
A Tocatta of Galuppi's

I have chosen to describe the neurological diseases last because these illnesses are intimately bound up with modern life. To address them properly, we must take stock of what it means to be modern and collectively ponder our future course. Mankind is distinguished from the animals in his ability to use tools and to manipulate matter by conscious thought. In our forward evolution, technology has reached a peak. The neurological diseases so endemic in this modern age represent a *de*-evolution, a regression specifically brought about by the application of modern technology to the areas of farming and food processing.

The diseases of the nervous system include seizure disorders, Attention Deficit Disorder, Alzheimer's disease, multiple sclerosis, Lou Gehrig's disease, Parkinson's disease and so forth, all of which are crippling and disheartening medical problems. Whole textbooks have been written about each one of these diseases. However, I will focus not on specific microscopic explanations but rather sketch an image or a picture of the phenomena that underlie them all.

In our discussion of heart disease, we noted Rudolf Steiner's perplexing statement that mankind's progress is impeded by his insistence on distinguishing between sensory and motor nerves. According to modern medicine, there are two types of nerve cells: the sensory nerves, which carry messages from a sense organ, such as the eye, to the brain, and the motor nerves, which carry messages from the brain or spinal cord to the muscles, causing them to contract and do their work. According to Steiner, all the nerves are sensory nerves, that is, nerves that carry impressions to the brain.

The evidence that there are, in fact, motor nerves as distinct from sensory nerves seems incontrovertible because if you put an electrical stimulation on a motor nerve, it will cause the muscle to contract. However, Steiner points out that this experiment does not in any way represent a normal physiological event and therefore is irrelevant.

Steiner's ideas about the nervous system may seem irrelevant, but I believe they are crucial to understanding and treating the various neurological diseases. Before we can make any progress with these diseases, we must understand that the nervous system exclusively serves as our organism's sense *receptor*. In Steiner's concept of the threefold man, the sphere of the head or nervous system lives in quiet and stillness as it carries out its vital role as the gatherer and integrator of all the various sense impressions that come to it. It does not initiate; it only senses and integrates. The impulses to action are the domain of the Metabolic sphere. Movement that seems to be initiated by the nervous system is, in fact, initiated and carried out by the muscular system and then *sensed* by the nervous system, not the other way around. While this may seem like a semantic distinction, it leads us to the important conclusion that musculo-skeletal disorders, such as polymyalgia (inflammation of the muscles) and rheumatism (inflammation of the joints), are disorders of the metabolism and will, while neurological diseases all have their origin in sensory stimulation. Therefore, we must look for the etiology of these various syndromes in the sensory input to which we are exposed. In fact, examination of this sensory input leads to some important and startling conclusions, which, as Rudolf Steiner suggested, have far-reaching effects on the future well-being of humanity.

As a result of many animal studies, we now know that there are two main pathways for nerve injury. The first is via the so-called excitotoxins, various external stimuli that cause excessive firing of the nerve cells. After intense short-term or chronic low-level exposure to these excitatory stimulators, the nerve begins to "protect" itself by forming scar tissue. This scar tissue then interferes with normal nerve transmission. The type of excitotoxin and the location of the scar tissue dictates the symptoms that eventually appear. For example, scarring of the "motor nerves" is associated with multiple sclerosis, and scarring of the *substantia nigra,* the black substance of the brain, is associated with Parkinson's. Some of the most common excitotoxins, shown decisively to cause nerve tissue scarring in animal studies, include monosodium glutamate or free glutamic acid (MSG), the artificial sweetener aspartame, neurotoxic proteins in breakfast cereals formed during the extrusion process, TV exposure and fluorescent light exposure.

The other main pathway of injury to the nerves is through substances like aluminum, alcohol, mercury and organophosphate agricultural chemicals, all of which can have adverse effects. Aluminum causes plaque or scar tissue formation in the cortex or higher brains of laboratory animals; alcohol is a chronic nervous system depressant; mercury interferes with nerve cell function; and organophosphate agricultural chemicals interfere with nerve transmission.

In their search for the causes of MS, Parkinson's, Alzheimer's, attention deficit disorder and other neurological syndromes, scientists are looking at the nerve cells and their transmission characteristics. This is like looking under a street lamp for a set of keys lost in a dark alley simply because there is light under the street lamp. Researchers are looking in the wrong place, and the answers are not there. The answers can be found only when one accepts the premise that the function of the nervous system is solely to gather and process sense impressions, sense impressions of all sorts. The solution to the tragedy of neurological diseases will be found by examining the sense impressions to which we are exposed, and discovering which part of the brain or nervous system they affect.

Consider MSG, a food additive that has been in widespread use since the late 1950s. The food processing industry uses MSG to impart flavor to products that would otherwise be dull and tasteless. Most people think it is only a minor additive, whereas in fact it is found in its various forms in virtually every packaged and boxed food that humans consume. Sometimes it appears on the label but usually it does not. Any product containing "flavors," "natural flavors," "spices," "citric acid" or "hydrolyzed protein" usually contains MSG. The food industry uses vast quantities of MSG in fast food, frozen dinners, sauce mixes, dried soups and bouillon cubes. Even baby food and baby formula contain MSG, disguised as "hydrolyzed protein." Anyone who does not eat in the way we are suggesting in this book is exposed to MSG and similar excitotoxins every day. Many children live almost exclusively on processed foods loaded with excitotoxins. In the short term these chemicals can cause overestimation of the nervous system leading to Attention Deficit Disorder. Long-term usage results in scarring and eventually Parkinson's, Alzheimer's and similar diseases later in life.

The light of TV screens and fluorescent bulbs can also cause overstimulation and then scarring of the nervous system. The work of John Ott and many others has revealed the mechanisms whereby these various artificial forms of light overstimulate various glands in our brain, such as the pineal gland. Even the stimulation caused by violent TV and movies can injure the sympathetic nervous system. These effects have been well documented in both human and animal studies during the past 20 to 30 years.

In biology we are taught that the various animal and human organs evolved in direct response to stimulation from the environment. The eye and the whole visual sensory mechanism evolved in response to full-spectrum visible light. Other parts of the light spectrum do not have the same biological effects as natural sunlight. It is not difficult to grasp that artificial light, which lacks some of the frequencies found in natural light, can cause overstimulation of the nervous system leading to injury. Even short-term exposure to fluorescent lights can cause fatigue and concentration problems in sensitive individuals.

Aluminum may be the culprit in Alzheimer's as it seems to cause the formation of neuro-fibrillary tangles characteristic of the disease. Sources of aluminum include aluminum cookware (which leach naked aluminum into cooked food), deodorants (which are absorbed through the skin) and antacid formulations. Until recently, most vaccines contained thimerosal, a mercury-based preservative that has been implicated as a major contributing factor to autism.

Organophosphate pesticides cause dramatic short-term neurological symptoms, which is no surprise since their mechanism for killing "pests" is to poison their nervous system. Organophosphate compounds affect the neuromuscular interface, the location where the nerves and muscles meet. These pesticides are ubiquitous in nonorganic foods—in fruits, vegetables, grains and the animals to which the grains have been fed. Direct exposure comes from the spraying of crops, lawns, golf courses, schools and houses.

Mercury is another well-recognized neurotoxic substance to which most of us are exposed—from tainted fish to amalgam fillings. Mercury seems to cause injury to the parts of the nervous system that control balance and coordination. Mercury that "out gasses" from dental fillings can be absorbed directly into the brain. Poisons can also develop in root canals and spread to various parts of the body, including the nerve cells.

Mrs. B. G., a woman in her early 40s, had suffered gradual neurological deterioration over a ten-year period. She had blurred or double vision, walked with a cane, suffered fatigue and was having difficulties with her bowels and bladder. These symptoms are typical of multiple sclerosis, but an MRI was inconclusive. The first step in her therapy was to have all her amalgam fillings replaced with a more inert composite material, and all her root canal teeth removed by a dentist skilled in proper ways of handling these situations. She then received intravenous treatments of a substance called DMPS to remove as much mercury as possible from her system. I also gave her herbs and an adrenal cortex supplement, along with suggestions for dietary changes. Within six months her vision was much improved, she could walk easily without a cane and she felt less fatigued than she had in years.

This case had a happy ending as the patient was able to improve, but it is important to keep in mind that the nervous system has the least ability to heal and regenerate of any system in the body. Frequently, injuries to the nerve cells are irreversible. For all the neurological disorders, prevention is the key, and prevention usually means major changes in life-style.

And the key to prevention involves the realization that the nervous system is the sensor and integrator of all sensory input to which we are exposed. In the chapter on digestive diseases we asked the question: "Is our food real?" So, too, we must ask about our sensory experiences, which are "digested" by the nervous system—are they real? Consider the difference between listening to birds, a choir or a live symphony compared to computer-generated music, or even a CD. The former provide full-spectrum sound that is real to the nervous system; the latter is "cold music," a simulation that tricks the listener. So, too, do fluorescent lights trick the viewer, and foods containing artificial flavors trick the palate.

Consider the difference in sensory experience between synthetic fabrics and the richness of silk, wool and cotton. Natural fiber has an individuality or uniqueness that the nervous system recognizes as something familiar, as something that is its proper food. Plastics and synthetics, with their numbing uniformity of texture, are like junk food for the nervous system—they stimulate but do not nourish. So, too, with the toys we give to children these days—uniformly stamped plastic, lifeless gadgets with none of the creativity, originality or even mistakes of the old doll made by Aunt Frances, or that leather baseball mitt carefully oiled throughout the years. Even the sense of smell has been invaded by imitation smells, from perfumes to air fresheners.

The care of the nervous system is really the hygiene of the senses. We are biologically programmed to have a rich sensory experience in life. Through the eyes we must see varied landscapes, bright colors, flowers, people and paintings, all in full-spectrum light. Through the ears we need the sounds of the animals, the wind, the trees, music, singing and human voices. The taste buds need the rich tastes and textures of natural foods, not imitation foods "flavor-enhanced" with MSG. The sense of touch wants natural fibers, the feel of the waves and cool lake water. We need human caressing and the touch of animals. And, with the sense of smell, we need to experience the natural perfume of flowers, ripening fruit, compost piles, human sweat, bread baking and stew simmering on the stove.

The prevention and treatment of neurological disorders can never be accomplished with a pill, nor even with herbs and natural medicines. It involves a complete change in environment and life-style, change in which all artificial sensory stimulation is replaced with genuine food for the senses. It calls for the replacement of all that is artificial with articles of genuine materials and the elimination of "cold music"—TV, radios, CD's and tapes—as much as possible. Instead go to concerts, put up a bird feeder, learn to play an instrument, join a choir, sing in the shower. If you must work in front of a computer or under fluorescent lights, do so in front of a window and take frequent breaks to be in the out of doors. Eat real food that has not been sprayed with pesticides. Put flowers and plants in your home and office, wear natural-fiber clothes, give your partner a massage, pet your dog, buy an original watercolor or oil painting from someone you know. This is the main therapy for both prevention and treatment of neurological disorders. Even if these measures do not bring a complete remission, they will put real quality into all aspects of your life and also may just alter the course of humanity as we enter the new millennium.

Communication also needs to be "real." For communication to be real it must be based on the truth. Mahatma Gandhi taught that no man is in possession of the absolute truth—absolute truth is the domain of the gods. Human truth lies in the connection, the relationship between one man and the other. Truth is a function of and is dependent on human relationships. Truth in relationships requires that one person listens to the other, straining to understand the other without prejudice and without judgment. Real communication requires acceptance of the fact that none of us has the truth; rather, truth will be found in our meeting together. As Jesus said, "When two or more are gathered in my name I (the truth) will be there."

Paradoxically, truth is intimately connected with the phenomenon of memory. Mark Twain, who was renown for his remarkable memory, even in his later years, was asked how he managed to have such a good memory. He response was, "I tell the truth." Think about it: if you are asked what color shirt you have on and you lie, you will have difficulty answering a question about the color of that shirt one month later. If you always tell the truth, without exaggeration, without down-playing the facts, you will have to remember nothing except what you have observed, and your memory will remain intact.

Punctilious devotion to truth in communication is especially important as a healing therapy for those suffering from Alzheimer's disease. In Alzheimer's disease the neurons form "tangles," in fact the brain resembles a tangled web, not unlike the communication patterns of a chronic liar who spins a tangled web of tales. So much that goes on in our culture, our media, our business community and especially our politics is nothing more than a tangled web of non-truths, half-truths and outright lies. Is it any wonder that we have so much Alzheimer's disease in our country?

The tragic condition called autism also finds solace in truthful communication. For years I have worked as the physician to a number of communities of "handi-capped" people who live in our area. Many of the residents are classified as autistic. While I have no doubt that there are "physical" problems with their nerve tissue, many from the influences I have described, a major issue with all the "autistic" people, like all those with Alzheimer's disease, is their struggle with the truth, their struggle to break out of their prison and find real human connection. Mr. Q., a 38-year-old fellow with profound handicaps was brought to my office one day to investigate why he had suddenly started wetting his bed. Perhaps it was a urinary tract infection, perhaps it was stress. To my knowledge, no one had ever heard him directly answer a question in understandable words, certainly I never had. He did say words, but they were completely unintelligible. On that day I decided to see what would happen if I assumed that his communication problem was not his inability to speak, but my inability to understand. As he paced the room in his usual fashion, I asked him questions. He would grunt, turn his head, pound his head, or otherwise respond in unintelligible ways. With each response I would say "Mr. Q, I am having trouble understanding what you mean when you grunt like that, does that mean yes?" Within half an hour I could understand the rudiments of his language.

At the end of the hour, I asked him, "What would make your life better right now?"

He replied in the clearest voice one could imagine, "Could I please go to the bathroom?" He went to the bathroom and came back into my exam room. I asked him whether he needed medicine for his urine; he shook his head no. I asked him whether he would have someone call me if his problem continued; he said yes. The next day the bed-wetting problem resolved and to my knowledge has not reappeared.

This startling event taught me a lot about the power of communication, the power of listening and the essence of love, which lies partly in the struggle to understand the other. To understand is to not judge, not to criticize, but to understand that the truth lies between us, not within only one of us. Telling the truth as Mark Twain suggests is the vehicle of understanding; it creates a basis for what is real in the world, and is the key to the creation not only of a good memory but also the attainment of love, which is our task on this earth.

Nutrition

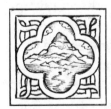 The diet outlined in this book is just as important for the nervous system as it is for all other parts of the body. The nerve cells, like every other cell in the body, need the right kinds of fats to function properly. Eggs should be emphasized as they are recognized as a brain food in Europe and Asia. Naturally, all processed foods should be eliminated as almost all contain MSG and other synthetic flavorings. Diet sodas and other products containing aspartame (Nutrasweet or Equal) are truly toxic and should be avoided completely. To avoid pesticides, eat organic food as much as possible.

Citrus fruit and juice, in particular, should be organic as citrus receives heavy spraying with organophosphate pesticides. The entire fruit is processed during the manufacture of orange and other citrus juices, so the juice is likely to contain high levels of potent neurotoxins. In fact, a recent study linked consumption of fruit and fruit juices with the development of neurological disorders. The investigators faulted the heavy load of pesticides used in fruit.

Calcium is a great protector of the brain and nervous system so calcium-rich dairy products and bone broths are a must. Ironically, MSG is used in sauces and soups to provide the flavor that should be provided by calcium-rich broth. When we consume imitation foods flavored with MSG, we not only poison the nervous system but also cheat ourselves of protective calcium. Remember that calcium cannot be absorbed without the fat-soluble vitamins A and D, found exclusively in animal fats.

Many nervous disorders often result from vitamin B_{12} deficiency. Most animal foods provide vitamin B_{12} but the best source is liver, which should be eaten at least once a week.

If you cannot bring yourself to eat liver, then take raw (dessicated) beef liver by Carlson Labs, 4-6 capsules per day. (Surprisingly, Carlson's beef liver capsules contain more B_{12} than the buffalo liver capsules.) Other supplements include cod liver oil and evening primrose oil, borage oil or black currant oil. These provide the long-chain fatty acids required for optimal neurological function. Extra vitamin D derived from cod liver oil may also be helpful, particularly in cases of multiple sclerosis.

Therapeutics

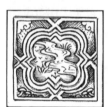

The therapies for neurological diseases mainly address those serious and frustrating illnesses like multiple sclerosis, Lou Gehrig's disease, Parkinson's and Alzheimer's. Obviously, each has its own specific etiology and causative factors, yet as pathologies of the nervous system, they share many features in common. One is a progressively downward course, as well as life-threatening and life-altering symptoms. In fact, the practitioner faces no more daunting task than the treatment of nervous system disorders, be she a conventional or alternative doctor. Because they are so difficult to treat, these diseases call for the same attention to detail required for the treatment of cancer.

The first step is to address the entire environment of the patient—the sensory environment, the diet and exposure to neurotoxic chemicals. The patient should avoid all artificial lights, television, electronic media and computers as much as possible while spending as much time as possible out of doors. All clothing should be made from cotton, wool, linen, silk, hemp or other natural fibers. Furthermore, all toxic chemicals should be totally removed from the house, including cleansers, detergents and so forth. This is the first and perhaps most crucial step—we must do all we can to remove the toxic load on the senses of the patient.

The next step is to take care of the dental situation. This means going to a dentist who is familiar with the removal of amalgam fillings and root canals, and the follow-up mercury detoxification protocols that are available. Again, this is a necessary step in decreasing the toxic load for the patient and allowing the nervous system to heal. (For sources of holistic dentists trained in the removal of amalgam fillings, see Appendix D.)

The third step is to intersperse periods of the normal *Nourishing Traditions* diet with 3-week periods of intensive detoxification. As neurological diseases are closely associated with exposure to neurotoxins, we must rely on the liver to clear these toxins from our tissues. The program I use for this is the Blessed Herb Internal Cleanse program, described in Chapter 4. During the cleanse, the patient consumes a traditional diet along with various herbal medicines taken sequentially to increase the detoxification abilities of our bodies, beginning with the bowels and progressing to the liver, lungs, kidneys and finally the blood. The program is thorough but gentle. At the end the good bacteria are restored to the intestinal tract. Many patients report increased energy and vitality with the cleansing program.

After the 4-week cleansing period, the patient resumes a normal course of supplements for five months and then repeats the detoxification program. This process continues until no further improvement is noted or until the patient's illness has remitted.

During the detoxification periods the patient uses no other medication or supplement except the Blessed Herb detoxification products. During periods between the cleanse programs, I prescribe a number of medicines. First is Neurotrophin PMG, the Standard Process protomorphogen for the nervous system. It is invaluable in the treatment of all neurological illnesses, because they all seem to have an immunological component. In the case of multiple sclerosis, we know that the immune system directly attacks the myelin sheaths of the nerves. By giving Neurotrophin as a decoy, we shunt this immune reaction away from our myelin and towards the medication. This kind of oral tolerance therapy has, in fact, shown great promise for the treatment of MS, especially when combined with the rebuilding and detoxification therapies included in this chapter. The dose is 1-3 tablets 3 times per day between meals.

Super EFF from Standard Process provides essential fatty acids in a form that is easily absorbed. These fatty acids work synergistically with cod liver oil and evening primrose oil to rebuild the nervous system. The nervous system actually contains the "fattiest" tissue type in our entire bodies. The myelin sheaths are basically lipid or fat coatings around the axons, the true nervous tissue. This explains why fat-soluble poisons in our environment accumulate in our nerve cells and are so toxic to the nervous system, and why the type and purity of our dietary fat is so crucial to the treatment of neurological illnesses. The dose is 2 capsules 3 times per day.

Livaplex by Standard Process provides nutritional support for the detoxification and elimination functions of the liver. In that sense it works as a follow-up and support to the 3-week cleansing program with a mild, more sustained detoxification. The dose is 1-2 capsules 3 times per day.

Catalyn by Standard process provides the broad-range nutritional support that is vital to any healing process. With its abundance of vitamins A, C and E from organic food sources, it helps the nervous system rebuild its tissue. The dose is 2 tablets 3 times per day.

Neurotrophin PMG, Super EFF, Livaplex and Catalyn can be given for all neurological disorders. I also prescribe specific herbal medicines for specific diseases.

For multiple sclerosis, which has a recognized auto-immune component, I give Rehmannia complex from Mediherb. This mixture contains rehmannia, which is an adrenal tonic herb that supports production of cortisone—a valuable substance in the amelioration of any chronic inflammatory or autoimmune disease. This preparation also contains bupleurum root which helps in liver detoxification, and hemidesmus root, a mildly immunosuppressive herb. Hemidesmus works in the same way as Neurotrophin PMG in that it damps down the excessive immune response, thereby allowing the assaulted tissue to regenerate and heal. The dose is 1 tablet 3 times per day.

With Alzheimer's disease, the benefits of gingko extract are well documented. We can understand the rationale of gingko both from the standpoint of its biochemical effects—it improves oxygenation of the tissues—as well as its metaphorical aspects. The gingko species has survived almost unchanged for over 150 million years, with some individual trees living longer than one thousand years. In fact, a lone gingko tree was the only survivor at ground-zero of the Hiroshima atomic blast, a profound testament to its astonishing hardiness and clearly a sign that it has learned in its being to withstand the ravages of aging, a phenomenon so intimately related to our nervous system. I use gingko extract from Mediherb at a dose of 1 tablet 2 times per day.

Finally, a combination of rosemary leaf, green tea extract, turmeric extract and grape seed extract called Vitanox from Mediherb can be given for all neurological illnesses at a dose of 1 tablet 2 times per day. Studies show that the procyanidins (OPCs) of grape seed extract penetrate the blood-brain barrier and protect the nerve cells from oxidation damage. Rosemary leaf extract protects vitamin E, a fat-soluble vitamin necessary for healthy nerve cell function. The catechins in green tea extract are recognized as cellular antioxidants. But, the most interesting ingredient in this formulation is extract of turmuric.

Researchers first became interested in turmeric as a medicine for the nervous system when they discovered that people who consume a lot of curry (which contains a lot of tumeric) have very low rates of Alzheimer's and other neurological diseases. A recent study found that high-dose turmeric extract gave good results with Alzheimer's patients.

The neurological benefits of turmeric are surprising since turmeric was traditionally used only as a choleretic, that is, as a medicine to stimulate the flow of bile. Turmeric extract was also used by Rudolf Steiner in a medicine he called Choleodoron, formulated to heal and balance gall bladder disease. How can we understand this paradox given our hypotheses that the fundamental cause of neurological illnesses is cellular poisoning? The answer can be found in the physical properties of turmeric for in this plant, the smell, color and activity is not in the flower but down in the ground, concentrated in its tubers. According to the anthroposophical perspective, the root of a plant corresponds to the nervous system while the flower and fruit correspond to the metabolic and reproductive realm of man. Thus, turmeric is telling us that it is active in the nervous system. But what about the traditional connection with the biliary system and the bile? This indicates the mechanism used for healing the nerves. Bile is the body's substance that carries poisons out of the body. To stimulate the flow of bile is to stimulate the removal of poisons from our cells. Bile is perfectly suited for this clearing because the substances that poison the nervous system are fat-soluble, and bile is the fat detergent or fat dissolution medium of the body. In this subtle and elegant way the humble, yet powerful spice called turmeric shows us not only a path towards healing, but if understood properly, it teaches us about the very nature of the disease we are confronting.

Movement

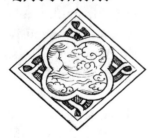

Nervous disorders benefit from gestures that still the head, such as the Tides, or that are graceful and rhythmical, such as swimming. Also helpful are exercises that work on the opposite pole, such as the Rice Paper Walk. People who suffer from nervous disorders or who are locked in their intellect often find great comfort in foot baths and foot massage. Sports that involve quick stops and starts, such as tennis, or that stress the upper parts of the body, such as fencing, are best avoided by highly nervous individuals.

Nervous disorders stem from our attempts to direct the world "out there" from the ivory tower of our central nervous system, a tendency shared by the vast majority of those living in the western world. To illustrate, try this simple experiment. Stand facing a light switch across a room. Have a companion watch as you slowly raise your hand. Stop at the point that you think would allow your hand to touch the light switch, should your hand extend across the room. Your companion will be able to judge where your hand would actually touch the opposite wall. For most people that point occurs on a spot much higher than the light switch. Now try the experiment again. Imagine that your hand is attached to the light switch by a string. Slowly raise your hand to the point where the string would lead your hand to the light switch. Most likely, your hand will stop at the proper height because you are allowing your actions to be shaped not by the intellect, but by the light switch, the world "out there."

People who suffer from depression and nervous disorders are people for whom most thoughts originate in the body. Of course, some of our thoughts must originate from the body, as the needs of the body require satisfaction. But when all of our thoughts originate in the body, we are locked in a narrow, limiting and self-centered mode of perceiving the outside world.

Some thirty years ago I was driving around lost, searching for Silver Saddles Riding Stables which I had heard was tucked away somewhere in the surrounding countryside. I stopped at a gas station to get directions. The attendant knew the riding stables well; he had been there many times himself. But he interrupted and restarted his own explanation no fewer than five or six times. His face reddened, forehead knitted and his neck swelled. Finally, exasperated, throwing up his hands, he said in all earnestness, "You just can't get there from here!" In that instant I knew I had just learned far more than I had been asking for. I had witnessed someone's thinking being clouded through a virtual collapse of the space around his head. Through his misplaced effort, he had inadvertently crowded himself—he got in his own way. This "cave-in" was so strong that at that moment he was the one who was lost. He was looking in his head for the location of the riding stables. The stables were located somewhere else, of course. Giving directions requires being simultaneously at the goal and where you are, and then being able to move between these two spaces. The attendant was caught in his head and that made him a prisoner of his own brain cells.

We have been taught that we think *in* our brains. In excess, this can be spacially invasive. We can think *with* our brains. This is spacially very different. In the second version the brain is a sense organ. Sense organs are designed to perceive something besides themselves. They are directed towards the object they are perceiving.

The best way to extend out of the body, and still remain centered in the head, is through one's hands. Movement and activity with the hands, particularly movement that involves extension and stretching, is a great antidote for a crowded mind. Highly distraught people often keep their hands close to the front of their bodies where they engage in fidgeting motions. The Magnet, the Personal Space Gesture and the Crest, in which the hands are directed outwards in response to objects or towards the external world can be highly therapeutic.

The Pulley is a very good movement for those suffering from neurological disorders, but it may require a preliminary movement from a seated position. Start seated, slowly relax your spine from the top down until your head is down between your knees. Stay there for five seconds, letting your head fill up with blood. Then slowly reverse the process until the head is upright again and the extra blood has flowed back down again. Build this up slowly by doing this exercise three times a day, spaced out over the day. Add five seconds a week until you are up to 20 seconds after a month. If you do not experience any dizziness, pain, or discomfort, then begin with the Pulley exercise. Regular "brain bathing" washes the cells with rich blood, dissolving and discouraging mineral deposits. This regular rhythmical filling and emptying the head with blood keeps the blood vessels elastic and the inner ear free of congestion that can cause dizziness. Well nourished with blood, the head can maintain the stillness that is its proper gesture.

All of us need to be open to ideas that come from the outside, that come from others. If we are constantly projecting our own thoughts onto other people, then we are not receptive but captive. The more stillness in the head that we can cultivate, the more broad-minded or open-minded we will be. The calm mind is receptive to new ideas. It sees the world for what it is and sees others living in the world for what they are. The Lemniscate Dynamic can help build the capacity of openness to the world "out there."

It is no exaggeration to say that in order to love, the mind must be still. For love is seeing something for what it is. The nervous, disordered, distracted, muddied mind cannot see clearly and therefore cannot experience the love that comes from the level of the soul.

The still mind that excels in the creative use of surrounding space finds peace and joy in doing things well. Every activity is experienced as full. Ancient cultures postulate that the gods have hidden themselves in the world. When we do things well, the gods reveal themselves; and when we do things well often enough, we acquire wisdom. Joy comes from uncovering the beings that are there in the world, but must remain hidden until we learn to deal with the world in a beautiful and loving way.

Meditation

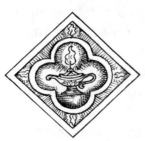

Remember that what we eat is "sensed" by the digestive system, and what we sense is "digested" by the sense organs and nervous system. Let the food for your senses be only that which is rich and real, which nourishes rather than merely stimulates. Allow yourself to relish the feasts of the senses through that quiet contemplation that properly belongs to the realm of the head. This ability to contemplate, to fully digest that which comes to us through the senses, is what makes us human. The human spirit needs real food. Otherwise it dies.

A major block to the proper nourishment of the nervous system is a sense of unworthiness. Many people feel that they are not "good enough" to enjoy rich sensory stimulation. Much religious education promotes the notion that humans are abject sinners who must deny themselves anything that gives them genuine pleasure. Bright colors, rich food, fine flavors, lush sounds, touching, back-scratching and massage are viewed as sinful indulgences. Therefore, your meditation should focus on restoring your sense of worthiness as a human being—not a sense of superiority to others but a sense of deservedness in which the entire human race participates. As you engage in the *Rückschau* Meditation, focus your attention on the various sense impressions you have received and contemplate your worthiness to receive the rich banquet God has laid before you to nourish your soul and mind.

Summary

Nutrition

✳	Avoid	All processed foods containing MSG
		All diet foods containing aspartame (Nutrasweet or Equal)
		Non-organic foods, particularly citrus and citrus juices

✳ Emphasize   Traditional fats

Eggs from pastured chickens

Dairy products and bone broths for calcium

Liver, at least once a week

✳ Supplements   Desiccated liver from Carlson Labs, 4-6 capsules per day

Cod liver oil to supply 10,000 - 20,000 IU vitamin A daily

Evening primrose oil, borage oil or black currant oil, 4 capsules per day

Carlson's vitamin D from cod liver oil, 2000 IU per day (See discussion on page 23)

Therapeutics

* Avoid all artificial lighting, particularly fluorescent lighting.
* Minimize exposure to TV, electronic media and computers.
* Avoid all pesticides and household chemicals.
* Wear natural fibers.
* Remove amalgam fillings and follow-up with mercury detoxification.
* Blessed Herb Internal Cleanse for a 4-week period alternating with 5 months of regular supplements.
* Neurotrophin PMG 1-2 tablets 3 times per day.
* Super EFF from Standard Process, 1-2 capsules 3 times per day.
* Livaplex from Standard Process, 1-2 tablets 3 times per day.

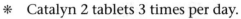

* Catalyn 2 tablets 3 times per day.
* Vitanox from Mediherb, 1 tablet 2 times per day.
* For MS, Rehmannia complex from Mediherb, 1 tablet 3 times per day.
* For Alzheimer's disease, gingko extract from Mediherb, 1 tablet 2 times per day.

Movement

* The Tides and the Rice Paper Walk.
* The Magnet.
* Space Finding Gesture.
* The Crest.
* The Pulley.
* The Lemniscate Dynamic.

Meditation

* Reflect on the nourishment of your senses and your worthiness to receive it.

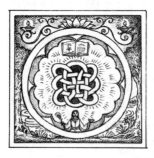

Post Script
How to Be a Patient

*T*he Art of Medicine includes the Art of Being a Patient. Let me explain with a story. Some time ago I spent a year in England with my family. My son was in his first year of kindergarten in the Waldorf School in Forest Row. His teacher was a man we called Christo. Christo really liked my son even though my son was always a bit reluctant to go to school and probably was a bit reserved while he was there. I had also had a number of very positive discussions and encounters with Christo, so I felt good about my son being in his class.

One day about three months into the year I brought my son to school and he refused to stay. He cried and cried saying he wouldn't stay. I started to panic as I had to get to work and it was getting later and later. Finally Christo came over and very warmly said, "Son, what's wrong?"

My son cried out, "I want to go home."

Christo thought a moment, then said, "Well, why don't we all walk to your house."

My son's face lit up. "Wow, you're all coming to my house?"

"Yes, he replied, "and I'm calling your mother right now."

That morning the whole class walked through the woods to our house, played games and had a snack in our garden. My son never has had trouble going to school again. (Well, he doesn't really like school now but that's different.) Later that week I asked Christo how he had come to this masterful solution since it was highly unusual and since he had never done such a thing before. He replied, "I knew you really trusted me to do the right thing, so I just felt your trust, stayed in the moment, and flash, it came to me—go to his house!"

This story contains a gold mine of information and perfectly describes the conditions necessary for healing. First there was rapport between the patient (in this case my son and me) and the healer (Christo). Then there was trust and then full disclosure. That is, the situation of my family was right out there, my son was hurting and

I didn't know what to do. Then came a moment of intuition and finally full resolution of the difficulty. When this happens between doctor and patient, true magic occurs but, alas, it is rare. Let us examine the components of this experience.

RAPPORT AND TRUST

You must feel some connection with your doctor—that is a given—a connection that will lead you, the patient, to trust his or her judgment and decisions. Here we walk a delicate line. Too little trust effectively cuts off inspiration and intuition from "higher sources." It sets up a conflict between doctor and patient and ultimately blocks many healing possibilities. Any sensitive doctor will sense a patient's lack of trust and will often (subconsciously) suggest a therapy to earn the patient's trust rather than to heal. However, too much trust can become blind faith leading to manipulation. The right amount of rapport and trust constitutes a fine line but when achieved, the result is most conducive to healing.

DISCLOSURE

The next step in the process is one of the most important and one I often find very frustrating—that is the need for full disclosure. As a doctor, I like it (that's an understatement!) when a patient comes to me and describes his or her situation very clearly and precisely. For example, "Dr. Cowan, I am here today because I have a funny feeling in my heart area. When I exert myself or even once when I sneezed my heart felt like it skipped a beat or started racing. When this happens I may feel dizzy." Then I can ask specific questions about other aspects of heart function, other types of symptoms, associations, causes, diet, exercise, emotions and so forth. In other words, the patient gives me a full and accurate report of his or her experience. That's what I want—the full description of the experience on all levels.

Contrast this with the following all-too-frequent encounter: I say, "Hello, what can I do for you today?"

The patient replies, "Dr. Cowan, I have a yeast problem. Do you have any medicine that will help this?"

I may ask, "Can you describe your symptoms (or experiences) that lead you to think you have a yeast problem?"

The patient replies, wary and frustrated, "Don't you know about yeast problems? I have all the usual symptoms and it has been going on for years and I need help."

This kind of introduction makes me feel as though I am being pushed into giving a treatment for yeast and not for a human being sitting in front of me asking for help.

INTUITION

This is the moment of magic, the moment when the doctor knows just what to do. But it cannot peek through if he lacks an accurate idea of the patient's situation. Intuition usually occurs as a result of meditation, and the patient's process of accurately describing his experience to a doctor is very similar to the process of meditation. The patient must know and describe his experience on multiple levels—physical, emotional and spiritual. In this way he objectifies his experience, looks at it, brings it up into the thinking realm and then, finally, offers it up to the physician so he can be guided and even healed.

If that exchange can come with a feeling of trust and rapport and a genuine willingness to make changes in your habits (food, exercise, inner work and so forth), then the results can be miraculous. This is a very different process from approaching a doctor with suspicion, presenting a diagnosis (I have yeast, cancer, heart disease, whatever), withholding the essential facts about your experience of life and then asking for a treatment. When this happens, I find that the patient usually rejects my advice because they think I am wrong or that what I said or suggested didn't make sense. Unfortunately, this model is the usual scenario in conventional medicine today—patient proclaims he has a disease—"I have prostate cancer"—doctor then removes the prostate. No magic, no healing, no intuition, nobody grows.

Many years of medical practice have taught me that I have no cures for any disease, and neither does any form of medicine. What I strive for is the ability to listen and unlock the wisdom and magic of each person's own inner healer. This means listening without interference, without judgment and without preconceptions. In other words, listening with love. I invite all to join me in this quest to remold the practice of medicine into an image of compassion, an image of true healing.

Appendices

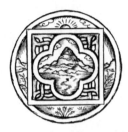

CHICKEN STOCK
Makes 4 quarts

1 whole free-range chicken or 2 to 3 pounds of bony chicken parts, such as necks, backs,
*   breastbones and wings or the carcass of a cooked chicken*
gizzards, feet and head from one chicken (optional)
4 quarts cold filtered water
2 tablespoons vinegar
1 large onion, coarsely chopped
2 carrots, peeled and coarsely chopped
3 celery sticks, coarsely chopped
1 bunch parsley

If you are using a whole chicken, cut off the wings and remove the neck, fat glands and the gizzards from the cavity. Place chicken or chicken pieces in a large stainless steel pot with water, vinegar and all vegetables except parsley. Let stand 30 minutes to 1 hour. Bring to a boil, and remove scum that rises to the top. Reduce heat, cover and simmer for 6 to 24 hours. The longer you cook the stock, the richer and more flavorful it will be. About 10 minutes before finishing the stock, add parsley.

Remove whole chicken or pieces with a slotted spoon. If you are using a whole chicken, let cool and remove chicken meat from the carcass. Reserve for other uses, such as chicken salads, enchiladas, sandwiches or curries. (The skin and smaller bones, which will be very soft, may be given to your dog or cat.) Strain the stock into a large bowl and reserve in your refrigerator until the fat rises to the top and congeals. Skim off this fat and reserve the stock in covered containers in your refrigerator or freezer. Use chicken stock for soups, sauces and gravies.

Note: you may also make this stock with turkey parts or a duck carcass.

BEEF STOCK
Makes about 4 quarts

about 4 pounds beef marrow and knuckle bones
1 calf's foot, cut into pieces (optional)
3 pounds meaty rib or neck bones
4 or more quarts cold filtered water
1/2 cup vinegar
3 onions, coarsely chopped
3 carrots, coarsely chopped
3 celery sticks, coarsely chopped
several sprigs of fresh thyme, tied together
1 teaspoon dried green peppercorns, crushed
l bunch parsley

Place the knuckle and marrow bones and optional calf's foot in a very large pot with vinegar and cover with water. Let stand for one hour. Meanwhile, place the meaty bones in a roasting pan and brown at 350 degrees in the oven. When well browned, add to the pot along with the vegetables. Pour the fat out of the roasting pan, add cold water to the pan, set over a high flame and bring to a boil, stirring with a wooden spoon to loosen up coagulated juices. Add this liquid to the pot. Add additional water, if necessary, to cover the bones; but the liquid should come no higher than within one inch of the rim of the pot, as the volume expands slightly during cooking. Bring to a boil. A large amount of scum will come to the top, and it is important to remove this with a spoon. After you have skimmed, reduce heat and add the thyme and crushed peppercorns.

Simmer stock for at least 12 and as long as 72 hours. Just before finishing, add the parsley and simmer another 10 minutes.

Remove bones with tongs or a slotted spoon. Strain the stock into a large bowl. Let cool in the refrigerator and remove the congealed fat that rises to the top. Transfer to smaller containers and to the freezer for long-term storage. Use beef stock for soups, sauces and gravies.

FISH STOCK
Makes about 3 quarts

3 or 4 whole carcasses, including heads, of non-oily fish such as sole, turbot,
    rockfish or snapper
2 tablespoons butter
2 onions, coarsely chopped
1 carrot, coarsely chopped
several sprigs fresh thyme
several sprigs parsley
1 bay leaf
1/2 cup dry white wine or vermouth
1/4 cup vinegar
about 3 quarts cold filtered water

Melt butter in a large stainless steel pot. Add the vegetables and cook very gently, about 1/2 hour, until they are soft. Add wine and bring to a boil. Add the fish carcasses and cover with cold, filtered water. Add vinegar. Bring to a boil and skim off the scum and impurities as they rise to the top. Tie herbs together and add to the pot. Reduce heat, cover and simmer for at least 4 hours or as long as 24 hours. Remove carcasses with tongs or a slotted spoon and strain the liquid into pint-sized storage containers for refrigerator or freezer. Chill well in the refrigerator and remove any congealed fat before transferring to the freezer for long-term storage. Use stock for fish soups, sauces and stews.

COCONUT SOUP
Serves 4

1 quart chicken or fish stock (page 349 or 351)
1 14-ounce can whole coconut milk
1/4 teaspoon dried chile flakes
1 teaspoon freshly grated ginger
juice of 1 lemon
sea salt
about 1 cup chicken (cooked or raw), fish or small shrimp
several green onions, very finely chopped (optional)
1 tablespoon finely chopped cilantro (optional)

Bring the stock to a boil, skim any foam that rises to the top and add coconut milk, lemon juice, chile flakes and ginger. Cut chicken or fish into small pieces. Add chicken, fish or shrimp to soup and simmer for about 15 minutes. Season to taste with sea salt. Ladle into soup bowls or mugs and garnish with optional onions and cilantro.

CREAM OF VEGETABLE SOUP
Serves 6-8

2 medium onions or leeks, peeled and chopped
2 carrots, peeled and chopped
4 tablespoons butter
3 medium baking potatoes or 6 red potatoes, washed and cut up
2 quarts chicken stock (page 349) or combination of filtered water and stock
several sprigs fresh thyme, tied together
1/2 teaspoon dried green peppercorns, crushed
4 zucchini, trimmed and sliced
sea salt and pepper
raw cream or cultured cream

Melt butter in a large, stainless steel pot and add onions or leeks and carrots. Cover and cook over lowest possible heat for at least 1/2 hour. The vegetables should soften but not burn. Add potatoes and stock, bring to a rapid boil and skim. Reduce heat and add thyme sprigs and crushed peppercorns. Cover and cook until the potatoes are soft. Add zucchini and cook until they are just tender—about 5 to 10 minutes. Remove the thyme sprigs. Purée the soup with a handheld blender.

If soup is too thick, thin with filtered water. Season to taste. Ladle into heated bowls and garnish with raw or cultured cream.

CRISPY NUTS
Makes 4 cups

4 cups raw nuts such as pecans, walnuts, cashews, macadamia nuts,
    skinless almonds or skinless peanuts, or a mixture
2 teaspoons sea salt
filtered water

Mix nuts with salt and filtered water and leave in a warm place for at about 7-8 hours. (Note: soak cashews for 6 hours only.) Drain in a colander. Spread nuts on a stainless steel baking pan and place in a warm oven (no more than 150 degrees) for 12 to 24 hours, turning occasionally, until completely dry and crisp. Store in an air-tight container at room temperature. (Note: walnuts should be stored in the refrigerator.)

BREAKFAST PORRIDGE
Serves 4

1 cup rolled oats
1 cup warm filtered water plus 2 tablespoons whey (page 354), yoghurt or kefir
1/2 teaspoon sea salt
1 cup filtered water
1 tablespoon flax seeds (optional)

Mix oats with warm water mixture, cover and leave overnight in a warm place. (Note: Those with severe milk allergies can use *lemon juice or vinegar* in place of whey, yoghurt or kefir.) Bring an additional 1 cup of water to a boil with sea salt. Add soaked oats, reduce heat, cover and simmer several minutes. Meanwhile, grind optional flax seeds in a mini grinder. Remove from heat, stir in optional flax seeds and let stand for a few minutes. Serve with plenty of butter or cream and a natural sweetener like Rapadura, date sugar, maple syrup, maple sugar or raw honey.

RAW MILK TONIC
Makes 2 cups

1 1/2 cups whole, certified clean raw milk, at room temperature
2 egg yolks, preferably from pastured chickens
1/4 cup molasses
1/2 teaspoon vanilla

Blend ingredients together with a whisk.

FRESH WHEY AND CREAM CHEESE
Makes 2 1/2 cups whey and 1 1/2 cups cream cheese

1 quart high-quality whole milk yoghurt or raw milk

If you are using raw milk, place the milk in a clean glass container and allow it to stand at room temperature 2-5 days until it separates. Line a large strainer set over a bowl with a clean dish towel. Pour in the yoghurt or separated milk, cover and let stand at room temperature for several hours (longer for yoghurt). The whey will run into the bowl and the milk solids will stay in the strainer. Tie up the towel with the milk solids inside, being careful not to squeeze. Tie this little sack to a wooden spoon placed across the top of a container so that more whey can drip out. When the bag stops dripping, the cheese is ready. Store whey in a mason jar and cream cheese in a covered glass container. Refrigerated, the cream cheese keeps for about 1 month and the whey for about 6 months.

CULTURED-MILK SMOOTHIE
Makes about 3 cups

1 1/4 cups wholemilk yoghurt or kefir
1 ripe banana or 1 cup berries (fresh or frozen)
2 tablespoons coconut oil
2 egg yolks
3-4 tablespoons maple syrup or raw honey or 1/4 teaspoon stevia powder
1 teaspoon vanilla extract (omit with berries)
pinch of nutmeg (omit with berries)

Place banana or berries in food processor or blender and process until smooth. Add remaining ingredients and process until well blended.

ICE CREAM
Makes 1 quart

6 egg yolks
1/2 - 3/4 cup Rapadura, Sucanat or maple sugar
1 tablespoon vanilla extract
3 cups heavy cream, preferably raw, not ultrapasteurized

Use an ice cream maker with a double-walled canister that is kept in the freezer. Beat egg yolks with sweetener for several minutes until pale and thick. Beat in vanilla extract and cream. Prepare in the ice cream maker, transfer to a shallow container and store in the freezer. About five minutes before serving, remove ice cream from the freezer and allow it to soften. Note: you may add 1 cup fruit puree and reduce the cream by 1 cup, omitting vanilla.

SAUERKRAUT
Makes 1 quart

1 medium cabbage, cored and shredded
1 tablespoon caraway seeds
1 tablespoon sea salt
4 tablespoons whey (page 354) (if not available, use an additional 1 tablespoon salt)

In a bowl, mix cabbage with caraway seeds, sea salt and whey. Pound with a wooden pounder or a meat hammer for about 10 minutes to release juices. Place in a quart-sized, wide-mouth mason jar and press down firmly with a pounder or meat hammer until juices come to the top of the cabbage. The top of the cabbage should be at least 1 inch below the top of the jar. Cover tightly and keep at room temperature for about 3 days before transferring to cold storage. The sauerkraut may be eaten immediately, but it improves with age.

GINGER ALE
Makes 2 quarts

3/4 cup ginger, peeled and finely chopped or grated
1/2 cup fresh lime juice
1/4-1/2 cup Rapadura, Sucanat or maple sugar
2 teaspoons sea salt
1/4 cup whey (page 354)
2 quarts filtered water

Place all ingredients in a 2-quart jug. Stir well and cover tightly. Leave at room temperature for 2-3 days before transferring to the refrigerator. This will keep several months well chilled. To serve, strain into a glass. Ginger ale may be mixed with carbonated water and is best sipped warm rather than gulped down cold.

KOMBUCHA
Makes 1 gallon

3 quarts filtered water
1 cup white sugar
1 tablespoon sea salt (optional)
4 tea bags of organic black tea
1/2 cup kombucha from a previous culture
1 kombucha mushroom (see Sources)

Bring 3 quarts filtered water to boil. Add sugar and optional salt and simmer until dissolved. Remove from heat, add the tea bags and allow the tea to steep until water has completely cooled. Remove tea bags. Pour cooled liquid into a 4-quart pyrex bowl and add 1/2 cup kombucha from previous batch. Place the mushroom on top of the liquid. Make a crisscross over the bowl with masking tape, cover loosely with a cloth or towel and transfer to a warm, dark place, away from contaminants and insects. In about 7 to 10 days the kombucha will be ready, depending on the temperature. It should be rather sour and possibly fizzy, with no taste of tea remaining. Transfer to covered glass containers and store in the refrigerator. (Note: Do not wash kombucha bowls in the dishwasher.)

When the kombucha is ready, your mushroom will have grown a second spongy pancake. This can be used to make other batches or given away to friends. Store fresh mushrooms in the refrigerator in a glass or stainless steel container—never plastic. A kombucha mushroom can be used dozens of times. If it begins to turn black, or if the resulting kombucha doesn't sour properly, it's a sign that the culture has become contaminated. When this happens, it's best to throw away all your mushrooms and order a new clean one.

Note: White sugar, rather than an unrefined sweetener, and black tea, rather than flavored teas, give the highest amounts of glucuronic acid. Non-organic tea is high in fluoride so always use organic tea.

A word of caution: Some individuals may have an allergic reaction to kombucha. If you have allergies, start with a small taste to observe any adverse effects. If you react badly, use beet kvass (page 357) several weeks to detoxify and then try again.

HAYMAKERS' OAT WATER
Makes 1 gallon

1 gallon filtered water
1 cup rolled oats
1 cup lemon juice or raw apple cider vinegar
1 cup molasses

Mix all ingredients and keep at room temperature several hours or overnight, stirring occasionally.

BEET KVASS
Makes 2 quarts

3 medium or 2 large organic beets, peeled and chopped up coarsely
1/4 cup whey (page 354)
1 tablespoon sea salt
filtered water

Beet kvass is an invaluable lacto-fermented tonic. It promotes regularity, aids digestion, alkalizes the blood, cleanses the liver and is a good treatment for kidney stones.

Place beets, whey and salt in a 2-quart glass container. Add filtered water to fill the container. Stir well and cover securely. Keep at room temperature for 2 days before transferring to refrigerator.

When most of liquid has been drunk, you may fill up the container with water and keep at room temperature another 2 days. The resulting brew will be slightly less strong than the first. After the second brew, discard the beets and start again. You may, however, reserve some of the liquid and use this as your inoculant instead of the whey.

Note: Do not use grated beets in the preparation of beet tonic. When grated, beets exude too much juice resulting in a too rapid fermentation that favors the production of alcohol rather than lactic acid.

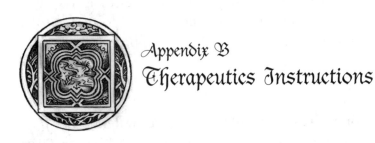

Appendix B
Therapeutics Instructions

BEE VENOM THERAPY

This therapy for osteoarthritis requires either live bees obtained from a local bee-keeper, which is the best, or injectable bee venom, obtainable through various suppliers. I will only describe the use of live bees, as this is more applicable to the home user. You will need bees in a jar, a pair of long tweezers, ice and an epinephrine kit, in case of an allergic reaction (don't use bee venom therapy if you are allergic to bees). Ice down the area of pain for a few minutes until it is numb. Using the tweezers, grab the bee around its midsection and place its hind-end on the numb area. It will immediately sting. Leave the stinger in about 1-2 minutes, then remove it carefully with the tweezers. I recommending applying bees to only one or two of the most painful areas per session but you can also do up to 20 stings in a session. A recommended treatment schedule is 1-3 sessions per week usually for 6-8 weeks, at which time there should be a significant improvement in symptoms.

BLESSED HERB INTERNAL CLEANSE PROGRAM

Through your health care practitioner obtain a copy of the cleanse brochure which explains the herbs and related procedures in excellent detail. The cleanse involves four steps, starting with herbs for the digestive tract. The second step cleanses the liver and gall bladder and helps remove parasites. The third step cleanses the lungs, kidneys and bladder. In the final step, herbs are taken to cleanse the lymph, blood and skin. You may eat normally during this period. All of the herbs in this program are organically grown or wildcrafted and are extracted using the most modern and effective concentration methods. At the end of the three weeks, most people notice a significant change in their health and in their ability to heal from their chronic illnesses.

BOWEL CLEANSING
The simplest method for bowel cleansing, especially for febrile illnesses, is to give 1-4 tablespoons of milk of magnesia before bedtime, 1 tablespoon for a child, 4 for a grown man. The other alternative is to give a full Dulcolax suppository at least 2 hours before bedtime.

CASTOR OIL PACKS
You will need good quality castor oil, a heavy wool flannel, a hot water bottle and a plastic sheet. Soak the flannel with the oil until it is saturated but not dripping. Place over the affected organ, cover with a thin towel, then the plastic and then the hot water bottle. Leave in place at least 40 minutes, lying quietly during this time. Remove the flannel and wash the area with diluted baking soda. You may store the flannel in a plastic bag for re-use. A recommended treatment schedule is 1-3 times per week until improvement is seen. Note: I recommend warm castor oil packs for the torso and abdomen or limbs, but when used on the head, omit use of the hot water bottle as the pack should be cool.

COD LIVER OIL AND HIGH-VITAMIN BUTTER OIL THERAPY
This therapy was developed by Dr. Weston Price. He used it to reverse tooth decay, to treat bone and growth problems and also to bring about rapid healing during bouts of acute illness. Both products are available from Radiant Life. For acute illness or a crisis situation, place alternating drops of cod liver oil and high-vitamin butter oil (also called X-factor oil) under the tongue for several minutes. For chronic illness you may take the two oils together, mixed with a little water, in the morning. Stir vigorously and swallow quickly. Use enough cod liver oil to provide the dose of vitamin A required (usually 10,000- 20,000 IU) plus 1/2 to 1 teaspoon high-vitamin butter oil. It is much better to take cod liver oil this way, rather than use capsules, which often cause indigestion.

EPSOM SALTS BATH
Add 1 cup Epsom salts to a warm bath. Sit in the bath for twenty minutes, dry off and get into a warm bed. Drink plenty of warm tea in bed, especially elder flower, linden flower, or peppermint tea to promote diaphoresis (intense sweating).

HYDROTHERAPY
This therapy will stimulate a fever in indulant colds and infections. Take a warm bath for 10-15 minutes, then stand under a cold shower for exactly one minute. Then quickly wrap up in a warm blanket and immediately get into a warm bed. As for Epsom salts baths, the same requirement for warm teas applies.

PINEAPPLE FAST

The pineapple fast can have an immediate beneficial effect on someone with recalci-trant back pain. Obtain organically grown pineapples, and make enough juice to last for one day (it takes about 2-3 pineapples per day). For three days eat nothing but the pineapple juice, plain water and an occasional herb tea with raw honey if you are feeling weak. Continue for no more than 3 days.

SITZ BATH THERAPY

Sitz bath treatment was widely used in former times as part of natural therapy for cancer and other diseases. The therapy requires two tubs (one can be a bath tub). Fill the bathtub with hot water and the smaller tub with cold water. (The cold bath should only cover the pelvic region.) Soak for about ten minutes in the hot bath, and then sit one minute in the cold, followed by one minute in the hot, and finally one minute in the cold bath. After this, wrap up warmly and get right into bed with a hot water bottle over the lower abdomen. These baths produce a dramatic warmth reaction in the area of the body that needs it most.

SALIVARY PH

Test the pH of the saliva using pH strips (see Sources). Place a strip under the tongue in the morning before eating and around 8 PM for a week straight. Record all mea-surements. Consistent readings of 6.8-7.0 indicate good mineral status and good general health. Readings below 6.6 indicate incipient or chronic health problems. Cancer patients generally have salivary pH levels in the range of 5.8.

VITAMIN D THERAPY

I usually test the 25(OH)D level about every 6-8 weeks until the value is consistently between 40-60. To supplement I often use the Carlson's 1000 IU vitamin D capsules increasing in 1000-unit increments until the therapeutic range is obtained. For those eating liberally of all the healthy, grass-fed animal fats described in this book, and taking cod liver oil and high-vitamin butter oil, additional supplementation with vi-tamin D is usually not necessary.

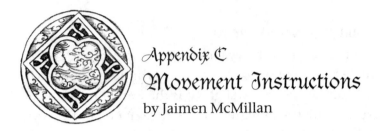

Appendix C
Movement Instructions
by Jaimen McMillan

The Spacial Dynamics exercises described in this section have been practiced by tens of thousands of people all over the world. Built on objective principles, the exercises have been successfully applied by people from diverse cultural backgrounds and every personality and body type under the sun.

Practiced in the manner suggested, these exercises are designed to help you to:

1. Move in an economical manner using the laws known to physics, engineering, and biomechanics to maximize your mechanical advantage, thus benefiting the Physical Body.
2. Increase your sense of well-being, thus supporting the Life-Force Body.
3. Move in a proportioned, balanced, and harmonious way that is beautiful, thus helping to heal the Emotional Body.
4. Enhance your consciousness, attention, and awareness, thus strengthening the Mental Body.
5. Integrate the Physical, Life-Force, Emotional and Mental Bodies into a dynamic relationship that contributes to health, wholeness and vitality through movement.

By practicing movement that provides wholeness to the Emotional Body, an individual will progress from a condition in which he is a pawn of fate, to one in which he is an architect of his relationships, goals and health.

Many of the conditions and illnesses described in these pages are serious and require proper medical attention. The Spacial Dynamics approach is not meant to replace but to augment any medical treatment that a patient may choose.

In addition to suggested movements for specific diseases, a program for maintaining wellness is provided on page 422.

Primary and Secondary Movement

BREATHING EXERCISE

Imagine you are sitting on the beach at the water's edge, looking out to the sea, with the waves rolling in. Exhale as a wave surrounds your legs and hips with swirling white foam flowing behind you. Pause ever so slightly as the water lingers, before it begins its return journey. Now create the dynamic of the forceful pull of the water back to the sea. Let your abdomen be drawn out with the departing wave, your lungs will fill with air as your belly silently widens with the swelling of the ocean. Pause as the next wave hovers, then exhale like a sigh as the new wave breaks at your feet yet again. You have joined in the cyclic drama of the rhythms of life.

Thus, there are four steps or phases to breathing. There are two still moments, the pauses between inhalation and exhalation, and there are two active moments, the in-breath and the out-breath. As breathing has four stages, so does the wave: the incoming breaking of the wave, the transitional period as the wave dissipates, the drawing back of the wave and the building of the wave again. We often think of a wave as having only two phases, but the in-between spaces in breathing and the ocean waves, although less noticeable, are what provide the rhythm. It is in these transitional, quiet spaces that the Emotional Body is enlivened. A day that has us panting to make it from one moment to the next stifles both the Physical Body and the Emotional Body.

Normally we conceive of the in-breath as being the active component and the exhaling the passive, but in this dynamic, the out-breath is active while the in-breath is the action that follows your relaxation. Your breathing then creates a countermotion to the waves of the sea—when the water goes out you inhale, and when the sea waves come in, you exhale.

Now do the exercise again, paying attention to the motions of your body. Did you feel your chest or shoulders rise up with the in-breath? If the answer is yes, your motions are actually counterproductive to breathing with maximum efficiency and ease. The shoulders and upper chest should remain where they are and the lower ribs, abdomen, and lower back should expand three-dimensionally. As you breathe in, the abdomen should expand because it is creating space for the air—just as the wave expands to become the sea again. Then when you exhale, the abdomen should contract and empty just as the ocean pours its water on the shore. Through this rhythmical breathing we can experience a release of unnecessary tensions and surges of renewed energy.

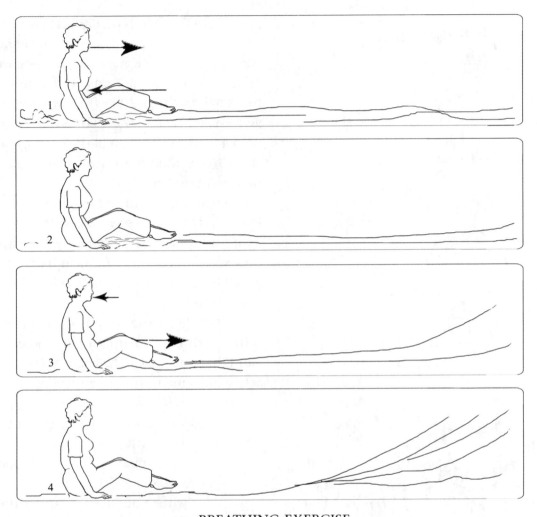

BREATHING EXERCISE

Imagine you are sitting on a beach and an ocean wave breaks and swirls in around you.

1. At this moment, allow the abdomen to draw in as the air exits.
2. As the water comes to a stop and prepares to change direction, gently pause in a moment of stillness and silence.
3. Then as the water moves out to sea and gathers into a new wave, inhale silently, allowing the air to fill the abdomen.
4. As the wave swells and prepares to come towards the shore again, enjoy another moment of stillness and silence.

This exercise has a calming effect on the Emotional Body and establishes a relationship between the inside and outside spaces. This is a fundamental exercise for any condition or disease, as breathing is the basic rhythm of life.

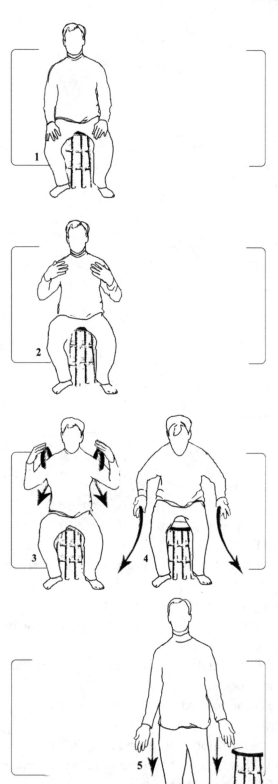

DOWNRIGHT-UPRIGHT

The simple acts of sitting down and standing up become graceful and when we add the opposite actions, the counter movements. In the Downright-Upright gestures, we balance the act of sitting down with an upward motion of the hands, and the act of standing up with a downward motion of the hands.

In sitting, the force of gravity on the lower body is balanced by a gesture of levity in the upper body; and in standing up, the expression of levity in the upper body is balanced by the force of gravity in the lower body.

Your "downright" position can be achieved through an upward lift and your "upright" posture can be achieved by the active movement of a downward pull.

To go from "downright" to "upright":
1. Sit on the front edge of your chair, your feet flat on the floor, shoulder width apart.
2. Bring your hands up to the shoulder area circling slowly behind and around your shoulders into a…
3-4. Large movement of the hands downward, performed simultaneously with the act of pushing down with the soles of your feet.
5. End with your hands down and your body upright. The body becomes "upright" as a countermotion to "standing down."

To go from "upright" to "downright":

1. Stand comfortably with your hands at your sides.
2. Your hands begin a small gesture behind your body.
3. Then swing your hands and arms forward and up in a large gesture while the hips pull the trunk down.
4. The hands are up—you have glided from the upright position to a sitting position. The upward movement of the hands and arms acts as a countermotion to the torso moving down. Your hands have reached their highest position at the moment that your weight is firmly on the stool.

These gestures help your Emotional Body experience the feeling of "getting back on your feet again." The exercise is helpful for arthritis (helping carry a person gracefully through a movement that is often painful); weight loss (as it helps a heavy person experience a feeling of lightness); osteoporosis (to practice the bone-building process of resistance); hypertension (as it creates a feeling of downward relief); problems of estrogen dominance (as it creates a grounding effect); and, especially, depression. Depression manifests as a gesture that is downward oriented. Practicing the dynamic of the opposite movement stimulates a dynamic balance that can be carried into all walks of life. Downright-upright helps the Emotional Body experience the sensation of "not having to give in to whatever may be going on."

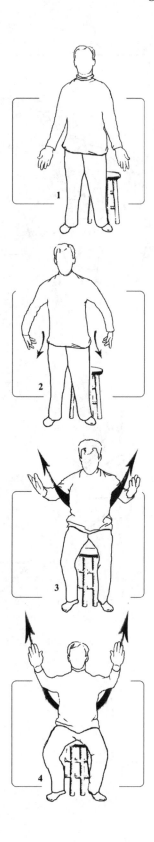

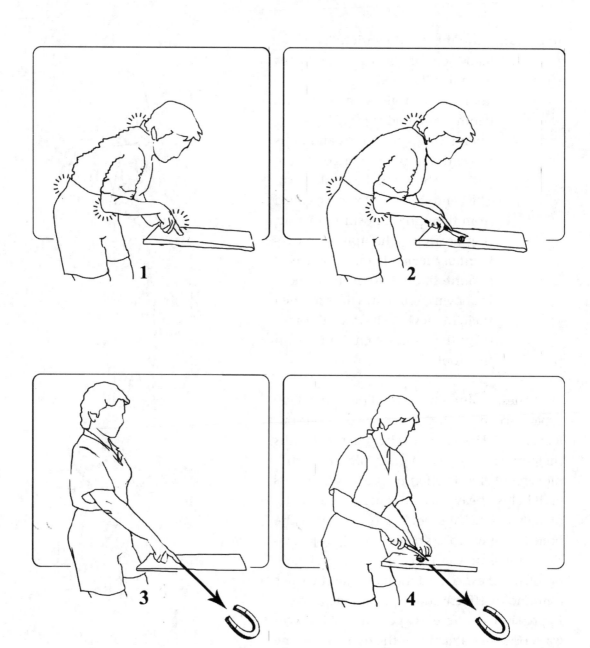

THE MAGNET

In practicing the Magnet, the Emotional Body experiences a response to a peripheral stimulus, independent of one's emotional state. It is particularly beneficial for neurological diseases because the body experiences the origin of a movement, not in the nerve but from an outside stimulus. The movement is a release rather than an effort.

1. Press your finger into the board with a constricted, pushing motion.
2. Place vegetables on a board and cut or chop them with a tense, pushing motion.
3. Then, visualize a magnet pulling your finger, noting the relaxation of tension in the shoulders, arms, back and neck.
4. Now, imagine a magnet underneath the board pulling the knife across the space between you and the vegetables, allowing the cutting to proceed with ease.

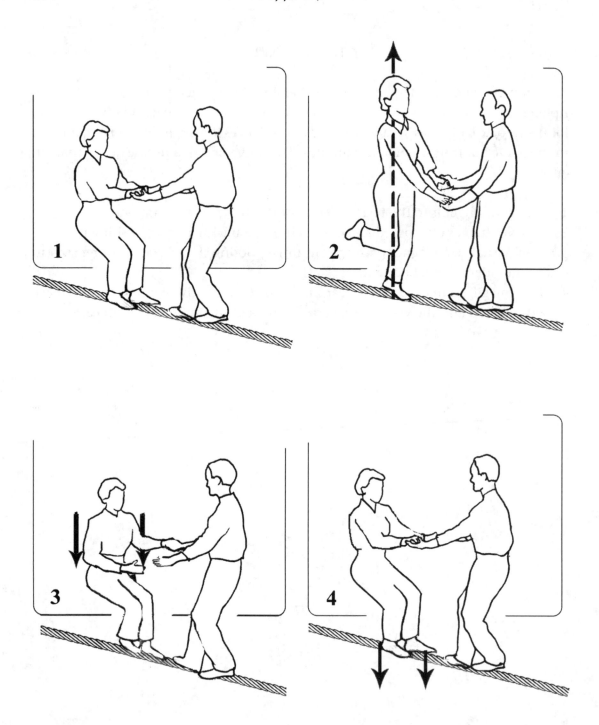

GROUNDING

The Grounding Exercise provides the Emotional Body with a sense of settling down, adding stability and strength in the growing connection with the earth. It is good for problems of estrogen dominance, hypertension, and cancer, as well as against timidity and losing your temper.

1. Place your feet one behind the other, as on a tight rope, and join hands with a partner. Create the spacial dynamic of mercury rising in a thermometer within your body as your partner and you slowly pull harder and harder.
2. As much as you try to stay on the tightrope, you will find your partner will easily pull you off balance when your mercury is rising. This movement is analogous to "being up-tight," "blowing your top," or "flying off the handle."
3. Then, begin again as in Figure 1. Release one hand and slowly move this hand in a downwards motion to indicate the spacial dynamic of the mercury sinking in the thermometer down through your feet and into the earth.
4. Join hands again. The partner will feel your strength increase as your mercury sinks. You will feel a quiet, "rooted" stability.

This is not "magic." Your body has taken the position of maximum mechanical advantage (best relationship to gravity, best angle of your joints, most advantageous muscle tension, etc.), all by adjusting the downward relationship of your space to gravity.

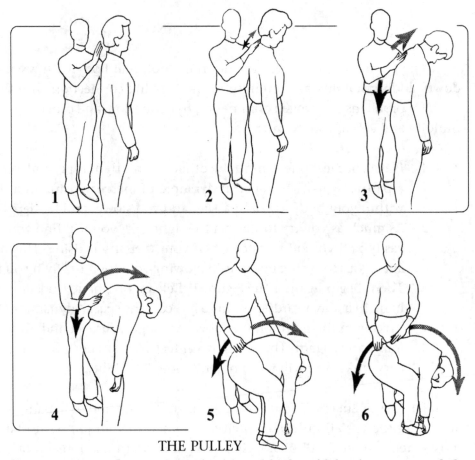

THE PULLEY

The Pulley juxtaposes the two basic building blocks of life, the curve and the straight line, as the body interacts rhythmically with the pull of gravity and the invitation of levity in balanced posture. You can do this exercise on your own, but it can be helpful to have a friend give you assistance in the beginning. The light touch of a friend moving his hand successively down the spine gives orientation from which you can relax as your head goes down. The friend now reverses this process and moves his hand from the sacrum slowly up. This time he pulls down on each successive vertebra like a pulley; and each vertebra comes into the column one by one.

In the Emotional Body, the rounded gesture at the moment of greatest release gives an experience of being protected and safe. The moment of reaching the upright lets you fully experience the feeling of having your feet on the ground, ready to face the world. In the Physical Body, this exercise creates increased circulation to the head, brain, and sinus cavities, and stimulates an increase of fluid in the discs between the vertebrae. The result is improved flexibility of the spine and improved blood supply to the entire body. The Pulley is suggested to prevent neurological diseases, and for hypertension, adrenal disorders (especially asthma) and chronic fatigue.

1. For Stage I, begin in a standing position
2. Create space between the first and second vertebrae.
3. Allow the head to become heavy and tilt downwards, much like the initial phase of dozing off during a lecture.
4-6. Repeat the release between the second and third and each following pair of vertebrae all the way down to the sacrum while relaxing the knees. The head changes from its vertical position to a hanging position through relaxing the small muscles between the respect segments of your spine.
7. For Stage II, begin by exerting downward pressure along the sacrum (analogous to tugging on the pulley rope).
8-10. The spine will begin to slowly unfurl, vertebra by vertebra, and approach a balanced upright carriage (8, 9, 10).
11. Keep the head relaxed and heavy until the very end. Resist the temptation to lift your head upwards in the accustomed manner.
12. Let the head, slowly take its position as a secondary movement, the result of the downward pulley effect of the shortening of the back muscles.

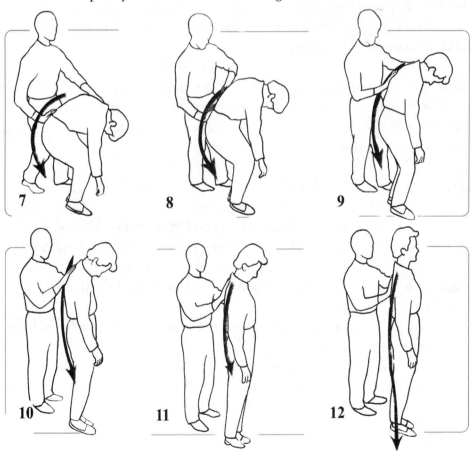

CARRIAGE DOWN/CARRIAGE UP

Proper posture also strikes a balance between gravity and levity. For the Emotional Body, the two wave-like gestures convey the feeling of life as a process. Attention to the carriage in this way can be helpful for all health conditions, but it is particularly useful for back pain; cancer (especially the Carriage Up gesture, which relieves the hardening process so characteristic of the cancer patient); hypertension (especially the calming Carriage Down gesture), adrenal problems; digestive disorders (especially the Carriage Up); men's diseases, rheumatoid arthritis and chronic fatigue.

The Carriage Gesture Down gives the spacial dynamic that aligns the head, neck, and shoulder girdle with the entire body. It eases headache, relieves tension in the neck and mitigates shoulder pain by integrating the arm into the large muscles of the rib cage.

1. Stand in an exaggerated bent-forward posture.
2. Imagine a spacial dynamic that begins in the front of the shoulder area, rises lightly and falls down around the shoulder blades and lower ribs.
3. Follow this movement from around the back, along the paths of the lowest ribs, continuing on forward and down.

The Carriage Up gesture gives the spacial dynamic that aligns the pelvic area with the rest of the body. It is a quickening gesture which awakens sluggish metabolism, enlivens forces of regeneration and reproduction, and alleviates lower back pain that comes from compression of the lower vertebrae.

1. Stand with the upper body slumped back and the abdomen thrust forward.
2. Follow a movement that begins on the ground in front of you. Let it rise up as a powerful wave, breaking behind the buttocks and lower back, slowing as it curves forward under the shoulder blades, continuing forward in front of the chest. The movement does not end, but rather it continues as if transformed into a fine mist. Care should be taken that the space around the head is not influenced by the rising wave.
3. The challenge is to experience the entire form and entire dynamics of both of these curves simultaneously:
   a. Each moment of a given curve.
   b. Both curves at the same time.

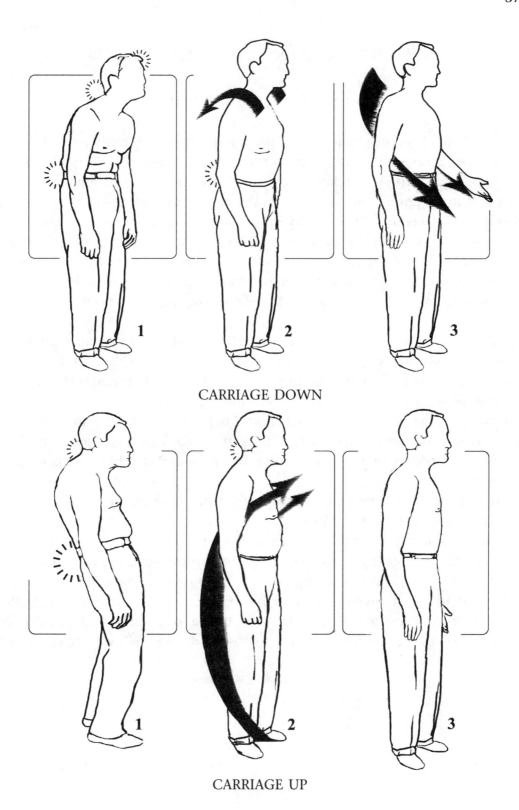

CARRIAGE DOWN

CARRIAGE UP

Learning to Live in Different Spaces

BODY SPACE IMAGINATION

The Body Space Imagination helps the Emotional Body by relieving unconscious gestures of tension and unnecessary control. It allows the sexual organs and the organs of reproduction to follow their natural rhythms, releasing any unnecessary control (constriction), while also clearing the head. This exercise lets every organ in every part of the body follow the rhythms of nature and gently releases them from the iron-clad grasp of intellectual tyranny. It is useful for women's and men's diseases (as it clears a space in the abdomen, releasing gestures of fear and frustration, digestive disorders (allowing for undisturbed peristaltic movement), and weight loss. (The relaxation following this exercise is as if you had just had a fine dinner.)

1. Sit in a comfortable position in a location that will give you a minimal number of distractions (phone off, radio off, television off, computer off) and close your eyes.
2. Now begin with the space within your head. Clear it. Experience it as a three-dimensional chamber like a crystal-clear lake within a cave.
3. Flow down the inside of the neck like a tributary undisturbed by any tensions or blockages. This streaming goes right under the collarbone and shoulder blades.
4. Fill the chest cavity with space that allows for rhythmical breathing that laps against the ribs.
5. The lower torso and reproductive organs allow the gentle tidal tugging of the moon downward from the other side of the earth.
6. Create a hollow space in the bones of your arms and legs.
7. Let the space beneath your limbs draw all the tension and knots from your shoulders, upper arms, hands, and fingers.
8. Now live in these different spaces you have created within your body, singly, then one after another; and then all at the same time as one vessel. With practice, you will be able to recreate and visit these spaces at will, even in the midst of everyday life.

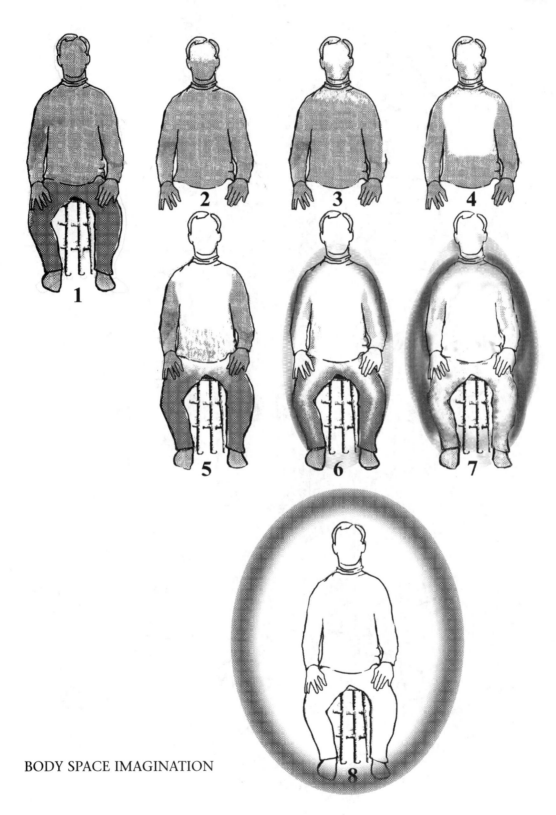

BODY SPACE IMAGINATION

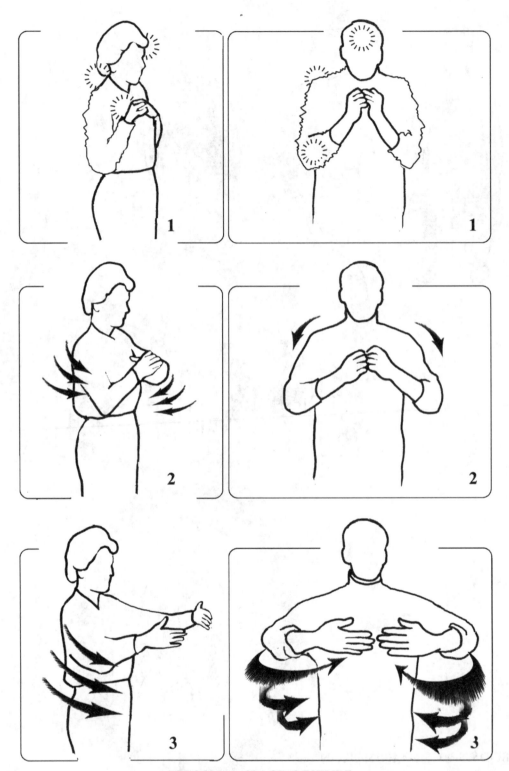

PERSONAL SPACE GESTURE

PERSONAL SPACE GESTURE

The Personal Space Gesture is a prerequisite for helping the Emotional Body define and enlarge the area we call our own. This new personal space allows you to meet what is coming to you from the outside world with confidence and grace. It is an excellent exercise for cancer, depression, problems of progesterone dominance, diabetes, weight loss and neurological problems.

1. Start with a tense and constricted gesture, hands to the chest, head tucked down and shoulders tense—the gesture of a fearful person with a very small personal space.
2. Then slowly relax the shoulders, arms and head, bringing the arms and hands down to describe a space swelling beneath them.
3. Use your arms and hands to define a new personal space about two feet in front of you, as though your arms are surrounding a large column. Imagine your ribs expanding to encircle this new space, as shown in Figure 3, a gesture of embracing.

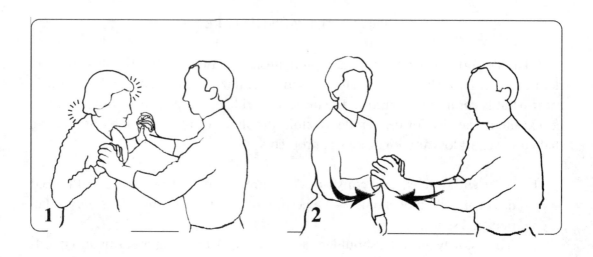

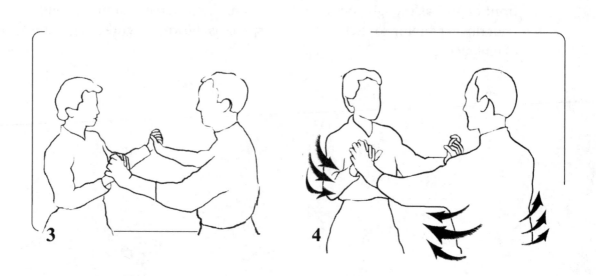

WRESTLING STANCE

WRESTLING STANCE

The Wrestling Stance helps us to define that personal space necessary for "two to know one." It strengthens the Emotional Body by preventing the invasion of the personal space, and helps you to meet what comes to you at the borders of your personal space. It is helpful for cancer (the Life-Force Body is given space to hover, not crowd), diabetes (the balance of the outer and the inner), weight loss (the body image is experienced as including the personal space and the full feeling is no longer dependent on large amounts of food), depression (the world is held at bay and gives you a fighting chance) and heart disease (especially for men as it helps counteract the feeling of "squeezing the heart," or for women of taking everything "to heart").

1. Two people lock hands. Here the man pushes forward to challenge his partner's ability to maintain personal space under pressure. If the one defending her personal space meets the "invasion" directly, with forward pressure, the "aggressor" easily comes into her personal space. The result is tension and strain.
2. Now round your arms to create a ring or circle between you and your partner.
3. Repeat the exercise, this time defining your personal space with your rounded arms.
4. You can now meet the other on equal terms, preventing invasion of your space.

Now repeat the exercise with the partners changing roles.

Then do the exercise again, this time as each partner simultaneously attempts to help the partner learn to maintain the personal space under pressure.

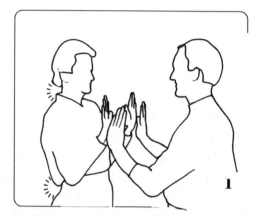

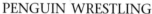

PENGUIN WRESTLING

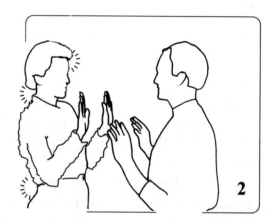

Penguin Wrestling helps the Emotional Body maintain its space under attack, with balance and ease. It is so named because of the humorous, balance-challenging Penguin-like position of the "wrestlers," feet together at an arm's length from each other. In this exercise one learns to deflect negative gestures, verbal attacks and unfortunate situations, without taking them personally.

The participant can either clap his partner's hands or remove his own hands quickly at any time. Besides helping those who are withdrawn to stand on their own two feet, it is an effective exercise for taming the "bull in a china shop." It creates the ability to "stand your own ground." Penguin Wrestling is excellent for cancer, heart disease, weight loss, depression and anxiety.

1. In Phase I, the woman demonstrates a practiced contracted personal space.
2. Even the thought of the challenge from the other brings on instability and fright.
3. They interact by clapping each other's palms with moderate force. The woman loses her balance and her "Penguin" feet retreat.
4. The challenge from the partner is experienced as a personal affront.

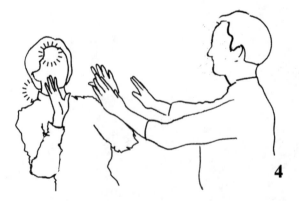

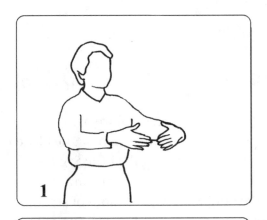

In Phase II, we do the exercise with an expanded personal space.

1. The participant first defines her space.
2. The participants interact again by clapping the palms.
3. This time she deflects the oncoming force like the prow of a ship that parts the water.
4. She no longer feels "invaded" or "injured." She meets the force objectively at the border of her personal space. She realizes that she can determine to what extent she takes things personally.

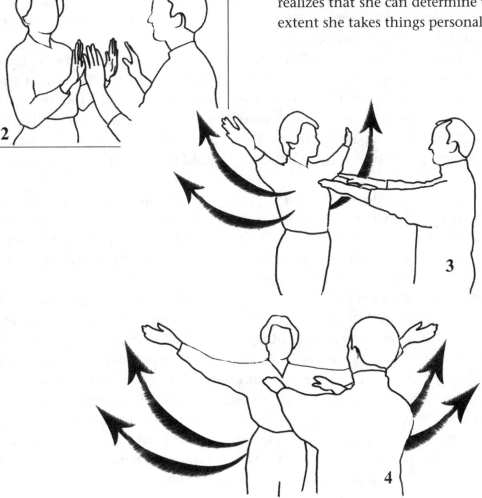

Qualities of Space

THE THREE PLANES

When we move, we actually sculpt all our bodies. The tool we use is space. The Physical Body is three-dimensional and can be divided by three planes. The plane that divides the body vertically into two symmetrical halves is called the Sagittal or **Symmetry Plane**. This plane gives the basis for concentration, focus and clarity, indeed it could be called the Judgment Plane. Here one weighs both sides of an argument before coming to a middle ground. When a judge signifies her decision with a tap of a hammer, or a king announces his decree with the downward motion of his sword, they are making a gesture that defines the Symmetry or Judgment Plane. When the communication between left and right sides of the body is poor, we can't "keep it together;" we are "beside ourselves."

The vertical plane that runs down the sides of our bodies, dividing the front from the back, is called the **Frontal Plane**. This plane divides the past—what you have put behind you—from the future which lies ahead of you. When we see a person who is stoop-shouldered or bends forward when he walks, we perceive that he has had a difficult life; his past weighs him down. The ideal carriage is perfect integration of memory (past) and anticipation (future), poised with balanced bearing in the present.

The transverse or **Horizontal Plane** has to do with our feeling life. The Horizontal Plane is very changeable and our feelings will vary according to where this plane ends up. For example, we speak of being "up," "high," "elated" or "on cloud nine." Rock musicians "get down," ballet dancers "go on point," and waltzers "meet in the middle." Similarly, we describe other emotions as being "down in the dumps" or "depressed" because we experience our emotions in relation to the Horizontal Plane. The horizontal position, such as swimming, lying on a beach, or even experiencing strong feelings of anger or aggression, can be conducive to a dreamlike quality.

The Symmetry and Frontal Planes are fixed. They are at ninety degrees to each other. The Horizontal Plane is moveable. The intersection of these three planes gives a single point, a focus of energy, awareness and possibility. Each activity we do requires a particular center. With practice you can learn to move and choose the relationship of these three planes according to the demands of what you are doing, and how the Emotional Body can best support that relationship. All three planes meeting in the heart area, for example, elicits feelings of interest, warmth and compassion.

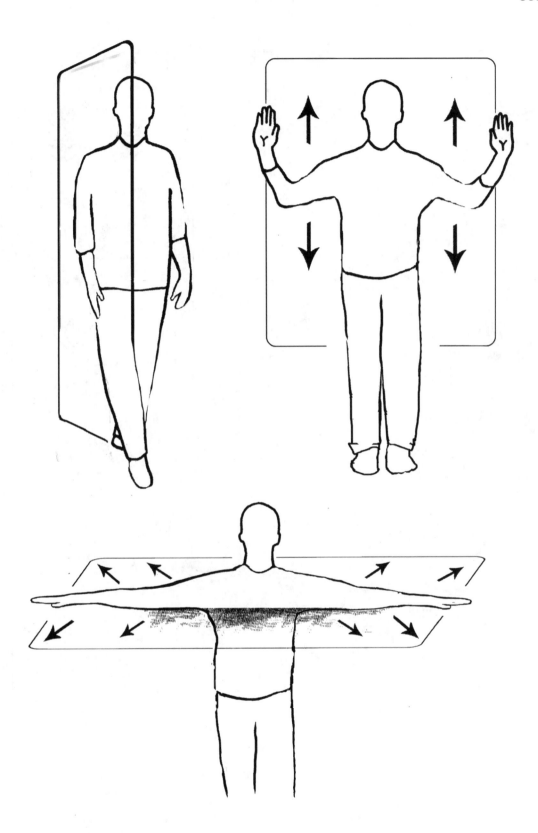

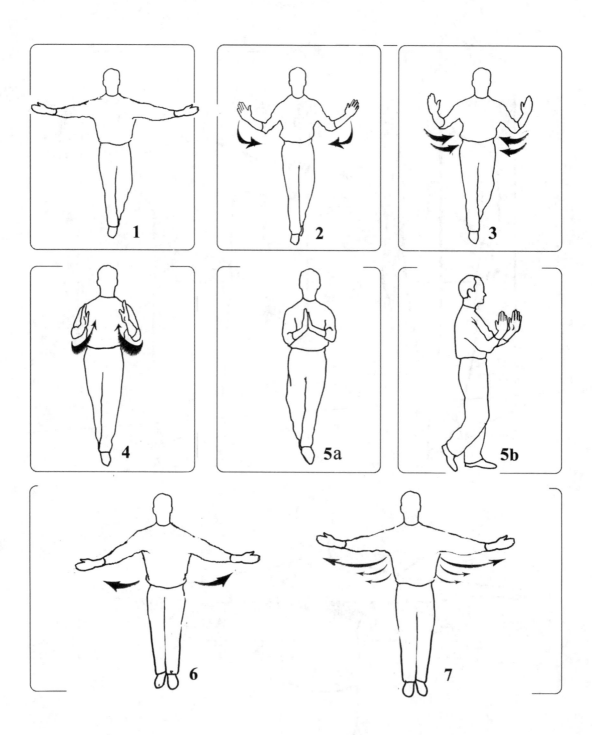

THE TIDES

The Tides helps us experience the clarity and exactness of the Symmetry Plane and the infinite expanse on either side of the arms at the same time. It helps slow the heart rate and the breath. For the Emotional Body, the exercise provides the juxtaposition of decisiveness and openness. This is an excellent morning exercise that will enhance attentiveness when concentration wavers.

Because of its quiet composure, the Tides is an effective gesture for infectious disorders, especially when inflammation and fever are out of control. Because of the rhythmical interplay between focused attention, release and opening wide, it is also useful for neurological disorders, problems of estrogen dominance, osteoporosis, back pain and rheumatoid arthritis.

Begin with your weight on the left foot and your arms hanging at your sides.

1. As you extend your right foot, reach out both arms.
2-4. Slowly bring both hands simultaneously towards an invisible midline.
5. At the moment when your weight is totally on the front foot, your hands arrive at the midline and are placed a hair's breadth apart on either side of the imagined midline (which defines the plane of symmetry), the left hand above the right.
6-7. As the hands release and wilt, the hands and arms are given weight and fall towards the ground; they then swing out, the arms extended and parallel to the ground.

Continue by extending the left foot forward. Both hands again move towards the midline as weight is slowly transferred to the left foot. At the moment when the hands are in the plane, the weight transfer is complete.

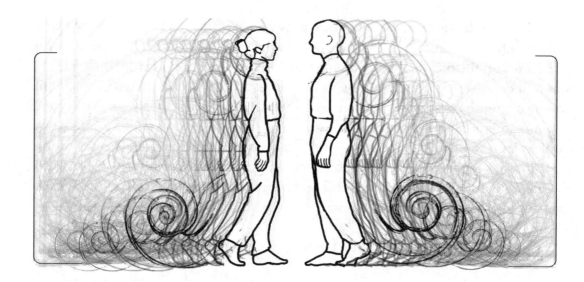

AUTUMN LEAVES

This exercise awakens both sides of the Frontal Plane. You can do it while walking anywhere. Imagine yourself strolling serenely down a path in the woods. A light wind is blowing towards you, and leaves are picked up and whirled behind you, spiraling around your feet.

In this exercise your Emotional Body practices "facing up to" what is coming towards you with equanimity. Autumn Leaves is useful for many diseases including adrenal disorders, chronic fatigue, depression, heart disease, and women's diseases (especially shortened cycle and cramping), particularly because you can practice playfully dissipating what you have put behind you.

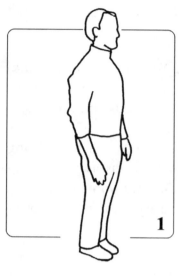
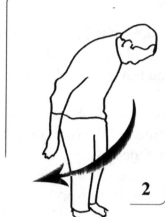
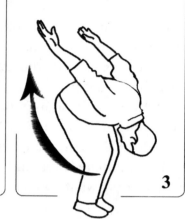

THE CREST

This exercise brings a rhythmical movement into play that alternates between hovering and falling in front of and behind the frontal plane. Through it the Emotional Body swings through the sensation of rounded heaviness and extension in lightness. It is thus good for back pain, adrenal problems, digestive disorders, diabetes, osteoporosis, neurological problems and weight loss (as the body feels the difference between weightless hovering and full heaviness).

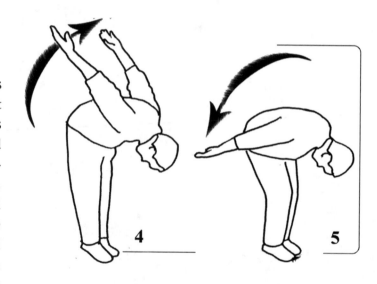

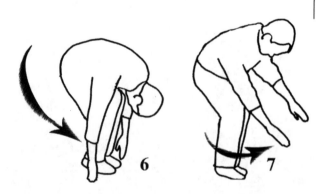

In this exercise, the arms describe the full 360 degrees of a circle.

1.   Stand with your feet together, arms hanging loosely at your sides.
2.   Release the vertebrae sequentially downwards.
3.   Let yourself gain momentum as you round the trunk and head together.
4.   Swing the arms together behind you, and upward slowly as they hover at about 11 o'clock.
5.   Then, let the arms fall, gaining weight and momentum.
6.   Sweep downward toward the floor.
7-9. Let the arms swing forward in an arc that rises, elongating the spine.
10. Continue moving the arms and lifting the body up, reaching backward to hover at about 11 o'clock with extended arms, keeping your balance with a counter movement through your legs and feet.

Now continue this cresting and falling motion (illustrated in the third to tenth frame) in a rhythmical fashion.

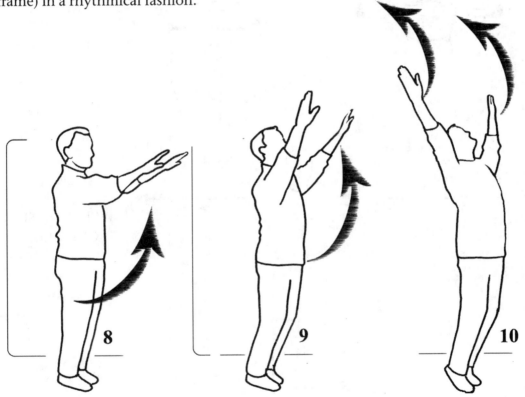

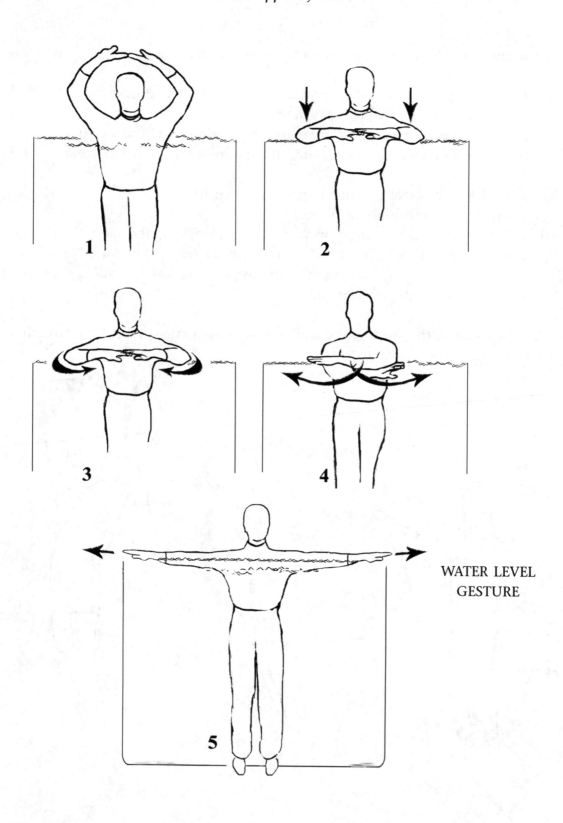

WATER LEVEL
GESTURE

WATER LEVEL GESTURE

This exercise helps define the Horizontal Plane, adjusting a "water level" that is either too high or too low so that you can keep your head above water. It supports the Emotional Body by clearing unwanted thoughts and putting you "head and shoulders above" a given situation. It creates the prerequisite for having a clear overview, of not being up to your eyeballs in clutter and confusion.

The Water Level Gesture is good for hypertension, adrenal disorders, conditions of progesterone dominance, depression, cancer, heart disease, impotence, back pain and rheumatoid arthritis.

1. Begin by making a circle around your head with your palms facing up, fingers touching.
2. Letting the elbows go out, bring the hands slowly down in front of the face, clearing the head space. The palms are now facing towards the ground and move against a slight resistance that is created with a spacial dynamic of condensing the area beneath the palms and arms.
3. The arms, now parallel with the ground, begin a motion across. . .
4. . . . the midline, while describing the widest possible sweep by reaching out and across toward the horizon on opposite sides.
5. Finally, the arms create two symmetrical arcs with accelerating rhythm that slows as the arms extend, parallel to the ground. The preceding motions are continued with the dynamic of an opening of the chest space, establishing the height of the water level.

The Different Centers of the Body

THE LEMNISCATE DYNAMIC

As Rudolf Steiner pointed out, in a healthy body, governed by healthy emotions, the space around the head is wide and the proper dynamic is one of material coming in, as shown above opposite. The arrows coming toward the head represent the "stuff" of the outside world that we perceive calmly and deliberately. At the same time, the proper motion for the abdomen is down and out, with arrows radiating from a central point. Steiner noted that the two gestures form a figure-eight or lemniscate, with the crossover point at the level of the solar plexus.

In the unhealthy body, in situations of pathology, the arrows are reversed. The head is not still but chaotic and muddied, so that it sends material out rather than receives what is coming in. This is the situation for the "estrogen dominant" or hysterical personality that cannot properly process and act on information from the outside world. Such individuals experience a chaotic character to their relationships and life-style. We say that they are "always on send."

The proper gesture for the energies of the abdomen is an outward flow, as in elimination, menstruation, birth and orgasm. If these energies are directed inward, as in the lower diagram, they become trapped there, resulting in colitis, constipation, digestive disorders and problems with the reproductive organs.

The Lemniscate Dynamic supports the Emotional Body by creating a pulsing relationship between taking in and giving out. It designates where those two gestures take place and intersect. It is good for reproductive problems (especially estrogen dominance), digestive disorders, hypertension, adrenal disorders such as allergies and asthma, cancer and neurological problems.

1. Hold your hands in a circular form around your head and imagine sense impressions towards you while you observe alertly and calmly.

2. Now imagine yourself "on send," "losing yourself," dispersing as a "space cadet." Note the sense of confusion in the head and the lack of warmth in the abdomen.

3. Repeat the first visualization, noting the sense of peace in the head and the sense of warmth in the abdomen.

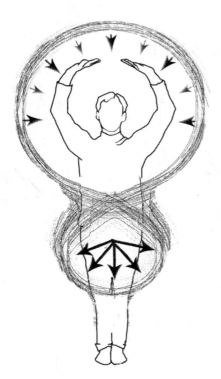

Figure 1
CONTINUOUS LEMNISCATE
Clarity above, power below

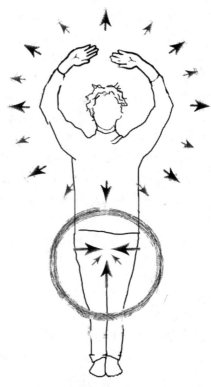

Figure 2
DISCONNECTED LEMNISCATE
"On send" above, constriction below

THE SILHOUETTE

The Silhouette gives a simultaneous experience of the form of the entire body. Remember, as a child, lying down, waving your arms and legs to make angels in the snow? Lie on the ground on a large piece of white paper and ask someone to trace the outline of your body with a crayon. Now stand up and step back from the outline and see the silhouette. This is a good exercise for people suffering from anorexia and other eating or body image disorders. It shows them the discrepancy between their perception of their Physical Body and objective reality. Alternately, you can create a silhouette made on a white sheet hung on a line with a light projected from behind your standing form. People find this phenomenon fascinating because the individual parts disappear while the entire form, the gestalt, appears as an entity in itself.

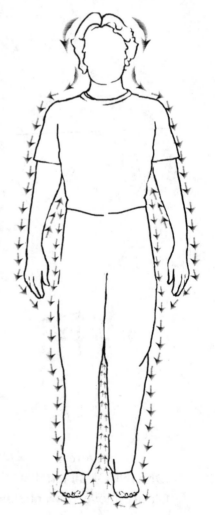

After having had visual experiences of your silhouette, ask a friend to stand behind you with both hands resting gently on the center of the top of your head. Then have them slowly "trace" or follow the contours of the body down—neck, shoulders, outside of the arms, hands, insides of hands and arms, rib cage, waist, hips, thighs, knees, calves, ankles and feet. You should have your eyes closed, and the motion should be done in a slow, flowing way so that it is possible to feel enveloped, encased, as a unit.

The Silhouette is a spacial dynamic that you can do at any time and in any place. With a bit of practice, it can be an effective aid to filling out and claiming your Body and Personal Spaces. As you imagine the silhouette, you will experience "gaps," one or more places that you skip over, or "holes" where the silhouette has sunken beneath the contours of the body. These are the places where disease is most likely to take hold. As you spacially fill in the silhouette, these "gaps" and "holes" will become "whole." The Silhouette is not only a healing exercise, but also a diagnostic tool that can be used prophylactically to prevent disease from manifesting.

The Silhouette fosters a sense of wholeness in the Emotional Body and is good for any disease condition.

COAT HANGER

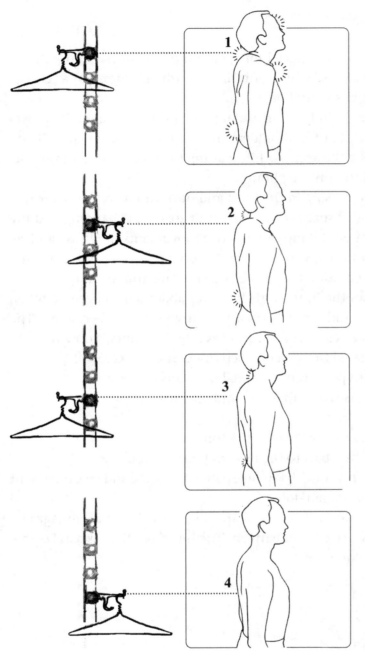

Our society provides us with pictures that often have more wisdom than we are aware of. We talk about someone having "hang-ups." In the Coat Hanger exercise, the Emotional Body practices the spacial dynamic of "relaxing our hang-ups." It is an excellent companion to the Water Level Gesture and is good for arthritis, back pain, adrenal problems and impotence.

1. Consciously overexaggerate the tension that one often feels at the nape of the neck while visualizing a hook placed too high, at the nape of the neck.
2. Move the hanger down one notch, to the top of the shoulders, while experiencing a release of tension.
3. Slowly relax the back muscles as if moving the hook sequentially down until it reaches the level of the middle back.
4. In this position, the shoulders will hang freely, and you'll be able to feel the weight of the arms and the increased blood flow into the hands.

LOWERING THE SAILS

This exercise is done using the spacial imagination of a Chinese ship, called a junk, which has "squarish shoulders," a horizontal boom with sails spread by a "chest," ribbed batten and a pelvic bowl-shaped boat form.

Although the arms are held in the horizontal plane in this exercise, the movement takes place in the muscles of the shoulders and the back. You can actually do this exercise without involving the arms—while waiting for a red light, for example, or when you have a telemarketer on the phone.

This movement relieves pressure in the head and neck and increases deep, diaphragmatic breathing. The head space is still, the chest space is expanding and the limbs are balanced. The Emotional Body can practice movements of release and relaxation. With your "sail" unfurled, you are open to receive possibilities. Lowering the sails provides a strong orientation of symmetry to the Horizontal Plane.

Lowering the Sails allows the lungs and the lower abdomen to become fuller, creating a feeling of "getting under sail," when formerly you were becalmed. The Emotional Body experiences a release of the intuitive "gut instinct," now freed to play its role, as distance is created from mental activity that is too cerebral.

The exercise is good for hypertension, adrenal disorders (especially asthma), for angina associated with heart disease, impotence and arthritis.

1. Start this exercise with the sails gathered at the top.
2. Now lower the boom (the crossbar) to the level of your collar bone.
3. Slowly unfurl the "sail" downwards. The rib-like battens separate and take on weight one by one until they draw the sail down.
4. Now let your chest expand out as well as you "spread your sails." Your rib cage will open, allowing more of its space to fill with air. The hips float like a boat. You are balanced in the center of a quiet sea.

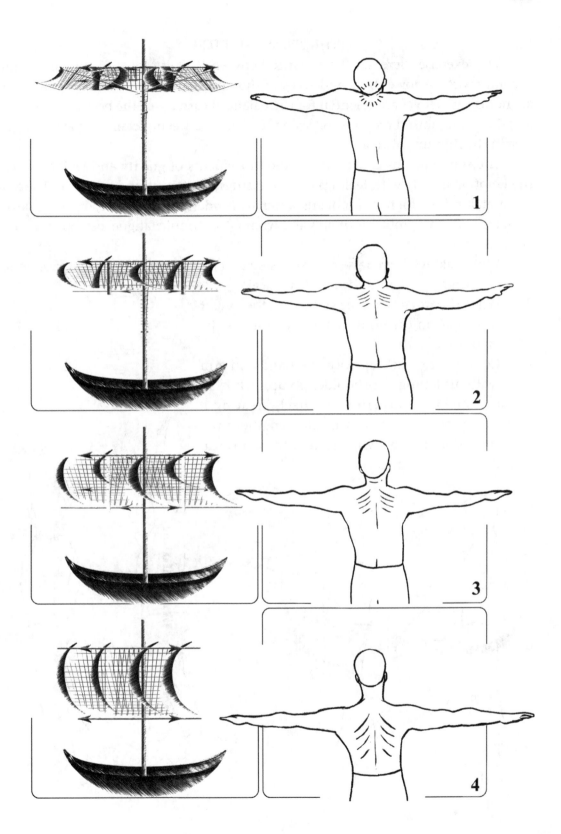

THE SPINAL STRETCH

This exercise increases the distance between the rib cage and the pelvic rim, decompresses the lower back and accesses the muscles on the side of the trunk that are not easily felt yet are essential for the balanced carriage of the body. The spine is lengthened in both directions, releasing tension and freeing cramping and congestion in the rhythmical area.

The simultaneous experience of the movements of gravity and levity provide the Emotional Body with feelings of steadfastness, certainty, and presence. The Spinal Stretch is good for back problems, adrenal disorders, heart disease, digestive disorders, reproductive problems (men's and women's), chronic fatigue, osteoporosis and arthritis.

1-2. While taking a step, raise the same-side arm forward by letting the space under the arm expand until the arm is vertical.

3. When the arm reaches the vertical, all the weight should be on the front foot and you should be on tiptoes.

4. Continue to reach up with the hand and arm (without letting the shoulder go up), while simultaneously lowering the heel, creating a stretch both up and down, that lengthens the entire side of the body, particularly the waist area. Repeat on the other side.

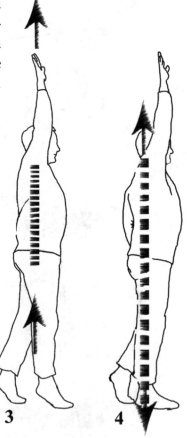

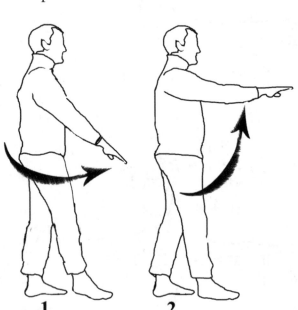

1   2   3   4

SHOULDER MUSCLE MAPPING

Shoulder Muscle Mapping allows the Emotional Body to experience the gesture of getting rid of a burden or getting that chip off your shoulder. Think of water flowing off a duck's back. Shoulder Muscle Mapping encourages a downward gesture, away from the hurried head and through the realm of rhythm into the slower pace of the metabolic sphere. It is good for hypertension, chronic fatigue, back pain, endometriosis, vaginitis, prostate problems, depression and arthritis.

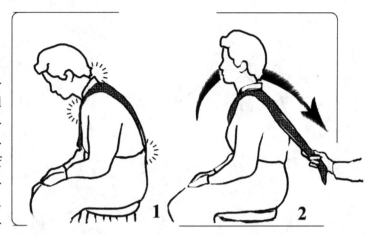

1. Sit in an exaggerated hunched over and cramped position with a scarf over the shoulder.
2. Have someone pull the scarf over shoulder.
3. Like the Carriage Down Gesture, the movement flows up over the shoulder, taking the shoulder blades down and giving them weight.
4. Now pull the scarf down, around and forward.
5. Balanced carriage and composure are achieved by releasing tension from behind and laying it in front of you at your feet.

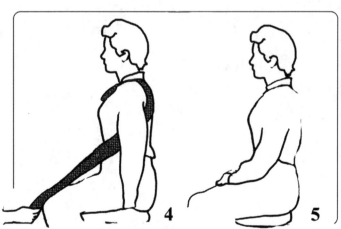

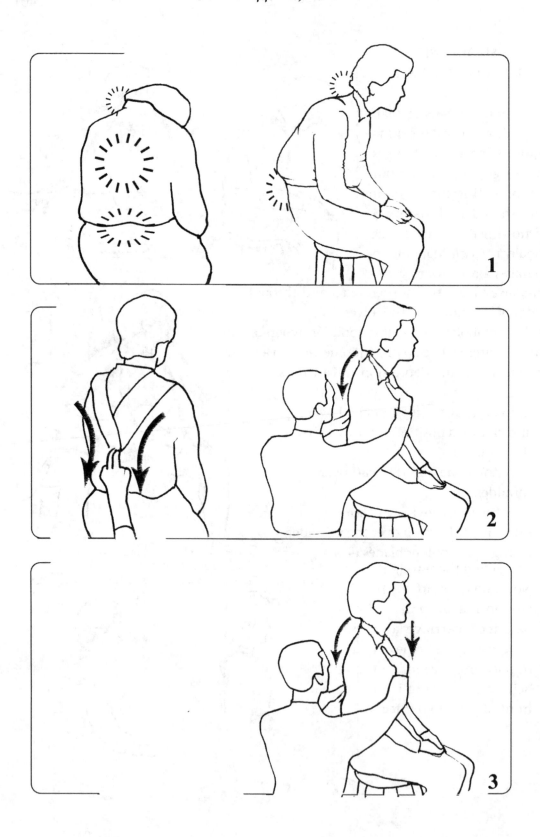

THE COWL

The Cowl gives the gesture of a cape-like garment. The trapezius muscles are called the "monk's hood" muscles in German. The Cowl's funnel-like form give the weight of the shoulders a vortex direction towards gravity. Your Emotional Body experiences a release from carrying the "weight of the world on your shoulders." The exercise gives a sense of being balanced between the past that lies behind you and the future that is before you. It is good for depression, adrenal diseases, cancer and chronic fatigue.

1. Sit in an exaggerated hunched-over position.
2. Have a partner gently trace downward from the nape of the neck to the middle of the back, while the torso straightens.
3. Notice that the spacial gesture of the cowl will remain long after the partner's hands have been removed. The goal is to be able to 'wear' the spacial dynamic that you choose.

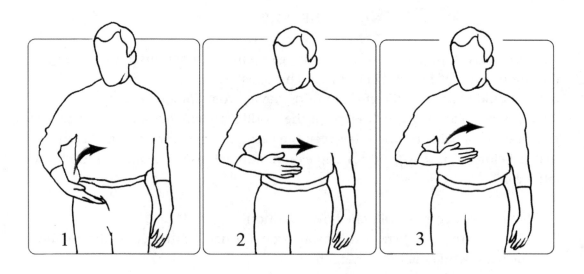

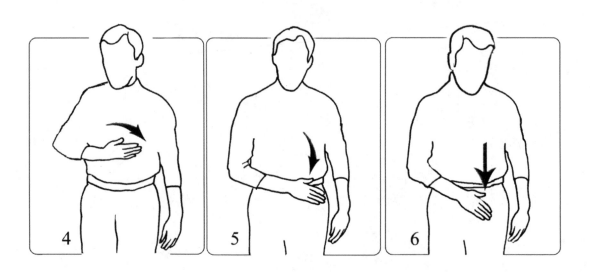

ABDOMINAL MASSAGE

ABDOMINAL MASSAGE

All motions here are done in a slow, undulating fashion. Take your time in between your pulsing massage movements. In the pauses when your hand does nothing, your intestines do the most. Performed rhythmically, the Abdominal Massage provides a palpitating flow of vitalization to the abdomen. It helps the Emotional Body by creating a glowing warmth that expands the space around the metabolic region. Increased regularity of the bowels provides a sense of well being that comes from a feeling of belonging to nature's cyclical patterns. The Abdominal Massage is good for constipation and other digestive disorders, reproductive problems, diabetes and chronic fatigue.

1. Place the right hand facing up at the bottom of the right side of the abdomen.
2. Following the direction of the peristaltic motion of the large intestine, as shown in these figures, lift the right hand and then turn the hand palm inward.
3-4. Move the hand gently across the middle abdomen from right to left.
5-6. Then, using gravity's pull, draw the hand down the left side indicating elimination.

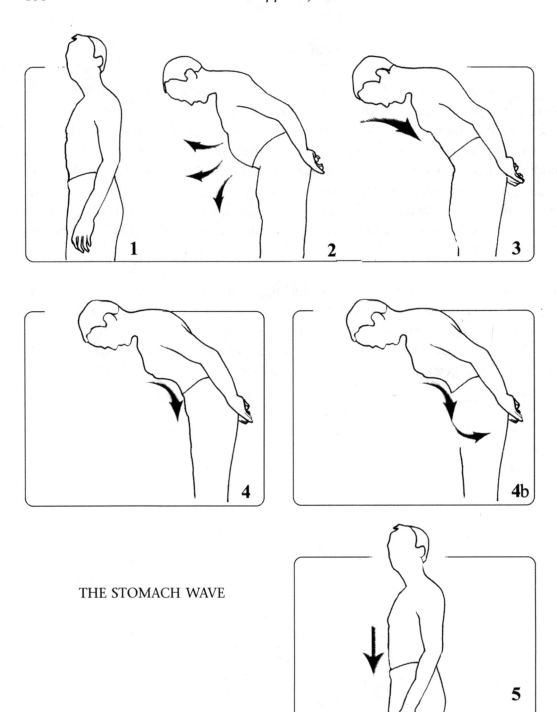

THE STOMACH WAVE

THE STOMACH WAVE

The Stomach Wave helps strengthen the abdominal and pelvic muscles, essential for the postural support of the trunk. It requires concentration and the sequential contraction of muscles that are controlled both consciously and unconsciously. The Stomach Wave involves a playful interaction between concave and convex forms.

This exercise allows the Emotional Body to experience a release of tension and an enlivening of the regenerative forces involved in metabolism and reproduction. It is good for all digestive and reproductive disorders as well as for chronic fatigue.

1.   Stand easily with arms to the side.
2.   Bend forward at about a 45-degree angle. Let your stomach muscles totally relax, protrude and round, making a potbelly.
3.   Then, initiate a motion at the end of the sternum (mid-abdominal area), contracting the abdominal muscles in a sequential wave downward.
4a. Continue the motion rippling from the bottom of the sternum to the top of the pelvic bone.
4b. The ripple moves all the way around the pelvic floor. All the abdominal and pelvic muscles are contracted simultaneously.
5.   Then allow a wave of release of the muscle contractions to begin at the starting point, the base of the sternum, and follow the path of the former wave of contraction with a downward releasing motion in front and behind while you return to a standing-up position.

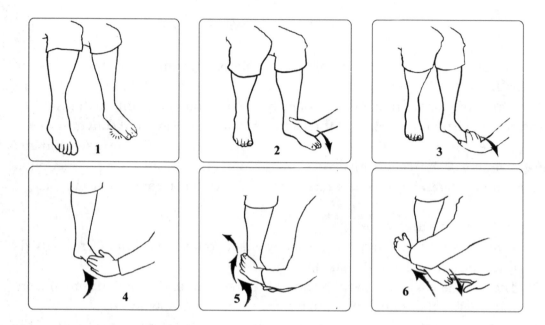

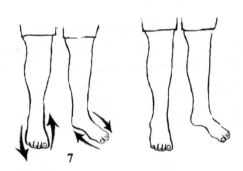

FOOT STREAMING

The foot works best with two complementary gestures. The anatomy and the function of the top of the foot need a gesture that radiates forward. The arch of the underside of the foot (the sole) can be re-formed by a gesture or a muscle stream coming from the front of the big toe, carving out a space beneath the foot and then flowing behind and away. These counter streams give the Emotional Body a firm footing in giving and receiving. Foot Streaming is good for depression, cancer, chronic fatigue, weight loss (providing someone who needs to lose weight with the experience of lightness on the sole of the foot), and adrenal problems, especially asthma.

1.   Sit comfortably and scrunch up the toes in an exaggerated cramped position.
2-3. Have a partner make a gentle forward motion along the top and outside of the foot.
4-5. Now the partner makes a gentle motion on the inside and bottom of the foot from front to back.
6.   Using both hands, the partner combines both gestures.
7-8. Stand up and experience the gesture of forward motion along the top of the foot and backward motion along the bottom of the foot.

KNEE MAPPING

The knee unites the lower and upper leg. Knee Mapping weaves and provides a rhythmical connection between gravity and levity. The upward surge of vitality is a source of nourishment and encouragement for your metabolic forces. It helps the Emotional Body experience the feeling of "picking yourself up by your bootstraps." Knee mapping is good for depression, fatigue, diabetes, digestion (especially constipation), back pain, reproductive problems in women, prostate problems and arthritis of the knee.

1. Begin in a sitting position; have a partner place his hands on the inside of your calf.
2. Draw slowly up on the inside of the knee to the inside of the thigh.
3. Then swoop across the thigh muscles.

4-5. This motion continues on, becoming slower and slower, over the "hip bone" and across the buttock. This map of muscle function is then anchored with strong downward pressure on the sacrum.

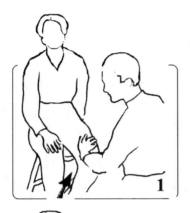

1

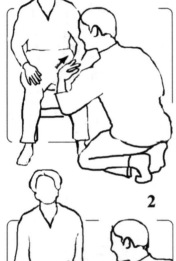

2

3

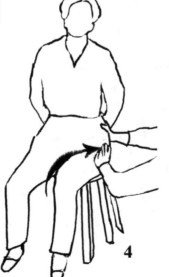

4

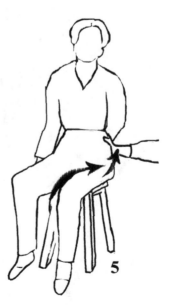

5

Integration

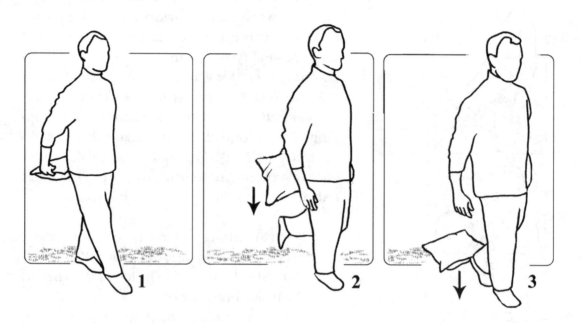

LETTING GO

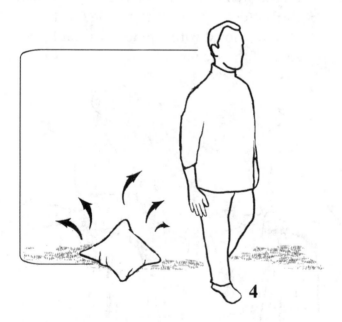

LETTING GO

Letting Go helps release tension and cramps in the abdomen. It has a warming effect on the hands and feet. The body learns to differentiate between the simultaneous movements: the arms that drop the object, the stepping of the feet, the forward motion of the torso, and the sovereign stillness of the head.

For the Emotional Body, this exercise elicits feelings of letting old baggage go, of releasing the past, of stepping towards the future, and of being balanced in the moment. It is good for heart disease, menstrual cramps, digestive disorders (especially constipation), fatigue or thyroid problems manifesting as cold hands and feet, and neurological problems manifesting as nervousness, headache, and obsessive-compulsive disorders.

1. In a standing position, comfortably reach back with the hands to hold a pillow or other soft object.

2. While slowly taking a step, release the hands and let the pillow "splash" on the ground behind the feet.

3. The weight transfer is accomplished when the splash is completed.

4. Imagine the pillow dropping into water. The hands "follow" the pillow while dropping and then also follow the "ripples" of the water into which the pillow has splashed. Repeat with the other foot, transferring weight while releasing the splash.

Appendix C

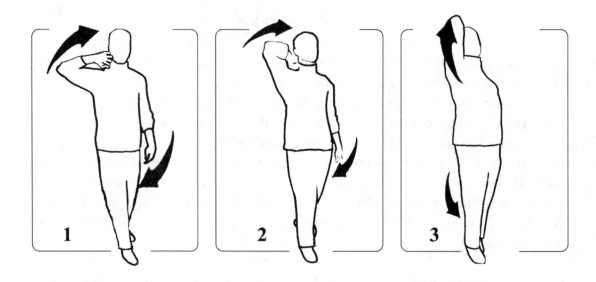

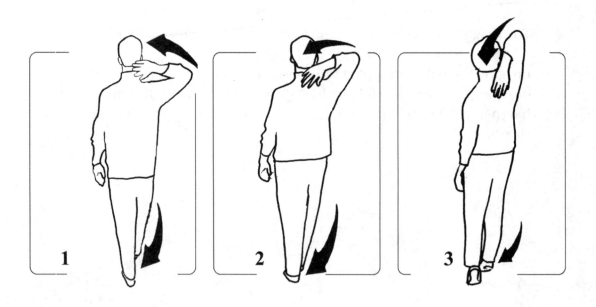

VICTORY STRETCH

VICTORY STRETCH

The Victory Stretch awakens the major muscle chains of the body, which leads to the subsequent enlivening of the back space. The Emotional Body experiences a celebration of the overcoming of obstacles, of self, of getting everything "off the chest." The exercise is good for cancer, back pain, diabetes, chronic fatigue, osteoarthritis and adrenal disorders, especially asthma.

1. Stand with your weight on your right foot, left foot un-weighted and the palm of your right hand against the nape of your neck.

2. Stretch up through the right elbow, twisting up and to the left while pushing down through your right heel.

3. You will actually describe a spiral that begins at your right foot, continues over your left thigh and across your lower rib area on the left, moves up underneath the right shoulder blade and along the outside of the triceps and elbow and continues up.

RICE PAPER WALK

Imagine that you are going through a rite of passage. Thin rice paper has been laid over an uneven surface. Your task is to move forward slowly without making a sound or any tears in the paper. This tracker-like walking exercise modifies our everyday strides into a series of slow, soft and silent steps. This gentle gait allows the soles of your feet to listen to the changing surfaces of the ground. They sense the center of the earth, the source of each still and certain step.

The Rice Paper Walk requires a quiet, consistent manner of moving. The trunk seems to glide smoothly through space without speeding up or slowing down. The exercise gives the impression of timelessness, of having no beginning and no end. The head and torso are transported regally as if in a slowly moving carriage. The feet move in such a way as to make this steady movement of the body possible. The Emotional Body experiences a feeling of comforting grounded-ness and quiet certainty, along with a feeling of sovereignty and openness. This is an exercise for hypertension, heart disease, adrenal disorders, infectious disease, neurological problems and also for digestive disorders and menstrual cramps. It is an excellent evening exercise before sleep or meditation.

1. Put all your weight onto the left foot, relieving the right foot of its own weight. The right knee will loosen and bend, moving slightly ahead of the left knee.

2. Then bring your right foot forward by extending this relaxed right leg, reaching with the ball of the right foot and extending it slightly beyond your comfort zone.

3. Give the right foot its own weight.

4. Now gently transfer the weight of the body forward until it is totally over the right foot. As the left knee relaxes, coming forward further than the right, the left foot will un-weight and peel slowly off the floor.

This process continues without accent or interruption. It is important to note that the Rice Paper Walk is accomplished without any pushing from the back leg. In fact, the body is drawn forward through the transferring of weight and relaxing of the back leg.

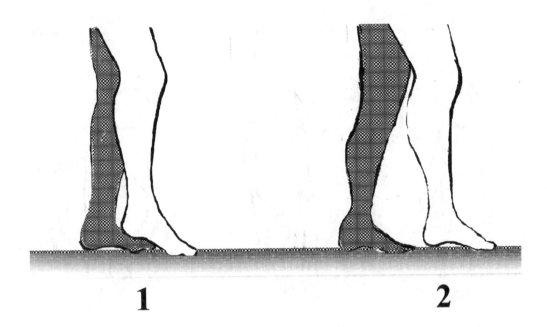

1   **2**

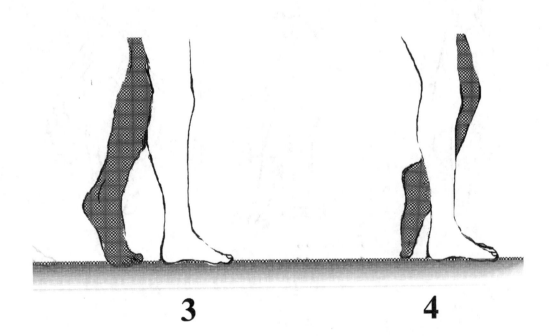

3   **4**

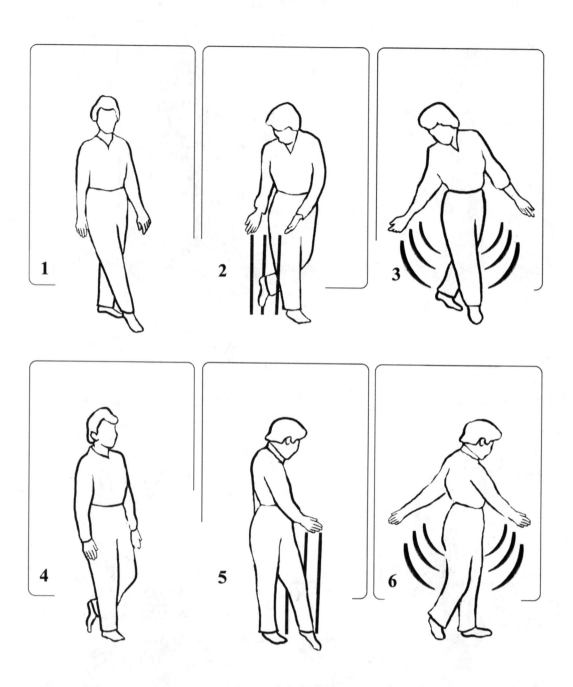

BESTOWING

BESTOWING

This exercise creates a serene movement of bestowal. The Emotional Body experiences a feeling of release, acceptance and letting go. It creates the understanding that something new can begin from nothing. Bestowing is excellent for all women's and men's diseases, hypertension, infectious disease and adrenal disorders.

When you gaze towards the space defined by your arms and hands, imagine that you are standing on top of a mountain; the floor is no obstacle to your vision. Imagine looking down into a river valley where a forest springs to life in the space between your hands, as if you are bestowing life upon the plants and trees.

1. Begin with the weight on the left foot, gazing straight ahead and reach forward with the foot of the extended right leg.

2. Pivot the upper torso 90 degrees to the right as you slowly transfer your weight onto the right foot. The palms should be facing together. The gaze is directed to the middle of the space that your hands are designating.

3. Open your hands out and allow the distance between them to slowly swell and increase to form two 45-degree angles to your right.

4. The trunk and gaze slowly return to their original positions.

5. Repeat the entire process on the other side. The weight is now on the right leg, and you reach forward with the left leg.

6. Transfer the weight to the left foot as you open the hands.

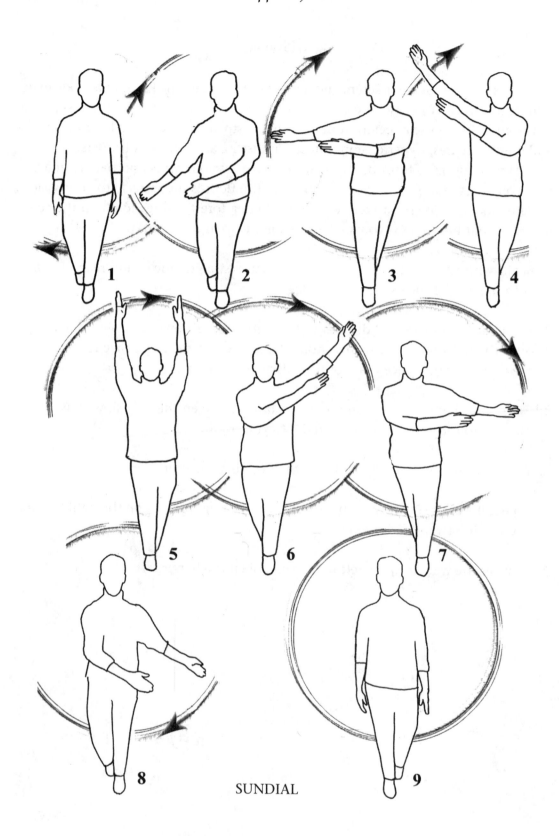

SUNDIAL

SUNDIAL

This exercise poses a coordination challenge for the arms and legs. It helps lengthen the entire spine, vitalize the muscles in the arms, shoulders and rib cage, and increase the range of motion for the rotator cuffs and shoulder blades.

In the Sundial, the Emotional Body experiences a feeling of being present as an individual as well as a friend, of creating space at our sides so that someone can stand by us. It is an excellent morning exercise before getting fully dressed.

Use the Sundial for depression, cancer, arthritis, diabetes and for conditions of anxiety, fear and anorexia that lead to adrenal fatigue.

In the Sundial or Frontal Plane Walk, your two arms remain parallel to each other the entire time. The full transfer of the weight will take place when the arms are either directly vertical or are hanging parallel at the sides. The arms describe two circles and designate two planes which are parallel to each other and a body width apart.

1. Begin with your arms at your side, weight on the forward left foot.
2. Keeping the arms parallel, move them towards the right side.
3. Still keeping the arms parallel, move them to a position horizontal to the ground, with the right foot now moving forward.
4. Move the arms higher while transferring the weight to the right foot.
5. The arms are now parallel above the head with the weight on your right foot.
6. Now the left foot comes forward as the parallel arms move down from the vertical towards the left.
7. As the weight comes forward onto the right foot, the hands are parallel to the ground.
8. Your hands come down and the right foot begins to come forward.
9. Now your arms are at your sides and your weight shifts to the right food as it comes forward.

Now repeat the exercise in the opposite direction. The Emotional Body will feel that it is possible to "turn back the hands of time" at any moment as the arms can move in the opposite direction as well. This allows the body to be stretched equally, resulting in a spacial balance.

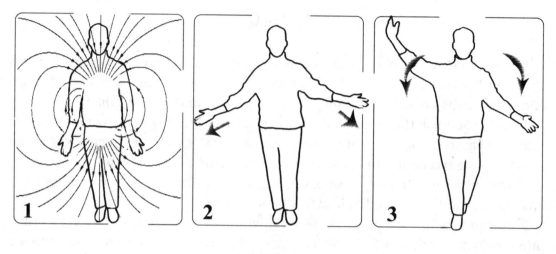

DIPOLE

In physics the word dipole is used to describe a pair of electromagnetic charges of equal magnitude but of opposite sign or polarity. Iron filings will arrange themselves over a dipole in the butterfly-like figure-eightish form. Open-lensed photography in the dark of someone doing this exercise while holding burning torches would reveal the form of the dipole and its unique magnetic field.

The Dipole provides the Emotional Body with a gesture of the symmetry axis, giving certainty and stability. The rhythmic, mirroring curves provide a feeling of fullness and a sense of belonging. The Dipole strengthens the rhythmical system, uniting the upper and lower parts of the body. Interestingly, women with estrogen dominance, or men experiencing impotence, are initially unable to move the fist into the lower part of the body (step 5)—instead their hands often stop at the belt line and have difficulty going further down. The Dipole is excellent for back pain (like the Victory Stretch, it helps the spine pull apart in two directions at the same time), diabetes, problems of estrogen dominance and impotence.

1. Start with the hands to the side, weight on both feet.
2. The arms go up and out.
3. The right foot comes forward while the right hand goes up and the left hand moves down.
4. The hands make fists and come together in front of the body.
5. With arms rounded and fists clenched, the right hand moves vertically up an invisible pole in front of the body while the left hand moves down the pole.
6. The right hand moves vertically up above the head while the left hand moves down to the reproductive area. The weight is now fully on the front right foot.

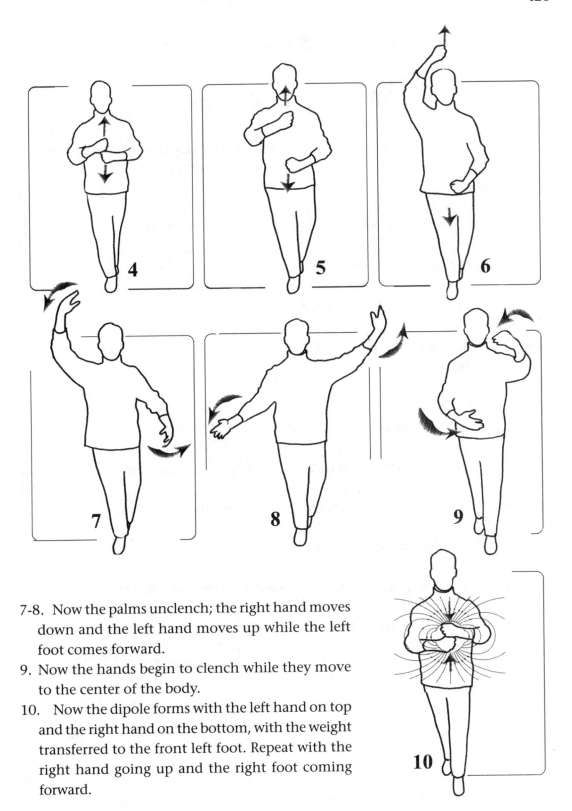

7-8. Now the palms unclench; the right hand moves down and the left hand moves up while the left foot comes forward.

9. Now the hands begin to clench while they move to the center of the body.

10.   Now the dipole forms with the left hand on top and the right hand on the bottom, with the weight transferred to the front left foot. Repeat with the right hand going up and the right foot coming forward.

Maintenance Program

These movement exercises help maintain good emotional and physical health when performed on a daily basis. A suggested maintenance program is as follows:

1.   The Breathing Exercise for enhanced vitality and resiliency.

2.   The Silhouette for the experience of the body as a whole.

3.   The Victory Stretch for increased core stability and balance.

4.   The Crest for suppleness of the spine and stimulating circulation in the head.

5.   The Abdominal Massage and the Stomach Wave for healthier metabolism, digestion and elimination.

6.   The Sundial for increased presence and peripheral awareness.

7.   The Tides for the rhythm between concentration and relaxation.

8.   The Dipole for integration of the cerebral with the metabolic poles.

9.   The Rice Paper Walk for the circulation in the feet and enhanced balance.

10. Bestowing for enhanced calm, tranquility and undisturbed sleep.

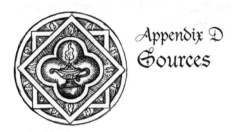

Appendix D
Sources

Adrenal Cortex Extract from Apothecure:
Available by prescription (800) 969-6601, apothecure.com.

Acerola Powder (natural vitamin C):
Radiant Life (888) 593-8333, 4radiantlife.com.

Amalaki Powder (natural vitamin C):
Bazaar of India (800) 261-7662.

Biotta Juices:
Available at most health food stores.

Blessed Herb Cleanse:
Blessed Herb, (508) 882-3839

Butter Oil, High-Vitamin (X-Factor):
Radiant Life (888) 593-8333, radiantlifecatalog.com; Green Pastures Dairy (402) 338-5551, greenpastures.org.

Castor Oil and Castor Oil Pack Supplies:
Heritage Store (800) 862-2923, caycecures.com

Cod Liver Oil:
High-vitamin cod liver oil from Radiant Life (888) 593-8333, radiantlifecatalog.com; Green Pastures Dairy (402) 338-5551, greenpastures.org; lemon-flavored regular-dose cod liver oil from Garden of Life (available in health food stores).

Dulcolux Suppositories:
Available at any pharmacy.

Estriol:
Women's International Pharmacy (800) 279-5708.

Kombucha Mushrooms:
Laurel Farms (941) 351-2233; G.E.M. Cultures (707) 964-2922; A. F. Kombucha (877) 566-2824, kombucha2000.com.

Kombucha (ready made):
A. F. Kombucha (877) 566-2824, kombucha2000.com.

Mediherb: Available through health care practitioners or through organicmadness.com. For practitioners in your area call (800) 558-8740.

Mercury Free Dentists:
International Academy of Oral Medicine and Toxicology, www.iaomt,com/findmember.cfm; talkinternational.com; or contact a local chapter of the Weston A. Price Foundation, westonaprice.org/chapters.

Non-Violent Communication (Center for):
cnvc.org

pH strips:
Premier Research (800) 325-7734 or Village Green Apothecary (301) 530-0800.

Raw Milk:
www.realmilk.com or contact a local chapter of the Weston A. Price Foundation, www.westonaprice.org/chapters, (202) 333-HEAL.

Rebounder:
Center for Cellular Health (800) 856-4863 or (435) 835-7393.